Head and Neck Manifestations of Systemic Disorders

Guest Editor

SIDNEY L. BOURGEOIS, Jr., DDS

ORAL AND MAXILLOFACIAL SURGERY CLINICS OF NORTH AMERICA

www.oralmaxsurgery.theclinics.com

Consulting Editor
RICHARD H. HAUG, DDS

November 2008 • Volume 20 • Number 4

SAUNDERS an imprint of ELSEVIER, Inc.

W.B. SAUNDERS COMPANY
A Division of Elsevier Inc.

1600 John F. Kennedy Blvd. • Suite 1800 • Philadelphia, PA 19103-2899

http://www.theclinics.com

ORAL AND MAXILLOFACIAL SURGERY CLINICS OF NORTH AMERICA Volume 20, Number 4
November 2008 ISSN 1042-3699, ISBN-13: 978-1-4160-6329-2, ISBN-10: 1-4160-6329-3

Editor: John Vassallo; j.vassallo@elsevier.com

© 2008 Elsevier ■ All rights reserved.

This journal and the individual contributions contained in it are protected under copyright by Elsevier, and the following terms and conditions apply to their use:

Photocopying
Single photocopies of single articles may be made for personal use as allowed by national copyright laws. Permission of the Publisher and payment of a fee is required for all other photocopying, including multiple or systematic copying, copying for advertising or promotional purposes, resale, and all forms of document delivery. Special rates are available for educational institutions that wish to make photocopies for non-profit educational classroom use.
For information on how to seek permission visit www.elsevier.com/permissions or call: (+44) 1865 843830 (UK)/(+1) 215 239 3804 (USA).

Derivative Works
Subscribers may reproduce tables of contents or prepare lists of articles including abstracts for internal circulation within their institutions. Permission of the Publisher is required for resale or distribution outside the institution. Permission of the Publisher is required for all other derivative works, including compilations and translations (please consult www.elsevier.com/permissions).

Electronic Storage or Usage
Permission of the Publisher is required to store or use electronically any material contained in this journal, including any article or part of an article (please consult www.elsevier.com/permissions). Except as outlined above, no part of this publication may be reproduced, stored in a retrieval system or transmitted in any form or by any means, electronic, mechanical, photocopying, recording or otherwise, without prior written permission of the Publisher.

Notice
No responsibility is assumed by the Publisher for any injury and/or damage to persons or property as a matter of products liability, negligence or otherwise, or from any use or operation of any methods, products, instructions or ideas contained in the material herein. Because of rapid advances in the medical sciences, in particular, independent verification of diagnoses and drug dosages should be made.

Although all advertising material is expected to conform to ethical (medical) standards, inclusion in this publication does not constitute a guarantee or endorsement of the quality or value of such product or of the claims made of it by its manufacturer.

Oral and Maxillofacial Surgery Clinics of North America (ISSN 1042-3699) is published quarterly by Elsevier Inc., 360 Park Avenue South, New York, NY 10010-1710. Months of issue are February, May, August, and November. Business and Editorial Offices: 1600 John F. Kennedy Blvd., Suite 1800, Philadelphia, PA 19103-2899. Customer Service Office: 6277 Sea Harbor Drive, Orlando, FL 32887-4800. Periodicals postage paid at New York, NY and additional mailing offices. Subscription prices are $271.00 per year for US individuals, $401.00 per year for US institutions, $125.00 per year for US students and residents, $313.00 per year for Canadian individuals, $478.00 per year for Canadian institutions, $362.00 per year for international individuals, $478.00 per year for international institutions and $170.00 per year for Canadian and foreign students/residents. To receive student/resident rate, orders must be accompanied by name or affiliated institution, date of term, and the *signature* of program/residency coordinator on institution letterhead. Orders will be billed at individual rate until proof of status is received. Foreign air speed delivery is included in all *Clinics* subscription prices. All prices are subject to change without notice.
POSTMASTER: Send address changes to *Oral and Maxillofacial Surgery Clinics of North America,* Elsevier Periodicals Customer Service, 11830 Westline Industrial Drive, St. Louis, MO 63146. Tel: 1-800-654-2452 (U.S. and Canada); 314-453-7041 (outside U.S. and Canada). Fax: 314-523-5170. E-mail: journalscustomerservice-usa@elsevier.com (for print support); journalsonlinesupport-usa@elsevier.com (for online support).

Reprints. For copies of 100 or more, of articles in this publication, please contact the Commercial Reprints Department, Elsevier Inc., 360 Park Avenue South, New York, NY 10010-1710. Tel.: 212-633-3812; Fax: 212-462-1935; Email: reprints@elsevier.com.

Oral and Maxillofacial Surgery Clinics of North America is covered in MEDLINE/PubMed (*Index Medicus*).

Printed in the United States of America.

Contributors

GUEST EDITOR

SIDNEY L. BOURGEOIS, Jr., DDS
Clinical Assistant Professor, Department of Oral and Maxillofacial Surgery, University of Texas Health Science Center, San Antonio, Texas

AUTHORS

SIDNEY L. BOURGEOIS, Jr., DDS
Clinical Assistant Professor, Department of Oral and Maxillofacial Surgery, University of Texas Health Science Center, San Antonio, Texas

VERNON P. BURKE, DMD, MD
Resident, Oral and Maxillofacial Surgery, Department of Oral and Maxillofacial Surgery, University of Texas Health Science Center, San Antonio, Texas

STEPHEN A. COFFEY, DDS
Chief Resident, Oral and Maxillofacial Surgery Training Program, University of Tennessee, College of Dentistry, Memphis, Tennessee

JULIANA DIPASQUALE, DMD
Chief Resident, Division of Oral & Maxillofacial Surgery, Department of Surgery, University of Florida, Health Science Center, Jacksonville, Florida

WENDELL A. EDGIN, DDS
Adjunct Associate Professor, Department of Oral and Maxillofacial Surgery, University of Texas Health Science Center; and Private Practice, San Antonio, Texas

RONALD E. GRIMWOOD, MD
Professor, Department of Medicine, Scott and White Division of Dermatology, Texas A & M Health Science Center, Temple, Texas

RAJESH GUTTA, BDS, MS
Assistant Professor, Department of Oral and Maxillofacial Surgery, University of Texas Health Science Center, San Antonio, Texas

LTC ROBERT G. HALE, DDS
Program Director, OMS Residency, Brooke Army Medical Center, Fort Sam Houston, Texas

MICHAELL A. HUBER, DDS
Associate Professor and Head, Division of Oral Medicine, Department of Dental Diagnostic Science, University of Texas Health Science Center, San Antonio, Texas

AARON LIDDELL, DMD
Resident, Department of Oral and Maxillofacial Surgery, University of Texas Health Science Center, San Antonio, Texas

STANLEY H. McGUFF, DDS
Professor, Department of Pathology, University of Texas Health Science Center, San Antonio, Texas

LANDON McLAIN, DDS, MD
Chief Resident, Department of Oral and Maxillofacial Surgery, University of Texas Health Science Center, San Antonio, Texas

TAYLOR C. PRATT, DDS, MD
Chief Resident, Department of Oral and Maxillofacial Surgery, University of Texas Health Science Center, San Antonio, Texas

DAVID B. POWERS, DMD, MD
Colonel, United States Air Force Dental Corps; Director, Facial Trauma Management Program, US Air Force Center for Sustainment of Trauma and Readiness Skills (C-STARS); and Assistant Clinical Professor of Surgery, R. Adams

Contributors

Cowley Shock Trauma Center, Department of Trauma Plastic Surgery, University of Maryland Medical Center, Baltimore, Maryland

JULIE ANN SMITH, DDS, MD
Assistant Professor and Predoctoral Program Director, Department of Oral and Maxillofacial Surgery, Oregon Health and Science University, Portland, Oregon

JAMES M. STARTZELL, DMD, MS
Associate Professor and Interim Chair, Department of Oral and Maxillofacial Surgery, and Program Director, Oral and Maxillofacial Surgery Residency Program, University of Texas Health Science Center, San Antonio, Texas

CPT DAVID I. TUCKER, DDS
Chief Resident, OMS Residency, Brooke Army Medical Center, Fort Sam Houston, Texas

LUIS G. VEGA, DDS
Assistant Program Director, Oral & Maxillofacial Residency Program and Assistant Professor, Division of Oral & Maxillofacial Surgery, Department of Surgery, University of Florida, Health Science Center, Jacksonville, Florida

LAWRENCE W. WEEDA, Jr., DDS
Professor and Chairman, Director, Oral and Maxillofacial Surgery Residency Training Program, University of Tennessee, College of Dentistry, Memphis, Tennessee

Contents

Preface   ix

Sidney L. Bourgeois, Jr.

Dedication   xi

Sidney L. Bourgeois, Jr.

HIV and AIDS in the Adolescent and Adult: An Update for the Oral and Maxillofacial Surgeon   535

Julie Ann Smith

> Human Immunodeficiency Virus (HIV) and Acquired Immunodeficiency Syndrome (AIDS) are among the most complex disease states in existence. HIV, AIDS, and their treatments have the potential to affect every system in the body, consequently influencing the oral surgery care of these patients. Additionally, patients often present to dentists and oral and maxillofacial surgeons with an oral lesion which may be an intial sign of HIV disease or evidence of worsening HIV disease. This article will provide an in-depth review of the pathogenesis of HIV, its systemic complications, antiretroviral therapies, and the oral manifestations of HIV and AIDS.

Sjögren Syndrome: A Review for the Maxillofacial Surgeon   567

Rajesh Gutta, Landon McLain, and Stanley H. McGuff

> Sjögren syndrome is a multisystemic condition that predominantly involves the salivary and lacrimal glands. Also known as sicca complex, the disease often is underdiagnosed and poorly understood. This article provides a comprehensive review on Sjögren syndrome, with an emphasis on diagnosis and treatment modalities.

Pemphigus Vulgaris and Paraneoplastic Pemphigus   577

Wendell A. Edgin, Taylor C. Pratt, and Ronald E. Grimwood

> Pemphigus vulgaris and paraneoplastic pemphigus are rare, chronic, life-threatening autoimmune mucocutaneous bullous conditions precipitated by IgG autoantibodies binding to desmoglein 1, desmoglein 3, and the plakin family of adhesion proteins. Oral lesions may be the only lesions or first to appear in these conditions, making it paramount that oral and maxillofacial surgeons are well-versed in diagnosis and treatment. Initial management almost always involves pain management, hydration, and tissue biopsy followed by corticosteroid therapy. Adjuvant therapy has greatly improved the safety and quality of life for these unfortunate patients.

Systemic Lymphoproliferative Diseases   585

Aaron Liddell and Sidney L. Bourgeois, Jr.

> This article focuses on lymphoma and subclasses that the oral and maxillofacial surgeon may encounter in practice. It elucidates a brief historical review of lymphoma,

including a basic review of classification schemes. Additionally, it will give a general overview of the pathology, pathophysiology, and current treatment modalities with specific attention paid to the head and neck manifestations and complications.

The Leukemias 597
Vernon P. Burke and James M. Startzell

This article reviews the major leukemia disorders, discussing their definitions, incidence, manifestations, and general treatment and prognosis, with additional description of oral findings common among or particular to the disorders. It reviews management of the most frequent oral manifestations of leukemia and the cautions required to provide oral and maxillofacial surgical services to patients who have leukemia.

Head and Neck Manifestations of Distant Carcinomas 609
Luis G. Vega, Juliana Dipasquale, and Rajesh Gutta

Metastatic lesions to the head and neck are rare entities. These lesions are often the first sign of systemic disease but are generally a sign of widespread systemic disease and poor outcome. This article discusses the general process of metastasis and describes the signs and symptoms of distant carcinomas (infraclavicular) to the oral and maxillofacial region.

Gastrointestinal Illnesses and Their Effects on the Oral Cavity 625
Michaell A. Huber

Many disease processes affecting the gastrointestinal (GI) tract may cause observable changes to the oral cavity. In fact, oral cavity changes may represent the first clinical manifestation of an underlying GI condition. Recognition and appropriate referral of a possible GI condition contribute to overall health and wellness in patients. Some of the more important GI conditions that may manifest oral cavity involvement include: reflux disorders, inherited GI polyposis syndromes, and inflammatory bowel disease. This article briefly reviews the aforementioned topics.

Head and Neck Manifestations of Tuberculosis 635
Robert G. Hale and David I. Tucker

Head and neck manifestations of tuberculosis (TB) are caused by the hematogenous or lymphatic spread of the bacteria to affect the larynx, oropharynx, maxillofacial structures, ear, mastoid, and cervical spine. Other cases of TB of the head and neck are from self-inoculation of open lesions of the aero–digestive tract with infected sputum. This article describes the history, epidemiology, bacteriology, pathophysiology, diagnosis, and treatment of TB with emphasis on head and neck manifestations of this systemic disease.

Wegener's Granulomatosis 643
Lawrence W. Weeda, Jr. and Stephen A. Coffey

Wegener's granulomatosis (WG) is a rare systemic disease associated with necrotizing granulomatous inflammation in the upper and lower respiratory tract, glomerulonephritis, and vasculitis. Generalized and limited forms are recognized, and both may present with nonspecific symptoms early in the process. Oral, sinus, and cutaneous findings commonly are seen at initial presentation and/or during the course of the disease. Early diagnosis and treatment are necessary to limit the potentially serious complications associated with WG. This article includes information pertaining to recognition, diagnosis, and management of WG to aid the clinician in early diagnosis and institution of therapy to limit these complications.

Systemic Lupus Erythematosus and Discoid Lupus Erythematosus 651

David B. Powers

Systemic lupus erythematosus (SLE) is an autoimmune disorder of unknown etiology that affects numerous organ systems including the renal, cardiovascular, gastrointestinal, and central and peripheral nervous systems. The practicing oral and maxillofacial surgeon needs to understand the potential complications of SLE and the alterations in treatment protocols which would be necessary to safely treat a patient with SLE. This article outlines the disease process, prevalence and presentation, and specific variants, and discusses treatment regimens available for incorporation into current practice.

Index 663

Oral and Maxillofacial Surgery Clinics of North America

FORTHCOMING ISSUES

February 2009

Complications of Cosmetic Facial Surgery
Joseph Niamtu III, DMD,
Guest Editor

May 2009

Current Controversies in Maxillofacial Trauma
A. Omar Abubaker, DMD, PhD and
Daniel M. Laskin, DDS, MS, *Guest Editors*

August 2009

Salivary Gland Infections
Michael D. Turner, DDS, MD and
Robert S. Glickman, DMD, *Guest Editors*

RECENT ISSUES

August 2008

The Neck
Eric J. Dierks, DMD, MD and
R. Bryan Bell, DDS, MD, *Guest Editors*

May 2008

Orofacial Pain and Dysfunction
Ramesh Balasubramaniam, BDSc, MS and
Gary D. Klasser, DMD, *Guest Editors*

February 2008

Practice Management
M. Todd Brandt, DDS, MD, *Guest Editor*

RELATED INTEREST

Dental Clinics of North America, January 2008
Management of the Oncologic Patient
Sook-Bin Woo, DMD, MMSc and Nathaniel S. Treister, DMD, DMSc, *Guest Editors*

Dental Clinics of North America, October 2006
Medical Conditions and Their Impact on Dental Care
James R. Hupp, DMD, MD, JD, MBA, *Guest Editor*

Both available at: www.dental.theclinics.com

THE CLINICS ARE NOW AVAILABLE ONLINE!

Access your subscription at:
www.theclinics.com

Preface

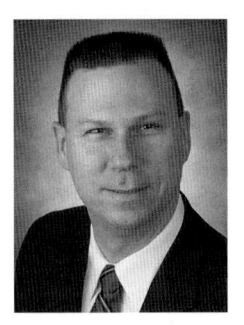

Sidney L. Bourgeois, Jr., DDS
Guest Editor

What does it mean to be a doctor? In one sense, it means being a teacher. I am grateful for the opportunity to work with such a fine group of oral and maxillofacial surgeons, and the opportunity to be Guest Editor of the *Oral and Maxillofacial Surgery Clinics*, as a means to reach out to our surgical community to fulfill that sense of being a teacher. In another sense, being a doctor means we are detectives. I do not mean to conjure up images of our television counterparts, but we do utilize multiple avenues and approaches to solve patients' problems if we can. Some problems are most certainly easier to solve than others. My vision for this issue was for it to be a review of systemic illnesses that have head and neck manifestations. There are numerous systemic illnesses that pose diagnostic and treatment challenges, for which we may be the first line of detection. Many systemic illnesses are undergoing revisions in prior treatment regimens as a new understanding of their pathophysiology and new medications and surgical treatments arise. It is my sincere hope that the articles in this issue will provide you with head and neck signs and symptoms and a review of the current medical treatment of some of these disorders.

Sidney L. Bourgeois, Jr., DDS
Clinical Assistant Professor
Oral and Maxillofacial Surgery
University of Texas Health Science Center
7703 Floyd Curl Drive, MSC 7908
San Antonio, TX 78229, USA

E-mail address:
bourgeois@uthscsa.edu

Dedication

This issue is dedicated to the memory of my wife, Samantha, who died suddenly on May 13, 2008. She was my soulmate, wife, and best friend. She was the kindest, sweetest, and most gentle soul I have ever known. I would not be the person I am today without her never ending love and support. She is missed in ways words cannot describe and loved with the deepest love possible.

Sidney L. Bourgeois, Jr., DDS

HIV and AIDS in the Adolescent and Adult: An Update for the Oral and Maxillofacial Surgeon

Julie Ann Smith, DDS, MD

KEYWORDS

- HIV • AIDS • Immunodeficiency • Antiretrovirals
- HAART • Oral manifestations of HIV • Oral candidiasis
- Oral hairy leukoplakia • Oral papilloma
- Oral herpes simplex • Linear gingival erythema
- Necrotizing ulcerative gingivitis
- Necrotizing ulcerative periodontitis
- Kaposi's sarcoma • Aphthous ulcer

Initially recognized as a disease in 1981, AIDS since has been one of the leading causes of death worldwide and in the United States. According to the Joint United Nations Programme on HIV/AIDS (UNAIDS) and the World Health Organization (WHO), approximately 33.2 million people worldwide are living with HIV infection; 15.4 million are women, and 2.5 million are children under the age of 15. It is estimated that 2.5 million people were newly infected in 2007 and that 2.1 million died of AIDS in 2007. Sub-Saharan Africa accounts for most current HIV infection cases, estimated to be 22.5 million, 61% of which are in women, a statistic that differs from other regions of the world, where most of the infected are males. North America accounts for 1.3 million of infected individuals. Although dramatic improvements in education and treatment of HIV have occurred over the years, the number of people infected worldwide is over 6800 people per day, and over 5700 people die every day from AIDS.[1] Various countries exhibit differing patterns of transmission. Some countries have a high prevalence of transmission between workers in the sex trade and their clients; some countries have a high rate of men having sex with men, and others have a high rate of transmission based on intravenous drug abuse. Of course, several behaviors leading to transmission may coexist. In the United States, homosexual or bisexual men comprise the largest group at risk, accounting for approximately 50% of infections. Intravenous drug abusers are the second largest group, comprising approximately 25% of infected individuals. Heterosexuals who engage in sexual activity with members of other at-risk groups make up about approximately 10% of the population. Nonhemophiliac and hemophiliac recipients of blood products (particularly before 1985) account for 1% and 0.5% of the infected population, respectively. In approximately 6% of cases, a risk factor cannot be identified.[2]

PATHOGENESIS OF HIV AND AIDS

HIV is a retrovirus well equipped to invade the T helper lymphocyte and subsequently self-replicate. The core of the virus contains several proteins, including p24 and p7/p9, two copies of RNA, and three enzymes: reverse transcriptase, protease, and integrase. The viral envelope exhibits two glycoproteins important for cell invasion: gp120 and gp41. The envelope glycoproteins may

Department of Oral and Maxillofacial Surgery, Oregon Health and Science University, 611 SW Campus Drive, Mail Code SDOMS, Portland, OR 97239, USA
E-mail address: smitjuli@ohsu.edu

exhibit considerable genetic variability, making the development of a vaccine difficult. Two genetically distinct forms of HIV exist, HIV-1 and HIV-2. HIV-1 is the most common, and when referring to HIV, it generally is implied that HIV-1 is being discussed. HIV-1 is subdivided further into M (major), O (outlier), and N (neither M nor O) groups. M viruses are most common (90%) and are divided into subtypes A through K. In the United States and Western Europe, subtype B is the most common, and subtype C is found most often in Africa, India, and Nepal.

HIV infection results in severe suppression of cell-mediated immunity. The immunosuppression results from loss of CD4+ T-cells and declining function of remaining T-cells. In addition to T-cells, HIV infection also affects dendritic cells and macrophages (which are also CD4+). During the first step of infection, the gp120 envelope glycoprotein of HIV binds to the CD4+ molecule on the CD4+ T lymphocyte. This leads to a conformational change, in which gp120 binds additional coreceptors, either CCR5 or CXCR4. This binding, in turn, results in additional changes in another envelope glycoprotein, gp41, allowing fusion of the cell membranes and subsequently the release of the HIV genome into the infected cell. A new classification of HIV drugs, fusion inhibitors or entry inhibitors, inhibits the fusion of the HIV virion to the T-cell by targeting either the gp41 receptor or the CCR5 co-receptor.[3-5] Once inside the cell, the RNA of HIV undergoes reverse transcription to form cDNA (proviral DNA), which can remain in the cytoplasm or enter the nucleus to be integrated into the host cell genome. The transcription into DNA is performed using the viral enzyme reverse transcriptase, which is the target of various antiviral medications (nucleoside reverse transcriptase inhibitors [NRTIs and non-nucleoside reverse transcriptase inhibitors [NNRTIs]).[6] This proviral DNA becomes integrated into the T-cell nucleus by the enzyme integrase, where it may remain latent even for years, or it may be transcribed into HIV RNA, resulting in the production of viral particles that are released outside of the T-cell. Newly approved integrase inhibitors target the integrase enzyme at this stage of the HIV lifecycle.[3-5] Successful viral particle assembly requires the translation of various genes within the HIV RNA genome and ultimately requires the function of viral protease to create viral proteins. The protease inhibitor (PI) drugs target this aspect of the HIV lifecycle. Currently, other transcription inhibitor drugs are in very early research stages.[3] The use of the - cell to manufacture additional virions in this manner ultimately results in the death of the T-cell. The loss of T-cells results in immunosuppression, which allows the development of other opportunistic diseases and eventually leads to the patient's death. As many as 100 billion new viral particles per day may be fabricated.[2]

CLINICAL COURSE OF INFECTION

As mentioned earlier, the first cases of AIDS were reported in 1981. Since then, significant advances in detection and treatment have influenced the natural history of the disease drastically. The first serologic test for HIV-1 was developed in 1985. The introduction of the first antiretroviral drug, zidovudine (AZT), in 1987, led the way in controlling the disease, and to the development of subsequent HIV medications. In 1996, drug combination therapy introduced as highly active antiretroviral therapy (HAART) revolutionized treatment and changed the natural progression of disease for those on HAART therapy. Fortunately, many people are diagnosed early and started on HAART, delaying the progression of disease. Diagnosis, however, may occur at any stage of disease, and in some cases, may occur in late stages. Oral and maxillofacial surgeons (OMS) must be aware of the stages of HIV illness, because they may see patients in early stages with signs and symptoms of HIV infection and if astute, may assist in making the diagnosis. Furthermore, an awareness of the manner of progression of this disease is essential in properly treating patients at various stages of their disease.

There are seven stages of HIV infection and progression. These stages include HIV transmission, primary (acute) HIV infection, HIV seroconversion, clinical latency period with or without lymphadenopathy, early symptomatic HIV infection, AIDS, and advanced HIV infection.[7] The first stage of HIV infection involves the actual transmission of the virus by means of exposure to contaminated fluids through a break in the skin or mucosa. The risk of transmission is higher when the infected patient has an elevated viral load. Once the virus is transmitted, the process of T-cell infection previously described occurs. Within 72 hours of virus transmission, infection occurs at the site of entry and the local lymph nodes.[8] The presence of the virus stimulates an immune response involving T helper cells and cytotoxic T lymphocytes, which ultimately are unable to completely contain the infection.[9] One week after transmission, the infection becomes systemic, as the virus infects massive numbers of CD4+ T cells. A few weeks after infection, T-cells of gut mucosa may be nearly depleted. This may lead to chronic activation of the immune system.[9] Within the first month after infection, HIV establishes long-lived reservoirs of virus in follicular dendritic cells and resting CD4+ T- cells. In fact, dendritic cells are felt to be important in initial and continued infection of CD4+ cells.[9] The virus integrates its genetic material into the DNA of the latent CD4+ cell, where it remains protected and dormant until the virus is activated. Integration into the host genome can protect and hide the virus from antiretroviral medications at this stage.[10]

Primary HIV infection describes the acute phase of HIV infection. Approximately two thirds of newly infected individuals develop symptoms of acute infection within 2 to 6 weeks postexposure. Studies have shown that an increased number and duration of acute HIV infection symptoms during this phase correlate with more progression of disease later in infection.[10] During primary HIV (also known as acute HIV infection or acute seroconversion syndrome), patients present with an illness similar to mononucleosis or influenza, with complaints of fever, rash, sore throat, malaise, mylagias, arthralgias, headache, nausea, vomiting, and/or diarrhea. These patients also may present to oral and maxillofacial surgeons with specific complaints or findings, such as oral ulcers, candidiasis, pharyngitis, neck lymphadenopathy, or cranial nerve palsies (especially involving the facial nerve).[10] It is of absolute importance that the OMS is aware of the possible association of these findings with HIV infection, as the patient may not have presented to his/her primary care physician, and rapid diagnosis and initiation of HAART are important in ensuring the best prognosis. The author recommends the inclusion of a thorough neck palpation examination and close evaluation of oral mucosa of all patients during any type of consultation. The author has had one asymptomatic patient who presented for third molar evaluation with generalized neck lymphadenopathy on initial examination, and work-up revealed HIV infection.

During the primary HIV infection phase, massive infection of CD4+ cells and rapid viral replication occur. The immune system becomes activated against the infection, with production of HIV-specific T helper cells. In most patients, however, the specific anti-HIV function of these CD4+ cells is weak or nonexistent because of dysfunction of these CD4+ T-cells on various levels.[9] The activation of the immune system often can cause the symptoms of acute HIV infection. In response to immune activation, the virus develops heterogeneity. As infection progresses, the viral load increases, often exceeding 100,000 copies/mL, and the CD4+ T-cell count decreases.[10,11] The decrease in CD4+ T-cell count is a hallmark of primary HIV infection. Laboratory findings during acute infection may include leukopenia (especially CD4+ leukopenia), mild thrombocytopenia, and liver function abnormalities. Anti-HIV antibodies may be detected by IgM-sensitive ELISA at 2 to 4 weeks after infection.[10] Viral load typically peaks at about 4 to 8 weeks after infection.[10,11] Subsequently, the viral load begins to drop, possibly because of decreased numbers of CD4+ cells and the appearance of anti-HIV cytotoxic CD8+ T-cells. Immune control of disease and HIV replication eventually balance each other, and a set point viral load is reached between weeks 8 and 24. At this time, that viral heterogeneity is at its peak, as the virus attempts to circumvent the immune system's attempt to control the infection. The more broadly that cellular and humoral responses are able to target the virus, the lower the set point will be, and thus, there will be slowing of CD4+ T-cell loss and slowing of the ultimate immune compromise and progression of disease.[10] Early antiretroviral therapy (ART) is recommended during primary HIV infection in order to prevent infection of nascent CD4+ T lymphocytes and to help limit the diversity of HIV. ART also reduces viral load and is felt to relieve some of the symptoms of the acute retroviral syndrome. Studies have shown that the institution of early ART can result in a decreased incidence of opportunistic infections (OIs), an increased level of CD4+ T-cells, and a delay in progression to AIDS. Antiretroviral drugs have the greatest potential if begun within the first 2 weeks of infection, making early diagnosis essential.[10]

Seroconversion, mentioned earlier, refers to the development of positive HIV serology documented by laboratory evidence. Seroconversion typically occurs within 4 to 10 weeks after exposure, and 95% of patients seroconvert within 6 months of infection. A small percentage (7% in one study)[12] of those who seroconvert are capable of demonstrating a strong enough immune response to spontaneously control viremia and may go on to have a nondetectable HIV RNA. These patients may experience long-term stability in their disease and may become long-term nonprogressors. The definition of long-term nonprogressors includes those who have been HIV infected for 13 years or longer, are asymptomatic, do not use antiretrovirals, maintain a CD4+ count above 600/mm^3, and have not had a decrease in CD4+ count for more than 5 years.[7]

Six months after infection, the acute or primary HIV infection phase is complete. During the ensuing clinical latency period, patients are typically asymptomatic except for possibly demonstrating persistent generalized lymphadenopathy. During this time, viral load remains fairly stable or may increase very slowly. The set point viral load is an important prognosticator of the progression of disease in early HIV infection, whereas the CD4+ count is a more important prognostic indicator in late-stage disease.[7]

In 1993, the Centers for Disease Control and Prevention (CDC) released a revision of the 1987 AIDS classification system. This system classifies patients according to their CD4+ count and their development of symptoms in various categories. Three categories of CD4+ counts are defined: greater than 500/mm^3, 200 to 499/mm^3, or less than 200/mm^3. Three clinical categories are defined: A, B, and C. Category A includes patients who are asymptomatic or only exhibit persistent generalized lymphadenopathy. Findings associated with Category B (symptomatic) include, but are not limited to oral-pharyngeal candidaisis, oral hairy leukoplakia (OHL), herpes zoster involving two episodes or more than one dermatome, idiopathic thrombocytopenic purpura, peripheral neuropathy, bacillary angiomatosis, persistent/difficult-to-manage vaginal candidiasis, cervical dysplasia, cervical carcinoma in situ, fever or diarrhea for more than 1 month, pelvic inflammatory disease (PID), or listeriosis. Category C includes AIDS- defining diseases, which are listed in **Box 1**.[13]

AIDS is defined as the presence of any of the category C diseases or a CD4+ count of less than 200/mm^3. Once patients have been defined as having AIDS, they remain in the AIDS category even after resolution of the original process that placed them in that category. Those who are symptomatic with only category B illnesses and who have a CD4+ count above 200/mm^3 are described as having early symptomatic HIV infection (once known as AIDS-related complex). Patients who progress to a CD4+ count below 50/mm^3 are considered to have advanced HIV infection, and median survival at this stage without ART is 12 to 18 months. Nearly all patients who eventually die of an HIV-related complication have a CD4+ count of 50/mm^3 or less.[7]

DIAGNOSIS

It is estimated that 25% of the more than 1,000,000 Americans infected with HIV do not even know they are HIV-positive.[14] Once a patient presents with possible initial findings of HIV infection, a thorough medical and social history is obtained. Symptoms frequently encountered during primary HIV infection include generalized lymphadenopathy, night sweats and fevers, unexplained weight loss, diarrhea, and oral candidiasis (OC).[14]

> **Box 1**
> **AIDS-defining diseases**
>
> Candidiasis of esophagus, bronchi, trachea, or lungs
>
> Invasive cervical cancer
>
> Extrapulmonary coccidioidomycosis, cryptococcosis, or histoplasmosis
>
> Intestinal cryptosporidiosis longer than 1 month
>
> Cytomegalovirus (CMV) disease in organs other than the liver, spleen, or lymph nodes
>
> CMV retinitis
>
> HIV encephalopathy
>
> HIV wasting
>
> Herpes simplex ulceration longer than 1 month or herpes simplex bronchitis, pneumonitis, or esophagitis
>
> Intestinal isoporiasis
>
> Kaposi's sarcoma (KS)
>
> Burkitt's, immunoblastic, or neurologic lymphoma
>
> *Mycobacterium avium* complex (MAC)
>
> *Mycobacterium tuberculosis*
>
> Other disseminated or extrapulmonary mycobacterium
>
> *Pneumocystis carinii* pneumonia
>
> Recurrent bacterial pneumonia
>
> Progressive multifocal leukoencephalopathy
>
> *Salmonella* septicemia
>
> Toxoplasmosis

A thorough intraoral examination may reveal evidence of significant immune suppression, such as KS, OHL, or oropharyngeal candidiasis. As mentioned earlier, neck lymphadenopathy also may be noted on initial presentation of acute HIV infection. Once HIV becomes part of the differential diagnosis, prompt referral to the patient's primary care provider for additional evaluation is paramount. During the primary care provider's assessment, a thorough physical examination will be performed to evaluate for the development of opportunistic diseases associated with an advanced stage of infection. This examination includes a skin examination looking for KS and a fundoscopic examination looking for CMV or toxoplasmic retinitis. Hepatomegaly or splenomegaly would indicate possible coinfection with hepatitis or disseminated mycobacterial infection. An ano–genital examination may reveal evidence of sexually transmitted diseases. Laboratory testing includes HIV antibody, quantitative HIV RNA level (viral load), CD4+ count, complete blood cell count (CBC), serum chemistry, fasting glucose, lipid screen, liver function tests, vaginal or anal Papanicolaou's smear, and testing for exposure to other infectious diseases such as hepatitis B, hepatitis C, *Toxoplasma gondii*, and syphilis.

The cornerstones of HIV testing since its introduction in 1985 have been strict adherence to providing confidential testing with informed consent and the provision of counseling.[15] HIV antibody testing traditionally has involved the use of ELISA as a screening test. If the ELISA test is positive, a second, confirmatory test, a Western blot, is performed. A positive Western blot then indicates HIV infection.[16,17] Recent advances in HIV testing have led to the development of rapid HIV antibody tests. Four such rapid tests are approved by the US Food and Drug Administration (FDA) and use samples either from oral fluids or blood.[18] A positive result with a rapid test requires confirmation with additional testing. Rapid tests have been helpful in providing greater access to testing and better communication with patients, as the results are available immediately. It has been estimated that 31% of people who tested positive for HIV in 2000 in the United States did not return to receive their results.[19] The availability of rapid testing should help decrease this number.

A baseline HIV RNA viral load provides important information about the patient's disease state and is predictive of outcome in patients who are untreated. Elevated viral load correlates with more progressive disease early in HIV infection.[14,20] In patients who exhibit symptoms of acute HIV infection, viral loads are often greater than 100,000 copies/mL.[10] Viral load is assayed during initial diagnosis, before changes in ART, and every 2 to 8 weeks after a change in therapy until stability is achieved. For patients on stable ART, viral load should be tested every 3 to 4 months, or as clinically indicated.[21] The desired result of ART is to reduce the viral load to an undetectable level (an ultrasensitive assay has a lower limit of 50 copies/mL).[14]

The CD4+ T cell count is also a very important indicator of the patient's cell-mediated immunity. Uninfected individuals may have counts in the range of 500 cells/mm³ to 2000 cells/mm³. Patients who have counts between 350 and 500 cells/mm³ rarely exhibit clinical findings of immunocompromise. Those who have counts between 200 and 350 cells/mm³ likely exhibit findings of immune compromise such as candidiasis, mucosal infections, and herpes zoster.[14] Patients who have CD4+ counts less than 200 cells/mm³ are defined as having AIDS according to the 1993 CDC classification system and may present with life-threatening OIs. Those who have CD4+ counts less than 50 cells/mm³ have advanced HIV disease.[13]

Evaluation of a CBC is essential, as cytopenias of all blood cell lines, anemia being the most common, have been reported in patients who have HIV.[22,23] A chemistry evaluation may reveal kidney dysfunction, as HIV nephropathy is a possible complication of HIV infection.[24] A fasting blood glucose, lipid screen, and liver function tests during initial testing are important, because many antiretroviral medications are associated with abnormal glucose metabolism, dyslipidemia, and hepatotoxicity.[14,25,26] Of course, additional testing for other communicable diseases such as sexually transmitted diseases, hepatitis, tuberculosis (TB), and *Toxoplasma gondii* are essential, as these individual entities also may require treatment. Evidence of advanced disease may indicate the need for additional testing such as radiographs or CT scans.

SYSTEMIC COMPLICATIONS OF HIV INFECTION

The advent of ART has changed the progression of HIV infection. Many of the systemic effects of HIV infection can be avoided or modulated with ART and other prophylactic therapy. Any of the systemic complications of HIV may exist, however, because of the development of resistance to antiretrovirals, lack of treatment, or eventual failure of treatment. A review of systemic findings follows, and a specific review of oral findings in HIV is found later in this article.

Infectious/Neoplastic

As immunodeficiency progresses, infectious and neoplastic complications not often found in the uninfected population appear. Infectious complications can include localized or systemic fungal infections caused by *Candidia albicans*, *Cryptococcus neoformans*, *Coccidoides immitis*, *Histoplasma capsulatum,* or *Pneumocystis jirovecii*.[27,28] *Pneumocystis carinii* originally was classified as a protozoan but was reclassified by means of DNA sequencing in 1998 as a fungus and was renamed *Pneumocystis jirovecii* in 2002.[28,29] Parasitic protozoan infections can include encephalitis caused by *Toxoplasma gondii* or gastrointestinal (GI) infection with *Cryptosporidium parvum* or *Isospora belli*.[13,27] Patients who have HIV are more susceptible to bacterial infections, especially those caused by *Streptococcus pneumoniae, Haemophilis influenzae, Salmonella* species, *Mycobacterium avium,* and *Mycobacterium tuberculosis*.[13,27] Viral infections that may appear include outbreaks of herpes simplex virus (HSV), varicella zoster virus, Epstein-Barr virus (EBV), and CMV.[13,27] Evidence of these viral infections may involve the mouth, head, and neck.

As the patient becomes further immunocompromised, several malignancies develop, most notably, KS, cervical cancer, and lymphoma. Up to 40% of patients who have HIV develop malignancy during their disease.[30] KS, the most common HIV-related malignancy, may present in a mucocutaneous form while the patient's CD4+ count is between 200 and 500 cells/mm^3 and progress to a visceral form as CD4+ counts decrease to between 100 and 200 cells/mm^3.[27,30] KS may involve the skin, oral cavity, GI tract, and even the lungs.[31] Approximately 35% of HIV patients with KS have oral lesions, and in 15% of patients, oral lesions may be an initial finding of KS. Evidence has shown that there may be an etiologic relationship between human herpes virus 8 and the development of KS. AIDS patients with KS have a median survival of 18 to 24 months.[30] First-line management for KS includes HAART. Several local modalities, such as radiation therapy, intralesional chemotherapy, surgical excision, laser treatment, cryotherapy, and photodynamic therapy, are options also.[30,31] Systemic chemotherapy is indicated in patients who have advanced disease. A discussion of oral KS will follow later in this article.

Cervical carcinoma in situ may be present early in HIV infection (1993 CDC category B finding), but progresses to invasive cancer once AIDS is present.[13] Women who have HIV are believed to be likely to have a higher rate of coinfection with human papilloma virus (HPV) and also have poor immune control of HPV because of immunosuppression, leading to a higher incidence of cervical cancer.[30] HIV-related cervical cancer is aggressive and carries a poor prognosis. Treatment recommendations are the same as those that are followed for non-HIV infected women who have cervical cancer.

Lymphomas found in patients how have HIV are most commonly non-Hodgkin's lymphomas (NHL), although there is also a high incidence of Hodgkin's lymphoma (HL). Approximately 70% of NHL is systemic, and 20% of NHL is primary central nervous system (CNS) lymphoma. The introduction of HAART has decreased the incidence of primary CNS lymphoma.[30] CNS lymphoma is a sign of very advanced HIV disease, with CD4+ counts usually below 50 cells/mm^3 at the time of diagnosis. Lymphoma is treated aggressively with intravenous chemotherapy and intrathecal chemotherapy, either prophylactically or therapeutically. AIDS-NHL carries a poor prognosis, and overall survival is 12 months.[30] HL also is managed with aggressive chemotherapy, and median survival rates up to 16 months have been reported.[30]

Other neoplastic diseases found in patients who have HIV include anal cancer, basal cell and squamous cell skin cancer, lung cancer, testicular cancer, and oral/head and neck cancer. Patients who have HIV are felt to be at greater risk for developing nonmelanoma skin cancers. Patients who have HIV are not at greater risk of developing lung cancer, but the features do differ from lung cancer in non-HIV infected patients. Patients who have HIV present at a younger age and more commonly with adenocarcinoma than non-HIV infected individuals. Over 70% present in an advanced stage or with inoperable disease. Testicular cancer found in patients who have HIV does not seem to be related directly to immune suppression and is managed in a manner similar to testicular cancer in non-HIV infected patients. Survival is good, and most patients can be cured of their testicular cancer.[30]

Skin

Mucocutaneous diseases are among the most common disorders of HIV. Cutaneous lesions generally may be classified into infectious (bacterial, viral, fungal), neoplastic, and reactive. Some skin lesions require biopsy for definitive diagnosis, and many different lesions have similar clinical presentation, also requiring biopsy for differentiation.

Infectious

Bacterial skin infections most commonly include *Staphylococcus aureus* infection and bacillary angiomatosis. Staphylococcal infections may be in the form of an abscess, ulcer, folliculitis, or cellulitis, and may involve methicillin-resistant *Staphylococcus aureus* (MRSA). These infections clinically may resemble viral infections such as HSV infection, and therefore, biopsy or culture should be performed whenever suspicious lesions are noted. Antibiotic treatment usually begins with an antibiotic active against methicillin-suseptible *Staphylococcus*. If the infection is recurrent or persistent, however, an antibiotic active against MRSA such as doxycycline, clindamycin, or trimethoprim-sulfamethoxazole should be used.[32] Complications of *Staphylococcus aureus* skin infection include staphylococcal scalded skin syndrome, bacteremia, and pruritis.[33] Bacillary angiomatosis lesions consist of vascular proliferations, which may be papular or nodular, multiple, single, or widespread. Clinically, these lesions resemble KS, and biopsy is essential to differentiate between these lesions, as their etiology and management differ. Bacillary angiomatosis is caused by infection with *Bartonella henselae* or *B quintana*. The histologic diagnosis is best made using Warthin-Starry staining to demonstrate the coccobacilli within macrophages and in the interstitium. Progression of this disease is potentially lethal, but it responds well to antibiotics (erythromycin or doxycycline).[33,34]

Viral skin infections in patients who have HIV include HSV, varicella-zoster virus (VZV), HPV, and molluscum contagiosum. HSV infections are among the most common viral infections occurring in patients who have HIV, with as many as 95% of HIV patients being seropositive for either HSV-1, HSV-2, or both.[35] Lesions are painful vesicles located on an erythematous base on the skin or mucosa. HSV lesions are more widespread, with more atypical presentation and more persistence in patients who have HIV.[36] HSV infections persisting longer than 1 month meet the 1993 CDC criteria for AIDS.[13] Diagnosis may be confirmed by means of biopsy, viral culture, or a Tzanck smear.[33] A Tzanck smear (or preparation) is obtained by unroofing a fresh (preferably less than 3 days old) vesicle and gently touching the fluid onto a slide. The slide then is fixed and usually stained with Giemsa stain. Classic histologic characteristics include multinucleated syncytial giant cells.[37] Management historically has involved five doses per day of acyclovir; however, recent studies have demonstrated equal efficacy with twice-daily doses of famciclovir (and likely better compliance).[35,38]

VZV remains latent in the sensory nerve ganglia after the primary infection with varicella has occurred. It may become reactivated in the form of shingles, resulting in a dermatomal distribution of vesicles on an erythematous base. In immunocompetent patients under the age of 40, shingles is rare, but it is fairly common in patients who have HIV.[36] Lesions in patients who have HIV also follow dermatomes, but are usually longer-lasting and are more likely to involve more than one dermatome in more advanced HIV.[33,36] In the head and neck, three types of VZV involvement may occur: trigeminal distribution (ophthalmic, maxillary, or mandibular division), VZV ophthalmicus or retinitis, or facial paralysis s/p VZV infection.[36] Ophthalmic/retinal involvement or facial paralysis in the setting of VZV infection is rare. Oral or intravenous (in the case of ophthalmic VZV) acyclovir has been the mainstay of treatment, but valacyclovir has better bioavailability and is used also. Care must be taken when treating immunosuppressed patients with valacyclovir, because there is a risk of hemolysis.[33]

Lesions caused by HPV are fairly common in individuals who have HIV, and these may appear anywhere in the mouth, cervix, or on the skin, primarily in the ano–genital region. The presence of HPV increases the risk of intraepithelial neoplasia and cancer, including anal intraepithelial neoplasia and anal cancer.[36,39] The lesions of HPV do not respond well to ART.[32] Treatment for the warts of HPV typically has consisted of local therapies, including surgery, cryotherapy, laser treatment, and intralesional interferon injections.[32,33]

Molluscum contagiosum is a cutaneously transmissible lesion caused by the poxviridae family of viruses. The lesions most commonly occur on the limbs, trunk, and neck. Molluscum contagiosum is typically not painful and results in raised, round papules with a central area of umbilication. Clinically, these lesions may resemble cryptococcosis or histoplasmosis, so biopsy is recommended. Treatment consists of surgery, cryotherapy, or topical tretinoin.[33,40]

Fungal skin infections in HIV include candidiasis, cryptococcosis, histoplasmosis, dermatophytosis, and arthropod infections. *Candida* infections are among the most common fungal infections in patients who have HIV and may involve the mucosa, skin, or nails. OC will be discussed later in this article. Cutaneous *Candida* typically involves intertriginous areas with erythematous patches and is treated with topical antifungals. Nail involvement usually is confined to the proximal nail, turning it white, and it is treated with a 12-week course of oral itraconazole. A risk of cutaneous *Candida* is that it can enter the blood stream, resulting in life-threatening fungemia.[41]

Infections with *Cryptococcus neoformans* most commonly affect the lungs, as this organism is found most commonly in the soil and in bird waste. Skin involvement does occur, however, and the lesions may be pustular, papular, nodular, verruciform, or granulomatous, usually involving the head and neck.[33,41] Clinically, these lesions resemble mulloscum contagiousum; therefore, biopsy of suspicious lesions is prudent. Management usually consists of systemic antifungal medication, as cutaneous lesions often are accompanied by disseminated disease.[33]

Isolated skin infections with *Histoplasma capsulatum* are rare, as the route of infection is inhalation of spores from the soil. Skin lesions of histoplasmosis may appear as ulcers, papules, macules, or pustules. Again, diagnosis is made best by means of either tissue culture or biopsy. Antifungal therapy with itraconazole, fluconazole, or amphotericin B may need to be life-long because of the disseminated nature of the disease.[41]

Dermatophyte infections with the fungal parasite, *Trichophyton rubruim*, are fairly common, especially in patients who have CD4+ counts of less than 100cells/mm^3, and these often affect fingernails and toenails.[42] Skin involvement produces scaly, erythematous annular patches. Ketoconazole often is used to manage dermatophyte infections.[33]

Neoplastic

Common skin neoplasias in patients who have HIV include KS, basal cell carcinoma, and squamous cell carcinoma. Cutaneous KS was discussed earlier in this section, and a discussion of oral KS will follow later. Both basal and squamous cell skin cancer seem to have a higher prevalence in patients who have HIV than in noninfected patients. The risk factors for development of nonmelanoma skin cancer are the same as for the general population—sunlight exposure, fair skin, and family history—but co-infection with HPV seems to be important also. Melanoma does not seem to be more common in HIV, but it may be more widespread at the time of diagnosis. Squamous cell carcinoma of the skin may be more aggressive in the HIV patient; therefore, wider excisions are recommended.[30]

Inflammatory

Common inflammatory skin conditions associated with HIV infection include seborrheic dermatitis, atopic dermatitis, psoriasis, pruritic papular eruption, photodermatitis, and drug reaction. Seborrheic dermatitis is one of the most common dermatologic manifestations of HIV, affecting up to 85% of patients who have HIV at some point.[33,41,43,44] Seborrheic dermatitis is characterized by epidermal hyperplasia with increased turnover resulting in erythema and scaling. It occurs in areas of dense sebaceous glands, especially on the face, scalp, back, and chest. Secondary infection by *Staphylococcus aureus* is a risk in affected areas. Treatment consists of ketoconazole shampoo/cream; topical corticosteroids, salicylic acid, coal tar, sulfur, or UV-B light.[33,41,43]

Atopic dermatitis and dry skin are very common in HIV patients who have HIV and is often severe. Clinically, the affected skin may exhibit lichenification and pruritis with excoriations that may become secondarily infected. Management usually consists of topical steroids, moisturizers, and antihistamines to relieve itching. Topical tacrolimus and pimecrolimus, both immunosuppressants used in immunocompetent patients to treat atopic dermatitis, should not be used in patients who have HIV because of immune dysfunction.[32,43]

Psoriasis is as common in the general population as it is in the HIV population, but psoriasis is more severe, difficult to treat, and has a higher prevalence of psoriatic arthritis in patients who have HIV. It is also more common for patients who have HIV to exhibit more than one subtype of psoriasis at one time (pustular, guttate, or erythrodermic).[41,43] Clinical findings include red plaques with silverfish scales. Patients who have HIV are more susceptible to streptococcal throat infections with subsequent guttate psoriasis development with small pink plaques with white scales.[41,43] Another manner in which psoriasis in HIV differs from the general population is that in patients who have HIV, psoriasis may present on unusual surfaces such as the underarm and sole of the foot rather than on extensor surfaces.[32] Immunosuppressive therapy that may be used in the general population should not be used in patients who have HIV. Instead, zidovudine, minimal ultraviolet phototherapy, or etretinate have been reported.[43]

Many previous reports had indicated that pruritic papular eruption (PPE) was an initial presentation of HIV; however, Boonchai and colleagues[45] found that PPE was found more often in patients late in HIV disease when CD4+ counts were below 50/mm^3. Clinically, PPE results in pruritic hyperpigmented papules found on the trunk, extremities, or face. Treatments include UV-B phototherapy, antipruritics, or pentoxifylline.[41]

HIV infection causes photosensitizing of the skin, and this may be compounded by the use of photosensitizing drugs such as trimethoprim-sulfamethazole. Management includes use of sunscreen, topical steroids, emollients, and antihistamines.[32]

Patients who have HIV are at particularly high risk of developing cutaneous drug reactions. This is because patients who have HIV take more medications than the general population, and the medications they take have a high rate of reactions. Additionally, HIV patients have been found to have decreased glutathione, resulting in a decreased ability to detoxify metabolites.[41] Morbilliform exanethem is the most common drug reaction in patients who have HIV, but urticaria, vasculitis, anaphylaxis, Stevens-Johnson syndrome, and toxic epidermolysis (TEN) may occur also. Trimethoprim-sulfamethoxazole, used for *Pneumocystis jirovecii* pneumonia prophylaxis, is the most common cause of cutaneous adverse effects, which occur in up to 60% of HIV patients taking this medication.[33] Cutaneous reactions are managed according to their severity using antihistamines, steroids, withdrawal of the medication, or intravenous immunoglobulin in cases of TEN.[41]

Genitourinary

Genitourinary complications of HIV include syphilis, HSV-1 or HSV-2, lymphogranuloma venereum, gonorrhea, HPV, cervical cancer, bacterial vaginosis, vaginal candidiasis, trichomoniasis, chlamydia, PID, testicular cancer, and anal cancer. HSV, HPV, cervical cancer, testicular cancer, and anal cancer have been discussed previously and will not be discussed in this section. Patients who have HIV often are coinfected with other transmissible diseases, including syphilis. *Treponema pallidum* is a spirochete bacterium that enters the body through intact mucosa or abraded skin, disseminates, has an incubation period of 3 to 90 days, and results in syphilis. Three stages are recognized: primary, secondary, or tertiary (neurosyphilis). Primary syphilis results in the development of a painless chancre, which is an ulcer with a raised, firm border. Secondary syphilis develops within a few weeks to months and results in a rash, fever, anorexia, arthralgias, and adenopathy. Secondary syphilis also may be accompanied by meningitis, nephritis or nephrosis, gastritis, or hepatitis. Tertiary syphilis develops 5 to 35 years after primary infection and consists of neurologic involvement, gumma involvement of bone or brain, and/or cardiac disease. In patients who have HIV, the progression through these stages may be accelerated. Standard screening tests for syphilis includes rapid plasma reagin (RPR) and VDRL tests. If one of these tests is positive, confirmatory tests are performed with *Treponema pallidum* particle agglutination (TP-PA) or fluorescent treponemal antibody absorption (FTA-ABS) tests. Treatment for syphilis includes intravenous administration of benzathine penicillin. Eradication of neurosyphilis in patients who have HIV is difficult, especially in those with low CD4+ counts and those who are not on ART. There is some controversy about the workup for those coinfected with HIV and syphilis. Some authors recommend lumbar puncture for all patients coinfected regardless of symptoms in order to evaluate for cerebrospinal fluid (CSF) abnormalities caused by syphilis. If CSF abnormalities such as elevated CSF protein, elevated CSF white blood cell (WBC) count, or a positive CSF VDRL are present, treatment for neurosyphilis is warranted. Other practitioners believe that decision to perform lumbar puncture should be based on clinical symptoms, CD4+ count, or syphilis titer.[14,46,47]

Infection with *Chlamydia trachomatis* may result in lymphogranuloma venereum (LGV), nongonoccal urethritis, or cervicitis, depending upon the serovar involved. LGV is caused by *Chlamydia trachomatis* serovars L1, L2, and L3 and is rare in the United States, because these serovars are endemic in Africa, Southeast Asia, South America, and the Caribbean. Presentation usually involves painful genital ulcers, inguinal or femoral adenopathy that may be fluctuant, and hemorrhagic proctitis or proctocolitis. LGV is treated with a 21-day course of doxycycline.[47,48]

Chlamydia trachomatis serovars B and D through K cause most cases of nongonoccal urethritis (NGU) and cervicitis. *Ureaplasma urealyticum* and *Trichomonas vaginalis* are other causes of NGU. Symptoms of NGU include urethral discharge, dysuria, and itching. Cervicitis may result in mucopurulent discharge, dysuria, pyuria, and increased urinary frequency. Both *Chlamydia trachomatis* and *Neisseria gonorrhoeae* can result in PID, which is a CDC category B (symptomatic) manifestation of HIV. PID is associated with endometritis, salpingitis, and pelvic peritonitis and carries a risk of sterility. *Neisseria gonorrhoeae* also causes urethritis, resulting in severe dysuria and purulent discharge, and cervicitis, resulting in a copious yellow discharge. Gonorrhea also may affect the anorectal area, the pharynx, and may become disseminated resulting in arthritis–dermatitis syndrome or septic arthritis. In fact, *Neisseria gonorrhoeae* is the most common cause of septic arthritis in those aged 16 to 50.[46] Chlamydial infection is frequently present concurrent with gonococcal infection, so treatment for both usually is administered using ceftriaxone and doxycycline or azithromycin.[46,47] As in the non-HIV infected female population, vaginal candidiasis, bacterial vaginosis, and trichomoniasis are common in women who have HIV. Specific treatment for these entities is similar to that for non-HIV infected patients, and usually the response is good. Vulvovaginal candidiasis that is persistent or does not respond well to therapy, however, is a 1993 CDC category B symptom.[13]

GASTROINTESTINAL

GI symptoms in patients who have HIV may worsen existing malnutrition and weight loss. Dysphagia and burning in the substernal region are common in patients who have HIV. GI symptoms often are accompanied by a CD4+ count of less than 50 cells/mm^3. These symptoms, especially when coupled with OC, may indicate the presence of esophageal candidiasis, which is an AIDS-defining finding.[13,27] Treatment with an antifungal such as fluconazole 200 mg per day on day one, followed by 100 mg per day, should result in an improvement of symptoms within 5 days. However, it is recommended that treatment continue for a minimum of three weeks. If antifungal treatment does not result in an improvement, esophagoscopy with biopsy of visible ulcers is indicated to rule out CMV, aphthae or HSV, which are responsible for 50%, 45%, and 5% of esophageal ulcers, respectively.[27] CMV ulcers are managed with gancyclovir or foscarnet; aphthae are managed with prednisone or thalidomide (except in pregnancy). HSV is managed with acyclovir.

Nausea and vomiting are common, especially in advanced disease. Frequently, this may be the result of antiviral or prophylactic medications, in which case, trials of drug holidays may be attempted. Additionally, H_2 blockers or antiemetics may be provided. If relief is not obtained, esophagoscopy usually is performed to further investigate the cause.[27]

Diarrhea occurs at some point for at least 50% of patients who have HIV.[27] Diarrhea in the patient who has HIV most commonly has an infectious etiology, but GI lymphoma is also a possibility. When no definitive etiology is determined, the term HIV-associated enteropathy is used. Histologically, HIV-associated enteropathy is characterized by villous atrophy. Patients who have persistent diarrhea should have fecal cultures, assays for *Clostridium difficile* toxin, and examination for ova and parasites performed. *Clostridium difficile* is the most common cause of HIV diarrhea and has been found by Sanchez and colleagues to be the etiologic agent in 54% of bacterially associated HIV diarrhea in a study that examined bacterial diarrhea in patients with HIV from 1992 to 2002.[49,50] Other common causes included *Shigella* species (14%), *Campylobacter jejuni* (14%), *Salmonella* species (7%), *Staphylococcus aureus* (4%), and *Mycobacterium* species (3.6%).[49,50] It also has been demonstrated that the incidence of diarrhea increases as immunosuppression worsens. Antibiotic exposure and frequent hospitalization are risk factors for *Clostridium difficile* infection. *Clostridium difficile* is the sole anaerobic bacteria which is communicable. Complications include loss of protein, resulting in hypoalbuminemia, ileus, toxic megacolon, anasarca, leukemoid reaction, renal failure, need for colectomy, sepsis, and death. Treatment for *Clostridium difficile* infection in the patient who has HIV is the same as for non-HIV infected patients, including cessation of the offending agent, administration of oral metronidazole or vancomycin, and supportive care.

In addition to bacteria, parasites or viruses also may be responsible for diarrhea. *Cryptosporidium parvum* and *Isospora belli* are the most common parasites infecting the GI tract in patients who have AIDS. Both cryptosporidiosis and isoporiasis respond well to ART.[27] Intestinal cryptosporidiosis and isosporiasis lasting longer than 1 month are both AIDS-defining criteria.[13] Additionally, the colon may be infected by HSV, cytomegalovirus, or MAC.

LIVER DISEASE

Liver function tests are frequently abnormal in HIV patients. There are many possible causes for this finding, including chronic active hepatitis B or C (HBV or HCV), medication-induced hepatic inflammation; infectious infiltration by MAC, CMV, or cryptosporidiosis; cholecystitis; or AIDS-associated sclerosing cholangitis.[27] Approximately 25% of patients who have HIV are coinfected with HCV.[51] Greater than 75% of people infected with HIV because of intravenous drug use are coinfected with HCV.[52] Most who are coinfected are intravenous drug abusers. HCV is so common that end-stage liver disease is now the most common cause of non-AIDS death in the United States in patients coinfected with HIV and HCV.[51] Kellerman and colleagues[53] found that in the United States, the overall rate of HBV coinfection in patients not vaccinated for HBV is 7.6%. HIV patients coinfected with HBV or HCV tend to have more rapid progression to cirrhosis and ultimately have shorter survival times than non-HIV infected patients who have HBV or HCV.[52,53] Cirrhosis may be characterized by ascites, GI bleeding, spontaneous bacterial peritonitis, hepatorenal syndrome, hepatic encephalopathy, esophageal varices, and hepatocellular carcinoma. The administration of HAART may slow progression of liver disease; however, HAART medications also can induce hepatotoxicity, so a balance must be achieved. From a surgeon's perspective, any patient who has coinfection with HBV or HCV should be assumed to have some liver dysfunction and should be expected to possibly have a coagulopathy in addition to the other risks of liver disease (especially GI bleeding or esophageal varix bleeding). HIV infection is no longer a contraindication to orthotopic liver transplantation because of the availability of HAART, and post-transplant survival rates are similar to those of non-HIV infected patients.

RENAL

Renal diseases in the HIV-infected population include those caused by comorbidities such as hypertension, diabetes, and hepatitis coinfection, in addition to HIV-associated nephropathy and nephrotoxicity of antiretroviral drugs and other medications necessary to treat HIV.[24] Approximately 30% of patients who have HIV are believed to have abnormal renal function.[54] Renal dysfunction is often asymptomatic; therefore, infected patients should have regular assessment of renal function, because the risk of drug toxicity is high.[55] Screening studies include urine protein quantification by means of spot-urine protein:creatinine ratio (not dipstick, which is inaccurate) and serum creatinine to estimate creatinine clearance or glomerular filtration rate (GFR). Finings of proteinuria greater than 500 mg or decreased GFR less than 60 mL/min/1.73 m^2 would prompt further evaluation with renal ultrasound and nephrology referral.[55,56]

HIV-associated nephropathy (HIVAN) is an important cause of renal failure almost exclusively found in those of African descent. HIVAN is characterized by very rapid progression to end-stage renal disease (ESRD) over a period of weeks to months; therefore, rapid diagnosis by kidney biopsy is essential. Histologically, HIVAN is associated with collapsing focal segmental glomerulosclerosis with tubular dilation and interstitial inflammation.[24] Treatment primarily consists of HAART, but dialysis, glucocorticoids, angiotensin-converting enzyme inhibitors, and angiotensin-II receptor blockers are used occasionally.[55] Renal transplantation also may be considered for ESRD.

Patients coinfected with HCV are at risk of developing membranoproliferative glomerulonephritis (MPGN), a complication of HCV infection.[55,57] HCV infection is estimated to account for 10% to 20% of all cases of MPGN, and approximately 30% of patients who have MPGN progress to chronic renal failure within 10 years of diagnosis of MPGN.[57] Drug-related renal dysfunction related to HAART medications and medications to manage HIV-related complications is common and will be discussed in a later section covering the medical management of HIV.

HEMATOLOGIC

Cytopenias of all blood cell lines can be associated with HIV infection, and the incidence of cytopenia is directly proportional to the level of immunosupression.[23] The most common HIV-associated hematologic abnormality is anemia. There are many causes of anemia in the patient who has HIV: infection, malnutrition, malignancy, renal failure, and medications. Mycobacteria and fungi may disseminate to the bone marrow, replacing normal architecture. Viral infections, such as CMV or EBV, also may suppress bone marrow function. The bone marrow may become infiltrated by lymphoma or KS. Nutritional deficiencies leading to anemia are common because of anorexia, GI dysfunction, and malabsorption. Several medications have be implicated in bone marrow suppression, especially zidovudine (AZT).[23] In general, use of HAART decreases the incidence and severity of anemia. A 1994 to 1998 study of women who had HIV identified four risk factors for the development of anemia:

Mean corpuscular volume (MCV) less than 80 fL
CD4+ cell count less than 200
HIV-1 viral load greater thana 50,000/mL
AZT use within the past 6 months[58]

Anemic patients are managed by addressing the cause of anemia and transfusion if necessary. If transfusion is performed in a CMV-seronegative patient, it is recommended that CMV-negative blood be used, or if not available, blood should be transfused through a leukocyte filtering system.[23]

Thrombocytopenia occurs commonly in patients who have HIV, presenting in about 40% of patients who have at some point during their illness.[22] In fact, in approximately 10% of patients, thrombocytopenia may be the presenting symptom of HIV infection. Thrombocytopenia in patients who have HIV is either primary or secondary. The most common cause of thrombocytopenia in these patients is primary HIV-associated thrombocytopenia (PHAT). PHAT seems to be the result of decreased platelet survival combined with decreased platelet production.[22] Secondary thrombocytopenia may be caused by malignancy, OIs, or medications. Management of thrombocytopenia starts with the exclusion of secondary causes. Primary management of PHAT is AZT. Retrospective studies have suggested that HAART can also increase platelet counts. In patients who require rapid correction of thrombocytopenia, intravenous immunoglobulin may improve platelet counts dramatically, which may be particularly beneficial in thrombocytopenic patients requiring surgery or for patients who are bleeding actively.[22] Other agents been used to treat PHAT include dapsone, short-term corticosteroids, and interferon alpha.[22]

Patients who have HIV may present with various coagulation system abnormalities including thrombosis, antiphospholipid syndrome, protein C and S deficiency, and thrombotic thrombocytopenic purpura. Thrombosis has been associated with malignancy, OIs, CD4+ count less than 200/mm^3, and elevated levels of factor VIII, homocysteine, or lipids.[22] The incidence of thrombotic thrombocytopenic purpura–hemolytic uremic syndrome (TTP-HUS) in HIV has been decreasing in the post-HAART era, but should be considered in HIV patients with thrombocytopenia and anemia.

CARDIOVASCULAR

Cardiovascular risk factors in patients who have HIV appear to be the same as those found in the general population—hypertension, diabetes, smoking, hyperlipidemia, advanced age, male sex, and family history of cardiovascular disease. It is felt that HAART contributes to an increased cardiovascular risk, but the overall increased risk conferred by HAART may be low.[59] In 2003, the results of the Data Collection on Adverse Events of Anti-HIV Drugs (DAD) were released. Their findings revealed that the use of combination of ART correlated with a 26% relative increased risk of myocardial infarction per year of antiretroviral use during the first 4 to 6 years of use.[60] This study did not find any correlation between this increased risk and duration of HIV infection, degree of previous immunodeficiency, or the amount of HIV RNA replication. HAART use has been associated with: hypertriglyceridemia, low high-density lipoprotein (HDL), hypercholesterolemia, and insulin resistance, which elevate cardiovascular risk.[61] For this reason, the lipid profile is followed closely, and modifiable risk factors such as smoking and diet are addressed. If nonpharmacologic management fails to address hypercholesterolemia, lipid-lowering agents are instituted.[14] An OMS has the opportunity to spend extra time counseling these patients on smoking cessation and diet and exercise management. Although use of HAART is associated with an increased risk of cardiovascular disease, the benefits of its use outweigh the cardiovascular risk.

PULMONARY

Pulmonary diseases in patients who have HIV are common and include pneumonia, TB, histoplasmosis and coccidioidomycosis, KS, and pulmonary hypertension. Until prophylaxis against *Pneumocystis jirovecii* (previously known as *Pneumocystis carinii*) became common, *Pneumocystis pneumonia* (still called PCP) was the most common life-threatening infection in AIDS patients in North America.[27,29] In addition to PCP prophylaxis with trimethoprim-sulfamethoxazole, use of HAART also has changed the patterns of pulmonary disease observed. Since the introduction of HAART, PCP has become less common, and bacterial pneumonia has become more common.[62] Patients who have HIV are 7.8 times more likely to have bacterial pneumonia than noninfected patients.[63] In addition to the fungus, *Pneumocystis jirovecii*, encapsulated bacteria such as *Streptococcus pneumoniae*, *Haemophilus influenzae*, *Pseudomonas aeruginosa*, and *Staphylococcus aureus*, in descending order, are the most common causes of pneumonia.[27,62,63] Recurrent bacterial pneumonia and PCP are both AIDS-defining events according to the CDC.[13] Important clinical findings differentiate PCP from bacterial pneumonias. Bacterial pneumonia has an acute onset and may be accompanied by a productive cough and rigors. Chest radiographs usually demonstrate lobar consolidation. Patients who have PCP report gradual appearance of symptoms including a nonproductive cough, fever, and shortness of breath on exertion. As symptoms progress, hypoxemia worsens with even slight exertion. Commonly, patients also present with coexisting oral thrush.[63] Any patient presenting to an OMS with new onset of OC who also has symptoms suggestive of PCP, should be referred to his or her primary physician for further evaluation. The chest radiograph in PCP may look completely normal or show an interstitial pattern.[27,62] The typical interstitial infiltrate is bilateral, diffuse, and exhibits a butterfly pattern.[63] Blebs may be present, so the finding of a pneumothorax in a patient who has HIV raises the suspicion of PCP. It has been estimated that 13% to 18% of patients with PCP have a coexisting pulmonary problem such as TB, KS, or bacterial pneumonia.[63] Prompt initiation of therapy is essential, as both types of pneumonia can progress to respiratory failure rapidly. Sputum Gram's stain is used to guide antimicrobial management in bacterial pneumonia, and PCP is diagnosed through the identification of *Pneumocystis* organisms in sputum or lung tissue. Because expeditious therapy is paramount, broad-spectrum therapy is initiated while awaiting results of laboratory assessment. Antibiotic selection for treatment of bacterial pneumonia mirrors that selected in the non-HIV infected population. High-dose intravenous trimethoprim-sulfamethoxazole is used to treat PCP, although it is associated with a high incidence of adverse effects including fever, rash, cytopenia, pancreatitis, nephritis, toxic epidermal necrolysis, and anaphylaxis. In patients who have severe reactions, alternative therapy with pentamidine or trimetrexate may be used. In patients who have significant hypoxemia with room air PaO_2 of 70 mm Hg or less, steroids are used.[62] Prophylaxis against PCP consists of trimethoprim-sulfamethoxazole and is initiated in patients who have a CD4+ count of less than 200 cells/mm^3, OC, or a previous history of PCP.[14]

Over the past few years in the United States, the numbers of *Mycobacterium tuberculosis* infections have been decreasing. Coinfection with HIV is common, however; in 1999 it was estimated that 10% of patients who had TB in the United States also had HIV. WHO has estimated that 11% of worldwide AIDS deaths are caused by TB. TB may be diagnosed at any level of immunosuppression, but those who have CD4+ counts less than 200 cells/mm^3 are more likely to have disseminated or extrapulmonary disease.[63] TB cases may be classified as either primary (infection occurring immediately after exposure) or reactivation of latent disease. Patients who have HIV should be skin tested for TB exposure, and those found to have latent infection should receive a minimum 9-month course of isoniazid.[14] Isoniazid prophylaxis also is recommended for HIV patients living in areas where TB is endemic. Chest radiograph findings in pulmonary TB include upper lobe fibronodular infiltrates with or without cavitation. As HIV disease becomes more advanced, lower and middle lobe and miliary infiltrates are more common, and cavitation is seen less frequently.[63] In TB, sputum culture is positive for acid-fast bacilli or *Mycobacterium tuberculosis*. A negative sputum culture in a suspicious case can be examined further by nucleic acid amplification tests to identify *Mycobacterium tuberculosis*. Optimal management of active TB in patients who have HIV involves susceptibility testing for the first-line drugs (isoniazid, rifampin, and ethambutol) and adjustment of drug regimen if necessary. Multiple drug therapy is provided for 6 to 9 months. Although HAART is associated with a reduction in TB rates, ART can result in a paradoxical worsening of TB symptoms associated with exaggerated inflammation.[63–65]

Histoplasmosis is caused by *Histoplasma capsulatum* acquired by inhalation, and it may be limited to the lungs or disseminated. Histoplasmosis affects approximately 2% to 5% of AIDS patients not taking HAART who live in areas where it is endemic.[63] The use of HAART has decreased in the incidence of histoplasmosis. Pulmonary histoplasmosis may occur in patients who have CD 4+ counts greater than 300 cells/mm^3, and the disseminated form (often involving skin and bone marrow) usually is found in patients who have CD 4+ counts less than 150 cells/mm^3. Coccidioidomycosis is caused by *Coccidioides immitis*, which is endemic to the southwestern United States and is transmitted by contact with disturbed soil. Coccidioidomycosis may be localized to the lungs or disseminated, and either disease can be seen in patients who have CD 4+ counts of less than 250 cells/mm^3. Most commonly, coccidioidomycosis presents as either disseminated disease or meningitis.[63] Chest radiographs of patients who have either histoplasmosis or coccidioidomycosis may demonstrate nodular infiltrates or a miliary pattern.[27] Primary management for both includes the administration of high-dose amphotericin B and subsequent oral azole therapy for prophylaxis.[27,63]

Aspergillosis is caused by *Aspergillus fumigatus* or other *Aspergillus* species and results in either respiratory involvement (semi-invasive pseudomembranous tracheitis or invasive pneumonitis) or CNS involvement. This organism tends to invade vascular endothelium, resulting in infarction as a common feature.[63] Semi-invasive pseudomembranous tracheitis may present with cough, dyspnea, and airway constriction, leading to airway obstruction. Invasive pneumonitis presents with cough, dyspnea, and hypoxemia. Chest radiographs reveal an interstitial pattern or wedge-shaped infiltrates indicating pulmonary infarction. Recommended treatment includes voriconazole or amphotericin B.

KS can involve the lungs and may be asymptomatic or present with a cough, shortness of breath, fever, chest pain, or hemoptysis.[31] Radiographic findings typically include pulmonary nodules or pulmonary effusion.[27] Bronchoscopy with biopsy is performed to confirm diagnosis, and treatment is with chemotherapy.

Pulmonary hypertension has been known to be associated with HIV infection both prior to use of HAART and since its introduction. The incidence in patients who have HIV has been reported to be 0.21%, and it must be considered in the differential diagnosis of dyspnea.[64] Pathogenesis is unknown, and it does not seem to be associated with other risk factors for pulmonary vasculopathy such as intravenous drug abuse and chronic HCV infection.[66] The development of HIV-associated pulmonary hypertension is an ominous sign. A retrospective review performed by Meha and colleagues[67] found that median survival time after diagnosis of HIV-associated pulmonary hypertension was 6 months. Most deaths were caused by right heart failure, cardiogenic shock, or sudden cardiac death. Treatment usually includes the use of pulmonary dilators such as calcium channel blockers or epoprosterol.

ENDOCRINE/METABOLIC

Patients who have HIV are at risk of developing type 2 diabetes, as are noninfected patients; however, HIV patients who are being treated with PIs are at greater risk of glucose metabolism disorders. Recent studies by the Multicenter AIDS Cohort Study (MACS) revealed that the prevalence of diabetes mellitus (DM) in HIV patients receiving HAART is higher than previously published incidence rates of 5% to 7%.[68,69] MACS found that the incidence of DM in HIV-positive men receiving HAART was 10%, compared with 3% in seronegative men.[68] Their study found that the PI ritonavir was associated with hyperglycemia or DM significantly.

Other metabolic abnormalities exist in patients who have HIV, including HIV lipodystrophy syndrome, in which patients exhibit a large posterior cervical fat pad, truncal fat accumulation, enlarged breasts, facial fat atrophy, and peripheral fat atrophy. This lipodystrophy syndrome sometimes is referred to as HIV-associated metabolic and morphologic abnormality syndrome (HAMMAS).[70] This fat redistribution is felt to have a multifactorial cause. Patients who have lipodystrophy are more likely to exhibit hypertriglyceridemia, low HDL, insulin resistance, impaired glucose tolerance, and DM. The cause of insulin resistance in these patients is unknown and may be related to ART or to HIV infection itself.[71] As a result, affected patients are at greater risk of cardiovascular disease and should be encouraged to address modifiable cardiovascular risk factors, such as diet, exercise, and smoking. Treatment for the lipid disorders and hyperglycemia are similar to treatment for the non-HIV infected population.[70]

Wasting syndrome or cachexia is a CDC AIDS-defining feature.[13] Wasting often occurs secondary to an infectious process, but may be caused by other factors. During advanced HIV disease, there may be increased production of tumor necrosis factor/cachectin, which may result in the wasting. Cachexia may be addressed with administration of ART, recombinant growth hormone, megestrol, or androgens.[27]

SKELETAL

Prior to the use of ART, the skeleton of patients who had HIV most commonly was affected by malignancy or infection. With longer life expectancies, however, osteopenia, osteoporosis, and osteonecrosis have become more common. Decreased bone mineral density has been reported in HIV-infected patients who are receiving ART and in those who are not. Various studies have produced conflicting data concerning the possible effect of ART on osteopenia and osteoporosis.[72] Ultimately, the cause is felt to be multifactorial, with ART being just one of many contributing factors. Ideal management has not been determined, but calcium and vitamin D supplementation, bisphosphonates, exercise, smoking cessation, and decreased alcohol use have been suggested.[65,72] Overall, osteonecrosis is an uncommon finding, but its incidence in the HIV-infected population has been increasing over recent years. The pathogenesis of osteonecrosis remains somewhat unclear, but it may be associated with the use of corticosteroids, and ART may have a permissive effect by prolonging life expectancy.[72]

NEUROLOGIC

Nervous system disorders are exceedingly common in the HIV population, ranging from mild cognitive changes to dementia, as well as involvement of the peripheral nervous system. Nervous system disease may be related directly to the effects of HIV, antiretroviral medication, infectious diseases, or neoplasia. Within the spectrum of neurocognitive impairment, there is a range of symptomatology and terminology for these disorders, which has resulted in confusion and has revealed the need for re-evaluation of this terminology.[73] Neurocognitive disorders generally have been categorized as HIV-associated neurocognitive impairment (HNCI) and AIDS dementia complex (ADC).[27,73–75] Recently, it has been suggested that the term asymptomatic neurocognitive impairment (ANI) should be introduced to describe patients with HIV who have slight impairment that is not overtly recognizable.[73] Impairment associated with HNCI includes forgetfulness and difficulty with concentration, attention, and memory. HNCI occurs in patients receiving ART and in those not receiving therapy. Although evidence suggests that antiretrovirals may not treat HNCI completely, it still is felt that initiation of antiretrovirals as early in the course of HNCI is beneficial. It also has been demonstrated that patients who are coinfected with HCV exhibit more neurocognitive impairment than those uninfected with HCV.[74] Other than optimal ARAT, there are few therapeutic options for patients who have HNCI.

ADC often is associated with late HIV infection. It may begin insidiously and subsequently progress over months to years. ADC results in impairment of three major neurologic functions: cognition, motor performance, and behavior. A five-step staging system based on clinical findings describes the severity of the disease. Stage 0.5 describes patients who exhibit mild cognitive impairment similar to HNCI. Mild motor symptoms such as abnormal reflexes may be found in stage 0.5 and stage 1. During stages 2 to 4, cognitive function worsens and interferes with activities of daily living. Motor dysfunction and behavioral issues become more evident. Ultimately, patients may progress to frank poverty of thought and action, disorientation to time and place, and severe difficulty with basic movement.[75] CT scanning of patients who have ADC reveals cerebral atrophy, wide cortical sulci, and vertricular enlargement. Because there are many other neurologic diseases associated with HIV, all patients who have neurologic symptoms must undergo a thorough evaluation to rule out possible infectious or neoplastic etiologies. The only treatment for ADC remains optimal ART, including at least two drugs that cross the blood–brain barrier, as HIV infection itself seems to be the primary cause of this disorder.[75]

The three most common focal neurologic lesions of the CNS are toxoplasmosis, CNS lymphoma, and progressive multifocal leukoencephalopathy.[27] In patients with HIV not treated with ART, approximately 33% of those seropositive for *Toxoplasma gondii* developed toxoplasmic encephalitis.[27,63] ART and *Toxoplasma gondii* prophylaxis have resulted in a dramatic decrease in the prevalence of this disease. *Toxoplasma gondii* infection rarely is observed in patients who have CD4+ cell counts greater than 200 cells/mm^3, and it is more common in patients who have CD4+ cell counts less than 50 cells/mm^3. Symptoms include headache, fever, lethargy, confusion, motor weakness, and with disease progression, seizures and coma.[62,63] CT scan findings include multiple ring enhancing lesions and edema. Once the presumptive diagnosis of *Toxoplasma gondii* infection is made, therapy with pyrimethamine and sulfadiazine is started. If neurologic symptoms worsen or do not improve, brain biopsy is indicated to rule out other infectious etiologies or CNS lymphoma. Patients remain on chronic prophylactic therapy after resolution of their initial symptoms.

Primary CNS lymphoma is the second most common cause of focal CNS disease in patients who have HIV. It is found late in HIV infection, most commonly when CD4+ cell counts are less than 200 cells/mm^3.[62] Approximately 3% to 6% of patients who have HIV develop primary CNS lymphoma, and nearly all cases demonstrate the presence of EBV within the lymphoma cells.[27,62] Of NHLs that develop in patients who have HIV, 20% are primary CNS lymphoma, most of which are diffuse large cell lymphoma.[30] Patients who have primary CNS lymphoma demonstrate headaches, memory loss, confusion, dysphasia, lethargy, paresis, seizures, and possible cranial nerve abnormalities. CT scan or MRI demonstrate contrast-enhancing hypodense lesion(s) with edema and mass effect. Unfortunately, the prognosis is very poor, and available therapy is limited to optimization of ART and possible radiation therapy.[62]

Progressive multifocal leukoencephalopathy (PML), also known as JC virus encephalitis (JCV-E) is an AIDS-defining disease that results in demyelination.[27,63,76] PML is caused by a papovavirus, JC virus, and is the only disease known to be caused by this virus.[63] Presenting symptoms include cognitive dysfunction, vision impairment, ataxia, dementia, cranial nerve dysfunction, paresis, or seizures.[27,63] Lesions are only visible on MRI as white matter lesions consistent with demyelination. Studies have recommended that optimal treatment may consist of ART and interferon beta. Although combination antitretroviral therapy has improved the prognosis of PML, the outlook is still dismal, with 50% mortality 6 months after diagnosis.[76]

Meningeal diseases found in patients who have HIV may be categorized as aseptic meningitis, chronic meningitis, or meningoencephalitis. Aseptic meningitis may be a sign of the acute retroviral syndrome early in HIV infection.[27] In patients who have previously known HIV infection, other viral causes should be considered, such as enteroviruses and herpes virus.[77] Patients complain of headache, but demonstrate a normal sensorium and neurologic examination. Viral meningitis usually is self-limited and follows a benign course.

Chronic meningitis typically presents with fever, headache, difficulty with concentration, and possible sensorium changes. Causes of chronic meningitis in patients who have HIV include *Cryptococcus neoformans, Coccidioides immitis, Histoplasma capsulatum,* and *Mycobacterium tuberculosis*.[27,63] *Cryptococcus neoformans* is the most common cause of chronic meningitis and the most common life-threatening fungus infecting the CNS in patients who have HIV.[27,62] Classic meningeal signs of neck stiffness and photophobia are sometimes not present. Diagnosis is made by identifying *Cryptococcus neoformans* in the CSF. The CSF WBC count is elevated; protein is slightly elevated, and glucose is low. Commonly, cryptococcal disease is disseminated, and pulmonary manifestations are found frequently. Treatment of meningeal disease focuses on two issues: managing the infection and treating the accompanying elevated intracranial pressure. Initial treatment utilizes amphotericin B and flucytosine for 2 weeks. Subsuquently, fluconazole is administered for an additional 8 weeks. The elevated intracranial pressure is managed with percutaneous lumbar drainage. Without treatment, cryptococcal meningitis is uniformly fatal, but with treatment, mortality is less than 10%.[63]

Coccidioidomycosis is caused by *Coccidioides immitis* and may result in disseminated disease or meningitis; it is more common in areas where this organism is endemic, such as the southwestern United States. Approximately 10% of patients who have coccidiodomycosis present with signs consistent with meningitis, including fever, headache, lethargy, confusion, or nausea and vomiting.[63] CSF usually demonstrates lymphocytic pleocytosis and glucose below 50 mg/dL. Treatment includes use of fluconazole both initially and as prophylactic therapy.[63]

Histoplasmosis is caused by *Histoplasma capsulatum* and most commonly is a disseminated disease occurring chiefly in areas where it is endemic, especially in the midwestern United States. Diagnosis of *Histoplasma capsulatum* meningitis may be difficult, because CSF cultures are often negative. The diagnosis often may be made in a patient with disseminated disease who exhibits CNS signs that otherwise cannot be explained. Amphotericin B is used for treatment, and lifelong prophylaxis may be provided with itraconazole.[63]

The CNS is one of the extrapulmonary sites of infection with *Mycobacterium tuberculosis*. *Mycobacterium tuberculosis* meningitis typically is found once CD4+ cell counts are less than 50 cells/mm^3. It is very rare in North America, but should be considered in chronic meningitis if CSF testing is negative for *Cryptococcus*.[27] Patients have a history of fever, stiff neck, and headache, which can progress to confusion and disorientation. Patients may exhibit hearing loss or other cranial nerve dysfunction caused by inflammation at the base of the brain.[77] The CSF reveals elevated white blood cells, very high protein, and low glucose, but often the smear for acid-fast bacilli is negative. Positive cultures may take weeks to grow, so treatment is presumptive with antituberculous agents.[77]

Aspergillosis typically is caused by *Aspergillus fumigatus* and results in either pulmonary disease or meningoencephalitis. CNS involvement results in fever and altered sensorium.[27] A primary feature of CNS involvement is vascular infarction.[63] Invasive aspergillosis usually is treated with voriconazole or amphotericin B. Neurosyphilis is another infectious disease of the CNS and was discussed in the genitourinary section.

Peripheral neuropathies are the most common neurologic disorders in patients who have HIV. There are several types of neuropathies, including distal symmetric polyneuropathy (DSP), inflammatory demyelinating polyneuropathy (IDP), mononeuritis multiplex (MM), progressive polyradiculopathy (PP), and autonomic neuropathy (AN).[78,79] Etiologies of neuropathy include direct HIV effects, OIs (especially CMV), antiretroviral toxicities, and nutritional deficiencies. DSP is the most common neuropathy and is the only one that can be caused by HIV infection directly or associated with antiretroviral use.[79] DSP often is found late in HIV infection and is considered to be associated with a deteriorating immune status. Symptoms include paresthesia, hyperesthesia, or burning sensations, and usually involve the feet first. Treatment includes cessation of neurotoxic drugs, use of anticonvulsants, analgesics, tricyclic antidepressants, and topical agents. IDP may result in weakness in addition to paresthesias and may respond to corticosteroids, IVIG, or anti-CMV therapy. MM may result in pain, facial weakness, other cranial nerve dysfunction, and foot drop and usually is treated with anti-CMV therapy. PP results in lower extremity weakness, sphincter dysfunction, and paresthesias and is managed with anti-CMV therapy. AN results in syncope, orhtostasis, anhidrosis, palpitations, urinary dysnfunction, impotence, and diarrhea and is treated by withdrawl of drugs that may be contributing, fluid and electrolyte replacement, and antiarrhythmic agents.[78,79]

Ocular findings are common in patients who have HIV. The ocular findings generally can be categorized into one of four groups: HIV retinopathy, OI (primarily with CMV), orbital or supporting structure involvement with neoplasm, or neuro–ophthalmic lesions. Retinopathy is the most common ocular finding in HIV and can be seen at any stage of HIV disease. It often is demonstrated by microangiopathy with cotton wool spots with or without intraretinal hemorrhages. This disorder is typically asymptomatic.[80] CMV retinitis is the most common intraocular infection in patients who have HIV, and when vision is lost, it becomes an AIDS-defining disease. Untreated, it can lead to blindness. Anti-CMV therapy includes valganciclovir, ganciclovir, or foscarnet.[63] Ophthalmic neoplastic involvement with KS or lymphoma is very rare. Neuro–ophthalmic lesions have been reported in as much as 8% of one study population and 10% to 15% of another study population.[80,81] These lesions frequently are associated with cryptococcal meningitis. Patients who have neuro–ophthalmic lesions most often exhibit cranial nerve palsies and papilledema from increased intracranial pressure, and vision loss from optic neuropathy.[80]

PSYCHIATRIC

Patients who have HIV are at risk of developing the same psychiatric disorders that are present in the general population. There are synergistic influences between HIV disease and psychiatric disorders, however. Pre-existing psychiatric disorders may lead to risk-taking behavior, which can result in HIV infection. Conversely, the presence of HIV infection may lead to psychiatric illness. The patient who has HIV with coexisting psychiatric illness may have greater difficulty following antiretroviral and OI prophylactic regimens, which ultimately leads to worsening of HIV disease. Additionally, new psychiatric symptoms may actually represent neurologic OI or neoplasia, so thorough evaluations of these patients must occur.

Furthermore, many patients with may have drug or alcohol addiction, which also plays a major influence in their psychological and physical well-being. Major depressive disorder (MDD) is the most common psychiatric illness in patients who have HIV.[82,83] At one time, MDD was felt to be no more common in the HIV-infected population than in the uninfected population, but reanalysis of previously published data revealed that MDD is twice as common in the HIV-infected population than in the uninfected population.[84] Some estimate that the lifetime prevalence of MDD in patients who have HIV ranges from 22% to 45%, compared to a range of 5% to 17% in the uninfected population.[82] Management of MDD in patients who have HIV is similar to that in the general population. Other psychiatric illnesses exist, such as bipolar disorder, psychotic disorders, and personality disorders. Management typically parallels that followed in the uninfected population, with the caveat that close attention is paid to possible interactions between psychiatric medications and HAART medications. Patients who have HIV are at greater risk of developing extrapyramidal symptoms; therefore, agents that cause this effect often are avoided.[82,83]

OTHER
Mycobacterium Avium Complex

Mycobacterium avium and *Mycobacterium intracellulare* are related bacteria that contribute to the disseminated infection of MAC. In over 95% of AIDS patients who develop MAC disease, the etiologic bacterium is *Mycobacterium avium*.[63] MAC bacteria are ubiquitous in the environment and are transmitted by means of inhalation or ingestion and survive in the gut and lungs until dissemination occurs. MAC typically is found in patients who have CD4+ counts less than 50 cells/mm^3. Symptoms include fatigue, fevers, night sweats, weight loss, abdominal pain, and diarrhea. Patients also may have anemia and lymphadenopathy.[63] Diagnosis is made by means of culture from the blood or bone marrow. Treatment typically consists of clarithromycin and ethambutol, with the possible addition of rifabutin or rifampin.[63,85] Patients also receive lifelong prophylaxis once MAC has been diagnosed. Patients should receive MAC prophylaxis once the CD4+ count reaches 50 cells/mm^3 or less.

Immune Reconstitution Inflammatory Syndrome

Immune reconstitution inflammatory syndrome (IRIS) is a syndrome that develops in a small number of antiretroviral-naïve patients upon initiation of ARAT during presentation with an OI. It is felt that the introduction of ART results in increased numbers of CD4+ and CD8+ cells and their cytokine release. Paradoxically, this can result in the worsening of the pre-existing OI, which can even be fatal. IRIS most commonly occurs with OI with MAC, *Mycobacterium tuberculosis,* and *Cryptococcus neoformans*.[62] In life-threatening IRIS, ART is discontinued until the OI is under control; then it is resumed.

ANTIRETROVIRAL THERAPY

The categories of antiretroviral medications include NNRTIs, NRTIs, nucleotide reverse transcriptase inhibitors (NtRTI), PIs, fusion inhibitors (FIs), and integrase inhibitors. The mechanism of action of these various medications was discussed previously. The use of antiretroviral therapies has revolutionized HIV medicine, although the disease is still incurable. In general, HAART has consisted of two NRTIs with either a PI or NNRTI.[86] This regimen, however, can vary. The Department of Health and Human Services (DHHS) Panel on Antiretroviral Guidelines for Adults and Adolescents recently published recommendations for the initiation of ART.[87] The panel recommends that ART be started in any patient who has a history of an AIDS- defining illness or a CD4+ cell count less than 350 cells/mm^3. The following patients should be started on ART regardless of their CD4+ cell count: pregnant patients, those who have HIV-associated nephropathy, and those coinfected with HBV in whom treatment for HBV is indicated.

The most common complications of antiretroviral medications include lactic acidosis, hypersensitivity, abnormal glucose metabolism, dyslipidemia, changes in body composition, and cardiovascular disease. Lactic acidosis most commonly is associated with NRTIs and it is felt to be caused by the poisoning effect on the mitochondria, resulting in anaerobic metabolism and lactic acid production. The incidence is approximately 2%.[25] Hypersensitivity reactions are common, most often involving NNRTIs. Ten percent to 17% of patients taking NNRTIs will experience a rash. Hepatotoxicity is a common finding along with the hypersensitivity.[25] Impaired glucose metabolism and diabetes mellitus occur most frequently with PIs, as was discussed earlier. Lipid changes include elevated triglycerides, decreased HDL, and increased low-density lipoprotein (LDL). PIs are associated most commonly with this finding, but NNRTIs also may be associated. Lipodystrophy, including lipoatrophy and lipohypertrophy, is very common and typically is associated with

NRTIs, but HIV infection without therapy also seems to be a risk factor for this complication.[25] Although the substantial benefits of ART outweigh the risk, it was demonstrated by Fris-Moler and colleagues[60] that combination ART was associated with an increased risk of 26% of myocardial infarction during the first 4 to 6 years of antiretroviral use.

Drug interactions are particularly concerning with antiretroviral medications. It is essential to recognize the common medications in each category. Commonly used NRTIs include: AZT, didanosine (ddi, Videx), zalcitabine (ddC, Hivid), stavudine (d4T, Zerit), lamivudine (3TC, Epivir), emtricitabine (FTC, Emtriva), and abacavir (ABC, Ziagen). A common combination medication in this category is Combivir, a combination of AZT and 3TC. Common NNRTIs include: nevirapine (Viramune), delavirdine (Rescriptor), and efavirenz (Sustiva). A commonly used NtRTI is tenofovir (Viread), and it is combined with emtricitabine to form Truvada. PIs include ritonavir (Norvir), indinavir (Crixivan), saquinavir (Fortovase), nelfinavir (Viracept), amprenavir (Agenerase), and lopinavir–ritonavir (Kaletra). The fusion inhibitor currently available is enfuvirtide (Fuzeon), and the entry inhibitor, a CCR5 antagonist, is maraviroc (Selzentry). The integrase inhibitor available is raltegravir (Isentress).[6,87,88]

PIs and NNRTIs are metabolized hepatically by the CYP system, resulting in many drug interactions with several commonly used medications including benzodiazepines, statins, azole antifungals, anticonvulsants, calcium channel blockers, oral contraceptives, and methadone. The most important of these interactions for the OMS is the interaction between PIs and NNRTIs and midazolam and triazolam. Midazolam and triazolam are substrates of CYP3A4; therefore, their metabolism is affected by PIs and NNRTIs. The use of these benzodiazepines in a patient taking PIs or NNRTIs could result in prolonged sedation.[87,89] NRTIs are not metabolized by the liver's CYP pathway and therefore, have fewer drug interactions than PIs or NNRTIs.[87] Pharmacologically significant drug reactions most commonly occur with other antiretroviral agents. In terms of oral surgery practice, there are some potential interactions between NRTIs and certain antibiotics (clarithromycin, ciprofloxacin, and bactrim), antifungals (fluconazole and ketoconazole), and antivirals (acyclovir and valacyclovir).[90,91] The available NtRTI produces renal tubular dysfunction in a few patients, and some studies have demonstrated mild renal dysfunction in patients treated with this medication.[92] Therefore, because of the risk of renal complications, the OMS should be cautious with the use of NSAIDS in patients taking tenofovir or Truvada (combination of tenofovir and emtricitabine). The currently available fusion inhibitor, enfuvirtide, does not interact with the CYP system, and therefore, has few significant drug interactions.[88,93,94] The CCR5 inhibitor maraviroc has few drug interactions. Those that may relate to OMS practice include clarithromycin and ketoconazole, both of which increase the plasma level of maraviroc.[91] One of the newest agents, the integrase inhibitor raltegravir, does not interact with the CYP system. A recent study evaluated the effect of raltegravir on midazolam metabolism and found there was no alteration.[95] The pharmacology of HIV treatment changes rapidly, and new information is forthcoming every day concerning drug interactions and adverse effects. A Web site is available at: www.hiv-druginteractions.org to keep up to date on the latest information concerning drug interactions with antiretroviral drugs.[90]

ORAL MANIFESTATIONS OF HIV

The OMS plays an important role in detecting and managing oral lesions associated with HIV. The presence of oral findings may represent an initial diagnosis of HIV or may indicate progression of existing disease or failure of antiretroviral agents. Several oral findings may be CDC category B or C conditions. Oral diseases consistent with a category B condition include bacilliary angiomatosis, oropharyngeal candidiasis, OHL, and herpes zoster involving two distinct episodes or more than one dermatome. AIDS-defining diseases (CDC category C) with oral findings include CMV, HSV greater than 1 month duration, histoplasmosis, and KS.[13] The presence of oral disease may impact the patient's overall health, especially if pain is preventing the patient from having adequate nutritional intake.

Studies have demonstrated a correlation between oral lesions and immune status. Patton[96] studied a population of 606 patients who had HIV and found certain oral manifestations to be associated with parameters for immunosuppression. Overall, 42% of the study population exhibited at least oral lesion, and 58.2% of those who did exhibit an oral lesion had CD4+ cell counts less than 200 cells/mm^3. OC and OHL were the most common oral lesions. The lesion associated with the lowest CD4+ cell count was KS (mean CD4+ count 33 cells/mm^3). The lesions found most predictive of a CD4+ cell count of less than 200 cells/mm^3 were OC, OHL, oral KS, and linear gingival erythema. In this population, necrotizing periodontal disease, oral warts, oral ulcers, and salivary gland disease did not predict CD4+

counts of less than 200 cells/mm^3. The positive predictive value of oral lesions for elevated viral load was somewhat less clear, but the presence of KS and pseudomembranous OC were associated significantly with a viral load greater than 20,000 copies/mL.[96] In a separate study, Patton and colleagues[97] found that patients who had OHL and OC were 1.8 times more likely to have a viral load greater than 20,000 copies/mL than patients without these findings.

In general, HAART decreases the likelihood of the development of oral lesions, especially of OC.[98–104] Various studies, however, have revealed somewhat different findings with respect to specific oral lesions. Ramirez-Amador and colleagues[99] performed a prospective study of 1000 patients who had HIV in Mexico between the years 1989 and 2001 and found a decrease of approximately 50% in the prevalence of most oral lesions during that time period, attributable to better care of HIV patients, earlier detection of HIV, and use of prophylactic and antiretroviral medications. KS did not decrease during this time, and there was no change noted in the prevalence of salivary gland disease or HPV oral lesions.[99]

Patton and colleagues[100] studied two cohorts of HIV patients. One group was evaluated from February 1995 through August 1996, before widespread use of PIs, and another group from December 1996 through February 1999, a period of greater PI use. Several patients in the earlier cohort used antiretroviral medications, but only 8.1% used PIs, versus 42.1% who used PIs in the later cohort. The overall incidence of oral lesions decreased from 47.6% in the earlier cohort to 37.5% in the later cohort, indicating the influence of PIs in preventing the appearance of oral lesions in general. Upon examination of specific oral lesions, this group found a significant decrease in the prevalence of OHL and necrotizing ulcerative periodontitis. There was an increase in the prevalence in salivary gland disease, and no significant changes were noted in OC, aphthae, warts, HSV, or KS.[100]

Greenspan and colleagues[101] studied 503 women who had HIV from the years 1995 to 2001 as part of the Women's Interagency HIV Study. Their findings revealed a significant decrease in OC once HAART was initiated. The incidence of erythematous candidiasis (EC) fell from 5.48% to 2.99%, and the incidence of pseudomembranous candidiasis (PC) fell from 6.7% to 2.85%. The incidence of either EC or PC fell from 7.35% to 3.43%. This study did not reveal a change in the incidence of hairy leukoplakia or oral warts in response to HAART.[101] In contrast, Ramirez-Amador and colleagues[103] found a decrease in not only OC, but also in hairy leukoplakia in association with antiretroviral treatment in their cross-sectional observational study of 850 patients between 2000 and 2003. Additionally, this group did not find a decrease in KS associated with ART.[103]

In a separate study, Greenspan and colleagues[102] performed a retrospective assessment of 1280 HIV patients between 1990 and 1999. This study specifically examined the relationship of ART to the incidence of OC, OHL, and oral warts. Furthermore, they examined the incidence of oral lesions in general over time. Over time, a decrease was noted in the incidence of OC, hairy leukoplakia, and KS, but there was no change in the incidence of aphthae. An increase in salivary gland disease and the incidence of oral warts was noted. Specific examination of the relationship of antiretrovirals and incidence of OC, hairy leukoplakia, and warts was evaluated with respect to whether the patient was on antiretroviral therapy that included PIs (HAART) or therapy which did not include PIs ART. After adjusting for CD4+ count, OC, hairy leukoplakia, and wart incidence was not affected by ART. After the introduction of PIs, however, a decrease in the incidence of OC was noted, but there was not an association between hairy leukoplakia and ART with or without PI. The prevalence of oral warts increased by a factor of three for patients on ART and by six for patients on HAART.[102] King and colleagues corroborated this finding.[104] This group studied a subset of 56 patients with oral warts from a group of 2194 patients who had HIV from 1997 through 1999. They found that an increased incidence of oral warts was associated with a decrease in HIV RNA level and with chronic or previous infection with HBV. The group did not find a specific association between warts and HAART, but did find that a significant reduction in viral load in the previous 6 months was related to an increased incidence of oral warts. It has been suggested that this phenomenon of increasing incidence of oral warts associated with a decreasing viral load may represent a form of immune reconstitution syndrome.[104]

In 1992, the EC Clearinghouse on Oral Problems Related to HIV Infection revised the previously published classification of the oral manifestations of HIV disease.[105] This classification divides oral findings into three groups based upon strength of association with HIV infection:

> Group 1 lesions are associated strongly with HIV infection and include erythematous and pseudomembranous candidiasis, hairy leukoplakia, KS, NHL, and

periodontal diseases including linear gingival erythema, necrotizing ulcerative gingivitis, and necrotizing ulcerative periodontitis.

- Group 2 lesions are associated less commonly with HIV infection and include *Mycobacterium avium-intracellulare*, TB, melanotic hyperpigmentation, necrotizing ulcerative stomatitis, salivary gland disease (xerostomia or gland swelling), thrombocytopenic purpura, ulceration NOS, and HSV, HPV, and VZV infections.
- Group 3 lesions are seen in HIV infection and include *Actinomyces israelii*, *Escherichia coli*, and *Klebsiella pneumoniae* infection; cat scratch disease, drug reactions, epithelioid (bacillary) angiomatosis, fungal infections other than candidiasis, neurologic disturbances, recurrent aphthous stomatitis; and CMV or molluscum contagiosum infections.

Each lesion has been described in terms of presumptive and definitive criteria for diagnosis. Presumptive criteria are used during the first clinical encounter with the patient and are descriptive terms for clinical findings that need further evaluation before definitive diagnosis is rendered. Definitive criteria describe the criteria necessary for absolute diagnosis.[105] Patton and colleagues reviewed this classification scheme was reviewed in 2002[106] to determine if the 1993 classification should be updated. Their findings confirmed that OC is the most common oral lesion found in patients who have HIV. They also reported that a new fungal infection is emerging in Southeast Asia, *Penicilliosis marneffei*. It was felt however, by the authors that restructuring the 1993 EC classification was not warranted.[106]

The oral manifestations of HIV infection can be categorized broadly as infectious, neoplastic, immune-related, and other categories. Those with an infectious etiology can be subdivided further into fungal, viral, and bacterial. A discussion of each of the major oral findings of HIV infection follows.

Infectious—Fungal

Oral candidiasis

OC is the most common oral lesion in patients who have HIV.[106–108] It has been reported that OC occurs in 17% to 43% of patients who have HIV and in more than 90% of patients who have AIDS.[108] Several studies have examined the usefulness of OC as a predictor for ART failure.[109–112] Miziara and Weber[109] followed 124 HIV patients receiving HAART for at least 6 months and assessed the association of OC and OHL with decreasing CD4+ cell count and increasing viral load. They found that patients with OC and OHL had a lower CD4+ count and higher viral load than patients without OC and OHL. This group calculated positive predictive values (PPV) for each of these associations and found that OC had a high PPV for a decreasing CD4+ cell count and a moderate PPV for an elevated viral load. The PPV of OHL for both of these associations was low. The authors concluded that OC is a better predictor than OHL for immune and virologic failure for patients on HAART.[109]

Ramirez-Amador and colleagues[110] examined the usefulness of OC as a predictor of elevated viral load in their nested case–control study of 1134 patients with HIV on HAART in Mexico. They found an 80% PPV of HIV- associated oral lesions for at least a single viral load measurement of at least 2000 copies/mL. The PPV of OC for virologic failure was 83%.[110]

The first study to provide statistical evidence that an elevated viral load is a stronger predictor of the presence of OC than a low CD4+ cell count was published in 2006 by Mercante and colleagues.[111] This was demonstrated in their study of 161 patients who had HIV utilizing two statistical methods to evaluate the association of viral load and CD4+ cell count and the presence of oropharyngeal candidiasis.

Flint and colleagues[112] performed a recent review of the use of oral lesions as markers of immunodeficiency. One of their conclusions was that oropharyngeal candidiasis (OPC) is a useful marker of HAART failure with one caveat. The reliability of OPC as such a marker is questionable when PIs are part of the HAART regimen.[112] PIs have been demonstrated to have in vitro and in vivo activity against a major virulence factor of *Candida albicans*, the secretory aspartyl proteinase (Sap) enzyme.[113] The ability of PI to inhibit Sap enzyme production in patients who have HIV was demonstrated in a subsequent study by Cassone and colleagues.[114] Patients who received only an NNRTI-based regimen with no PI did not exhibit inhibited Sap production. Therefore, the failure of a PI- containing HAART regimen might not be heralded by an increased risk of appearance of OPC.[112]

There are three common presentations of OPC: PC, EC, and angular chelitis (AC).[105] Hyperplastic candidiasis was removed form the EC Clearinghouse classification of HIV-associated oral lesions in 1993, because it was rare.[105] PC is characterized by yellow or white plaques that wipe away, leaving behind a red and sometimes bleeding surface. (**Fig. 1**) EC (**Fig. 2**) may occur simultaneously

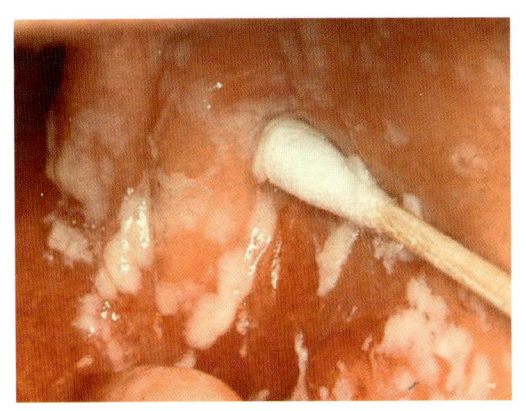

Fig. 1. Pseudomembranous candidiasis. (*Courtesy of* Joseph L. Konzelman, Jr, DDS, Augusta, GA.)

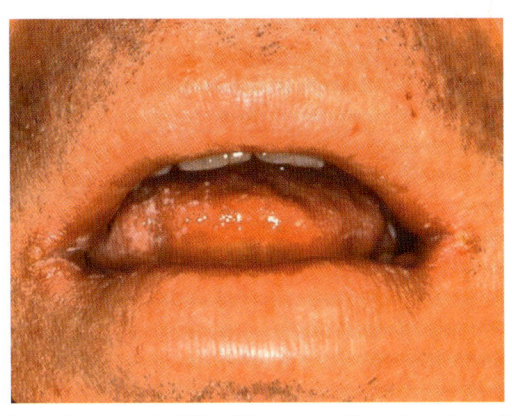

Fig. 3. Angular cheilitis. (*Courtesy of* Joseph L. Konzelman, Jr, DDS, Augusta, GA.)

as PC and is characterized by red areas on the palate or dorsal tongue, although they may occur anywhere throughout the oral mucosa. AC presents with fissuring or erythema at the commissures (**Fig. 3**).

Patients may complain of burning or changes in taste. Typically, *Candidia albicans* predominates, but *Candida tropicalis, Candida glabrata, Candida krusei,* and *Candida dubliniensis* may be responsible for OC also.[115,116] Diagnosis is based mostly on clinical suspicion, but may be confirmed by obtaining a cytologic smear that reveals hyphae. Diagnosis also often is made based upon demonstration of response to antifungal therapy. Antifungal resistance has developed over the years, and some species that are inherently azole resistant, such as *Candida glabrata* and *Candida krusei,* may be involved. Topical agents typically are recommended for patients who are on HAART and have a CD4+ count greater than 50. Those who are not on HAART with CD4+ counts of less than 50 should receive systemic antifungal therapy and most likely should be coordinated by the patient's primary care provider, as there is the potential for drug interactions with HIV medications and the development of resistance patterns. It is recommended that prolonged suppressive therapy be avoided to decrease the likelihood of development of resistant strains. Recommended topical agents include clotrimazole troche, nystatin suspension or pastille, amphotericin B, or chlorhexidine.[108,115,117] Amphotericin B lozenges are not available in the United States. Clotrimazole troches, nystatin pastilles, and nystatin suspension should be used with care, because they are cariogenic. Nystatin vaginal troches and chlorhexidine may be used and are not cariogenic (**Table 1**). Topical creams may be applied to areas of angular chelitis four times per day. Systemic antifungals that may be used include fluconazole, itraconazole, ketoconazole, voriconazole, and amphotericin B.[108,115,117] With all therapies, treatment must continue for at least 2 weeks to reduce organism colony-forming units sufficiently to prevent recurrence.[117]

Deep fungal infections

Deep fungal infections with organisms such as *Histoplasma capsulatum, Penicillium marneffei, Aspergillus* species, *Cryptococcus neoformans,* and *Geotrichum candidum* are rare and are in the EC Clearinghouse group 3 classification of oral lesions in HIV.[33,105,116] Histoplasmosis, aspergillosis, and cryptococcosis may present in a nodular, ulcerative, or necrotic manner (**Fig. 4**). Geotrichosis is pseudomembranous in appearance. Histologic examination is required for

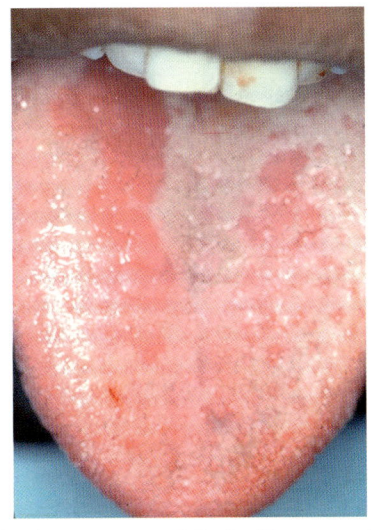

Fig. 2. Erythematous candidiasis. (*Courtesy of* Joseph L. Konzelman, Jr, DDS, Augusta, GA.)

Table 1
Oral candidiasis treatment

Drug	Dose
Clotrimazole troches	10 mg dissolved in mouth 5 times per day for 14 days
Nystatin pastilles	100,000–200,000 U dissolved in mouth 4–5 times per day for 14 days
Nystatin suspension	500,000 U per 5 cc; swish and swallow (optional) 5 cc 4 times per day for 14 days
Nystatin vaginal troche	100,000 U dissolved in mouth 3–6 times per day for 14 days
0.12% Chlorhexidine	Rinse and spit 5 cc 3 times per day; may debride with soaked gauze

diagnosis of these infections, and they usually are managed with intravenous amphotericin B.[33]

Infectious—Viral

Oral hairy leukoplakia

OHL is the result of EBV infection and in patients who have HIV; it commonly is associated with a CD4+ count below 200 cells/mm^3. In 1994, Glick and colleagues[118] reported the positive predictive value for a CD4+ cell count below 200 cells/mm^3 of OHL was 70.1%. Patton[96] reported this figure to be 66.3% in 2000. OHL may be associated with immunosuppression unrelated to HIV infection also. It is characterized by white patchy corrugations that may appear hairy, usually located on the lateral border of the tongue. (**Fig. 5**) Rarely, it

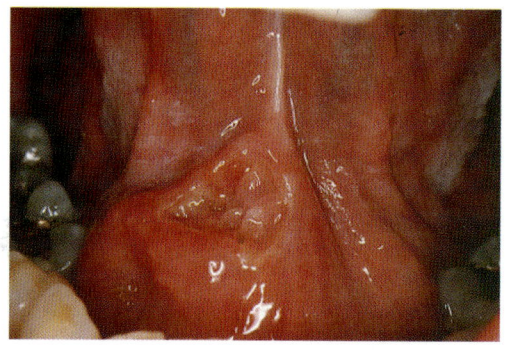

Fig. 4. Histoplasmosis. (*Courtesy of* Wendy Bernstein, MD, Bethesda, MD.)

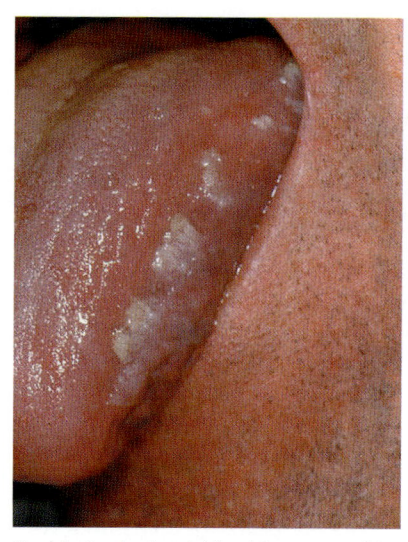

Fig. 5. Oral hairy leukoplakia. (*Courtesy of* Joseph L. Konzelman, Jr, DDS, Augusta, GA.)

can occur on other aspects of oral mucosa. It may be unilateral or bilateral and is distinguished from candidiasis by the fact that OHL does not rub off. OHL is usually asymptomatic, but on occasion, a burning sensation may be reported.[119]

Becauses OHL is suggestive of worsening immunosuppression, a definitive diagnosis should be pursued, and an evaluation of the patient's immune status should occur. A provisional diagnosis can be made based on clinical appearance and nonresponsiveness to antifungal therapy. Although *Candida* may be isolated from up to 80% of OHL lesions, antifungal therapy will not eradicate the OHL even if the *Candida* is cleared.[119] A presumptive diagnosis may be provided by histologic demonstration of hyperkeratosis, acanthosis, and koilocytosis without an inflammatory infiltrate. Definitive diagnosis requires identification of replicating EBV.[105,119] OHL is not premalignant and is not likely to convert to squamous cell carcinoma.[119]

Treatment often is not required unless the patient feels the lesion is unsightly. Surgical removal and antiviral therapy have been recommended, but topical therapy seems to have the most support.[120] Recurrence has been reported after surgical or antiviral therapy, in which case, prophylactic treatment with acyclovir 200 mg/d has been recommended.[108] One recommended topical agent is podophyllin, an extract of roots and rhizomes of *Podophyllum peltatum*, a topical chemotherapeutic agent with few systemic effects. A recent study by Moura and colleagues[120] evaluated the efficacy of topical podophyllin versus podophyllin and acyclovir cream. One year after completion of treatment, they found all 24 of 24 lesions of

OHL treated with the combination therapy maintained lesion resolution, while 18 of 22 lesions treated with podophyllin only demonstrated lesion resolution.

Human papilloma virus

As mentioned earlier, several studies have shown an increase in the incidence of oral warts related to HPV infection since the introduction of ART.[102,104,117,121] Therefore, the OMS may see an increasing number of patients with HPV-related warts. There are more than 50 genotypes of HPV, and the gross appearance of oral lesions can exhibit significant variability. The more common appearance of cauliflower-like lesions may be caused by genotypes 2, 6, 7, 11, 16, and 18. A more unusual type of wart seen in patients who have HIV is a flat, firm, sessile wart caused by HPV types 12, 13, or 32.[115,122] These flat papule-like warts are described as focal epithelial hyperplasia and may exhibit dysplasia. (**Fig. 6**) HPV warts primarily occur on the labial mucosa, but they can be present anywhere inside the mouth or on the lips. Definitive diagnosis is determined by biopsy.

Treatment may be sought because of the unsightly appearance of the warts. Typically, they are widespread and difficult to treat. CO_2 laser ablation is not recommended, because HPV particles may become dispersed and lead to nasal warts in the patient or the provider.[123] Multiple other modalities have been described, including topical podophyllin, interferon-alpha injection, and topical 5-flurouracil.[108,117,122,124,125] In general, there have not been well-controlled studies to evaluate the optimal management of oral HPV lesions; therefore, surgical excision is the most widely used treatment modality.[124,125] Even with surgical excision, the recurrence rate is high. There have not been reports of malignant transformation.[115]

Herpes simplex virus

HSV infection was discussed under the systemic complications section under "Skin—infectious." Intraoral HSV infection presents with shallow ulcerations with raised white borders that occur on nonkeratinized tissue such as buccal and labial mucosa.[108] In HIV-negative patients, these surfaces usually are unaffected by HSV, with most oral lesions being on the lips; however, patients who have HIV may have lip lesion also. Lesions in patients who have HIV usually are ulcerated and painful for a longer duration than similar lesions in HIV-negative patients.[108] Definitive diagnosis requires biopsy, as these lesions can resemble recurrent aphthae and CMV infection. Successful systemic treatment has included acyclovir, famciclovir, and valacyclovir.[124,125] Acyclovir resistance is on the rise, and patients who have HSV lesions resistant to acyclovir should be referred to their primary care physician for possible intravenous therapy.[108,124,125]

Varicella zoster

Varicella zoster was discussed earlier in the systemic complications section under "Skin—infectious." Prompt initiation of treatment with acyclovir or valacyclovir is essential in order to prevent postherpetic neuralgia.

Cytomegalovirus

Oral CMV infection is uncommon, but must be diagnosed definitively if suspicious lesions appear, because oral CMV almost always is associated with disseminated CMV infection that can lead to retinitis and meningitis.[108,115] Oral lesions of CMV appear as deep ulcerations of the buccal or labial mucosa and may closely resemble HSV or aphthae. Biopsy with viral identification is essential, and identification of CMV must result in immediate referral to the patient's primary care provider so potential disseminated CMV infection can be addressed. High-dose acyclovir is often the treatment of choice.[33]

Infectious—Bacterial

Linear gingival erythema

The three periodontal diseases associated with HIV are categorized as bacterial infections, although bacteria may not always be involved. These diseases include linear gingival erythema, necrotizing ulcerative gingivitis, and necrotizing ulcerative periodontitis. Some have reported periodontal diseases as being a spectrum of worsening disease, beginning with linear gingival

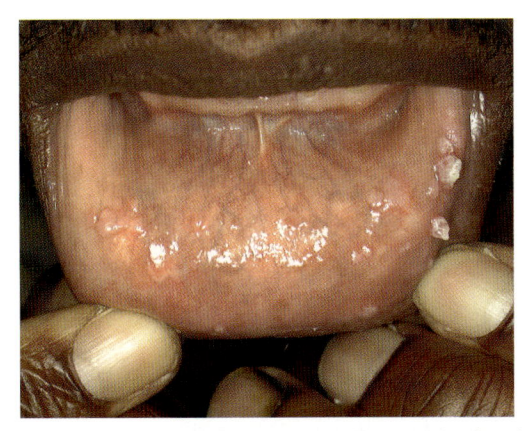

Fig. 6. Cauliflower-like human papilloma virus (HPV) lesions on patient's left and flat HPV lesions on patient's right.

erythema progressing to necrotizing ulcerative gingivitis, then necrotizing periodontitis, and occasionally culminating in necrotizing stomatitis in which nonalveolar bone also becomes involved.[107] Decreased CD4+ counts have been linked with more severe loss of periodontal attachment.[116] Despite this observation, gingivo–periodontal condition does not seem predictive of severity of HIV disease. Linear gingival erythema, formerly known as HIV-associated gingivitis, presents as an asymptomatic 2 to 3 mm band of erythema at the margin of the gingiva. (**Fig. 7**) Strikingly, there is often a lack of associated local factors such as plaque or calculus present. Histologically, there is little evidence of inflammation. Scaling and root planning should be performed, but usually this does not result in resolution.[33] Chlorhexidine gluconate 0.12% rinses may reduce the erythema.[108]

Necrotizing ulcerative gingivitis
Necrotizing ulcerative gingivitis (NUG) is a painful condition in which the gingival papillae and margin may become crater-like, ulcerated, and necrotic. The gingiva may slough and be accompanied by a foul odor. Fever and cervical lymphadenopathy also may be present. At this stage, there is no loss of periodontal attachment or involvement of alveolar bone.[33,88,105] Diagnosis is based on clinical appearance.[105] Involved microbiota included aerobic and anaerobic organisms and occasionally may involve more atypical pathogens.[107,125] Treatment involves debridement of teeth and necrotic tissue as necessary and optimization of oral hygiene and home care. Topical agents such as 10% povidone–iodine and 0.12% chlorhexidine gluconate have been used with some success. Additionally, systemic treatment with metronidazole 1 g/d for 4 to 5 days may be necessary.[33,107,125] Alternatively, clindamycin or amoxicillin may be used.[107]

Necrotizing ulcerative periodontitis
Necrotizing ulcerative periodontitis (NUP) can appear clinically similar to NUG, but it is accompanied by the rapid loss of periodontal attachment and alveolar bone. The gingiva is ulcerated, necrotic, and bleeds, and the bone destruction leads to intense deep bone pain. Bone necrosis may be so severe that bone becomes exposed intraorally. As in other periodontal diseases of HIV, NUP is a diagnosis made based on clinical evaluation. There may be minimal periodontal pockets because of the simultaneous loss of soft and hard tissue.[105] The involved periodontal flora has been reported to be similar to that seen in non-HIV infected patients, and the importance of bacteria in the etiology of NUP is questionable.[33,108,115] NUP usually is found in more severely immunosuppressed individuals, usually with CD4+ counts of less than 200 cells/mm^3.[33,108,117] Because of its association with severe immunosuppression, prompt referral to the patient's primary care provider is essential, so further evaluation of the patient's immune status can be undertaken. Treatment must include pain management so as to allow the patient to maintain nutrition. Treatment should include narrow-spectrum oral antibiotics such as metronidazole; alternative antibiotics may include clindamycin and amoxicillin.[108,117] In addition, removal of calculus and necrotic tissues should be performed. Topical therapies include 0.12% chlorhexidine gluconate and 10% povodine–iodine rinses.[108,117] NUP may progress, and once the supporting bone is involved, necrotizing ulcerative stomatitis develops. (**Fig. 8**) Microbiologic evaluation often fails to reveal a specific bacterial cause.[105]

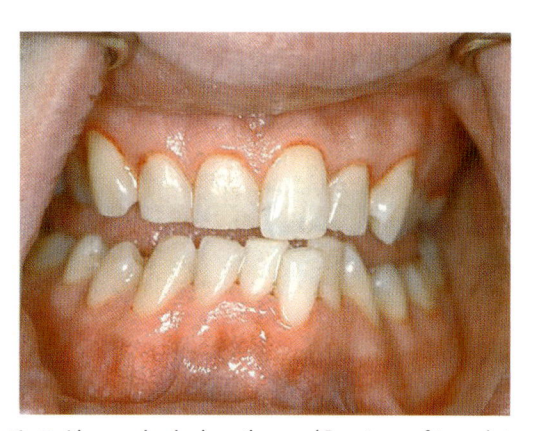

Fig. 7. Linear gingival erythema. (*Courtesy of* Joseph L. Konzelman, Jr, DDS, Augusta, GA.)

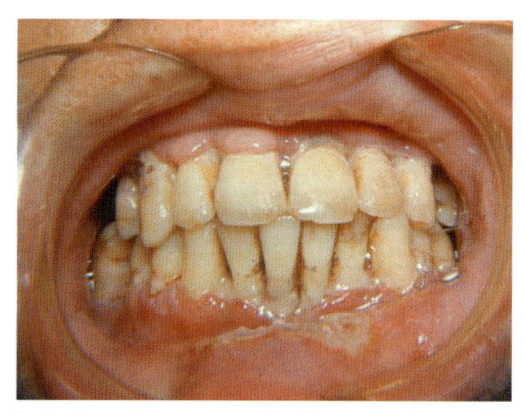

Fig. 8. Necrotizing stomatitis. (*Courtesy of* Joseph L. Konzelman, Jr, DDS, Augusta, GA.)

Bacillary epithelioid angiomatosis
Bacillary epithelioid angiomatosis was discussed earlier in the section on systemic manifestations of HIV in the section entitled "Skin—infectious." It is important to remember that this lesion clinically may resemble KS and pyogenic granuloma, making definitive diagnosis by biopsy essential.

Syphilis
Syphilis, which may have oral lesions, was discussed earlier in the section of systemic manifestations entitled "genitourinary".

Neoplasms

Kaposi's sarcoma
An introduction to KS was in the section entitled "Systemic complications of HIV infection—infectious/neoplastic." KS is the most commonly found oral malignancy in patients who have HIV and has been reported to be decreasing in the antiretroviral therapy era.[117] Up to 60% of patients who have KS may have oral involvement, and about 45% may have both oral and cutaneous lesions.[116] As with cutaneous lesions, human herpes virus 8 (HHV 8) is felt to be important in the etiology of oral lesions. Oral lesions are red or purple in color and are macular or nodular and may be ulcerated (**Figs. 9–12**). Earlier lesions tend to be flat and red and become darker as time passes.[117] Most common sites of involvement include the palate, attached gingiva of the alveolus, and the tongue. Alveolar involvement can lead to bone and tooth loss. Differential diagnosis includes bacillary angiomatosis, NHL, hemangioma, oral pigmentation from antiretrovirals, and pyogenic granuloma.[108,115] Biopsy is required for definitive diagnosis.

The appearance of oral KS lesions is an ominous sign, as it is associated with elevated mortality compared with patients who have cutaneous lesions alone.[126] Rohrmus and colleagues[126] studied 138 patients with KS who were not receiving triple ART. They found that patients who had KS with CD4+ counts of less than 150 had higher mortality risk (relative hazard 3.6) and shorter survival than patients who had CD4+ counts greater than 150, regardless of the location of their KS lesions. They also found that patients with oral KS had shorter survival than those who had cutaneous lesions, regardless of CD4+ count (24 month median survival for oral KS patients versus 72 months for cutaneous KS patients).[126] Therefore, any patient who develops oral KS should follow closely with his or her primary care provider, because this may indicate more serious progression of disease.

Treatment of oral KS often becomes necessary because of appearance and discomfort. If the patient is not already on HAART, initiation of HAART may cause regression of oral KS.[116] Various treatment modalities have been described, to include surgical excision, intralesional or systemic

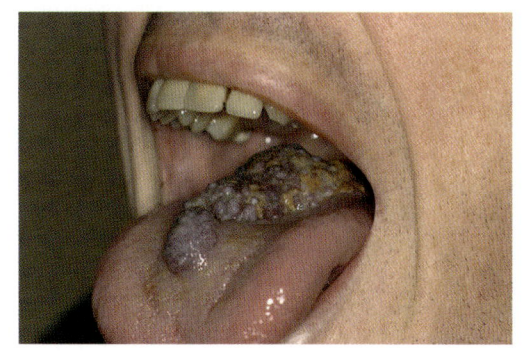

Fig. 10. Nodular Kaposi's sarcoma. (*Courtesy of* Robert Yarchoan, MD, Bethesda, MD.)

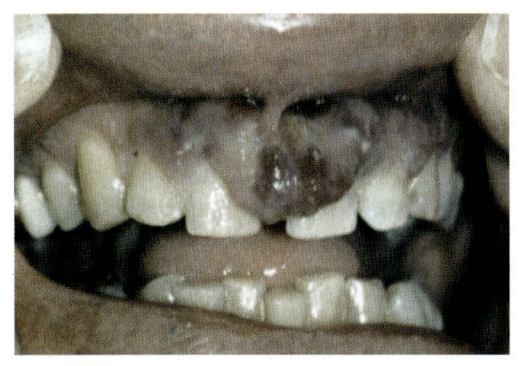

Fig. 9. Kaposi's sarcoma. (*Courtesy of* Naomi Aronson, MD, Washington, DC.)

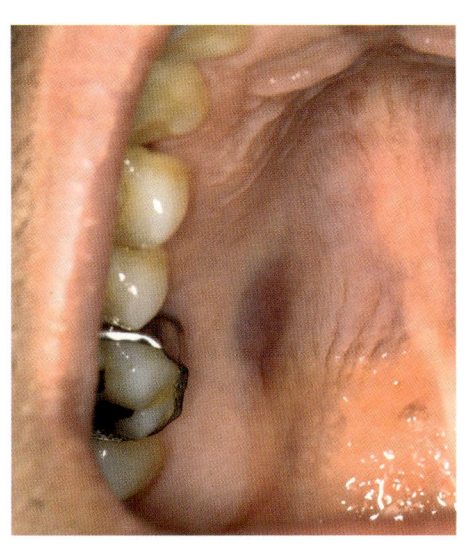

Fig. 11. Macular Kaposi's sarcoma. (*Courtesy of* Robert Yarchoan, MD, Bethesda, MD.)

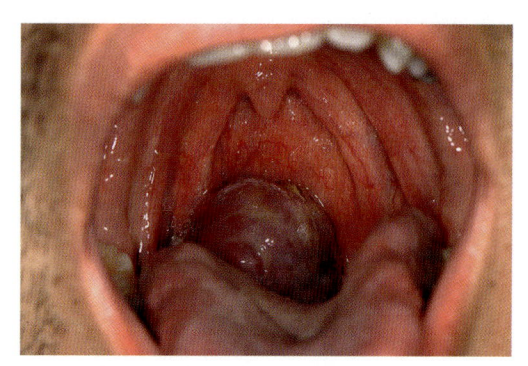

Fig. 12. Pharyngeal Kaposi's sarcoma. (*Courtesy of* Robert Yarchoan, MD, Bethesda, MD.)

chemotherapy, sclerotherapy, or radiation.[108,116,117] Intralesional injections of vinblastine or sodium tetradecyl sulfate 3% have been used. Patients who have extraoral lesions in addition to intraoral lesions may benefit from systemic chemotherapy. Radiation therapy is reserved for larger or multiple lesions.

Non-Hodgkin's lymphoma
Lymphoma was discussed in the sections on infectious/neoplastic and neurologic manifestations of HIV. NHL is the second most common head and neck malignancy in patients who have HIV. Clinically, intraoral NHL lesions present as a rapidly enlarging mass on the palate or attached gingiva. It may be ulcerated or plaque-like and may appear similarly to KS, necessitating biopsy for definitive diagnosis. Patients may have bony involvement, which can lead to significant pain and a widened periodontal membrane. Progressing paresthesia may be a feature also.[33] NHL usually occurs when the patient is fairly immunocompromised, with CD4+ counts of less than 100 cells/mm^3. Multidrug chemotherapy is the treatment of choice, but prognosis remains poor, with a mean time of survival of less than 1 year.[108]

Immune-Mediated
Aphthous ulcers
With a prevalence of 2% to 3%, major aphthous ulceration is the most common immune-mediated oral lesion in patients who have HIV.[108] Aphthae in patients with HIV have a similar appearance as in HIV-negative patients, and most commonly occur on nonkeratinized surfaces. In HIV who have HIV, however, these lesions may last longer, are larger, and are more therapy-resistant.[33,108] Because these lesions may appear in a similar manner as other virally mediated lesions, biopsy may be necessary for definitive diagnosis. For mild cases, treatment may consist of topical steroids such as dexamethasone. Severe cases may require systemic steroids such as prednisone.[108,117] Such treatments must be used cautiously, because they can lead to superinfection with *Candida*, reactivation of TB, or worsened KS.[108] Thalidomide has been evaluated for treating recurrent aphthous ulcerations (RAU), and in doses of 200 mg/d, it has been found useful, but because of its side effects, it is not recommended for prophylactic use.[124,125,127]

Neutropenic ulceration
Neutropenic ulcers may develop with absolute granulocyte counts of less than 800/μL. These ulcers are very painful, large, and fulminant-looking and cannot be explained otherwise; they should prompt appropriate referral for management. Such patients may be administered granulocyte-stimulating factor to address the neutropenia.[117]

Other
Salivary gland disease
Most commonly the parotid gland, but occasionally the submandibular gland, can become infiltrated by lymphoproliferative cells or benign lymphoepithelial cysts, leading to gland enlargement and diminished salivary flow. The etiology of this disease is unknown, although a relationship to CMV has been suggested.[108] Because malignant infiltration also can cause gland enlargement, needle aspiration has been suggested. Aspiration of yellow mucous type of fluid is suggestive of HIV-related salivary gland disease.

Xerostomia
Xerostomia may be related to salivary gland infiltration, or it may be an adverse effect of antiretroviral or other medications. This may result in significant dental decay, an increased risk of oral candidiasis, oral pain, and decreased oral intake. It is estimated that as many as 30% to 40% of patients who have HIV experience moderate-to-severe xerostomia.[117] Saliva substitutes, fluoride treatment, and pilocarpine may be offered for patients with some residual salivary function.[108]

SUMMARY

HIV and AIDS are among the most complex disease states affecting the worldwide population. OMS and other care providers should have a good understanding of the myriad of systemic effects of this disease and its treatment. This disease affects every system in the body, and in order to provide the best care to these patients, a basic knowledge of this disease process is mandatory.

The OMS has the potential to assist in the initial diagnosis of HIV and in recognition of worsening disease. Research continues to examine new treatment modalities, and the search for a vaccine continues. Until a cure is found, the stark statistic seen on bumper stickers remains: 40,000,000 infected. 0 cured.

REFERENCES

1. 2007 AIDS epidemic update. UNAIDS, WHO7; 2007. p. 1–60.
2. Abbas AK. Diseases of immunity. In: Kumar V, Abbas A, Fausto N, editors. Robbins and Cotran: pathologic basis of disease. 7th edition. Philadelphia: Elsevier; 2005. p. 245–58.
3. Aids medications. Available at: www.aidsmeds.com. Accessed April 6, 2008.
4. Aids information. Available at: www.aidsinfo.nih.gov. Accessed April 6, 2008.
5. Treatment of HIV infection factsheet. National institute of allergy and infectious diseases. Accessible at: www.niaid.nih.gov/factsheet/treat-hiv.htm; November 2007. Accessed January 18, 2008.
6. Wolfe PR. Practical approaches to HIV therapy. Postgrad Med 2000;107(4):127–38.
7. Bartlett JG. The stages and natural history of HIV infection. Up to Date; 11 August 2006. p. 1–9.
8. Zhang Z, Schuler T, Zupancic M, et al. Sexual transmission and propagation of SIV and HIV in resting and activated CD4+ T cells. Science 1999;286(5443):1353–7.
9. Rychert JA, Rosenberg ES. Immunology of HIV-1 infection. Up to Date; 14 September 2007. p. 1–11.
10. Zetola NM, Pilcher CD. Diagnosis and management of acute HIV infection. Infect Dis Clin North Am 2007;21(1):19–48.
11. Yu K, Daar ES. Primary HIV infection. Postgrad Med 2000;107(4):114–22.
12. Madec Y, Boufassa F, Porter K, et al. Spontaneous control of viral load and CD4 cell count progression among HIV-1 seroconverters. AIDS 2005;19(17): 2001–7.
13. Castro KG, Ward JW, Slutsker L, et al. 1993 Revised classification system for HIV infection and expanded surveillance case definition for AIDS among adolescents and adults. MMWR 1992; 41(RR-17). Available at: http://www.cdc.gov/MMWR/preview/MMWRhtml/00018871.htm. Accessed January 26, 2008.
14. Cohen DE, Mayer KH. Primary care issues for HIV-infected patients. Infect Dis Clin North Am 2007; 21(1):49–70.
15. Baggaley R, Dhaliwal M, Petrak J. Scaling up HIV testing and counselling services: a toolkit for programme managers. UNAIDS, WHO; 2005. p. 1–135.
16. HIV/Western blot. National Library of Medicine/National Institutes of Health. Available at: http://www.nlm.nih.gov/medlineplus/print/ency/article/003538.htm. Accessed January 26, 2008.
17. Guidance on provider-initiated HIV testing and counselling in health facilities. UNAIDS, WHO; 2007. p. 1–60.
18. Greenwald JL, Burstein GR, Pincus J, et al. A rapid review of rapid HIV antibody tests. Curr Infect Dis Rep 2006;8(2):125–31.
19. Centers for Disease Control and Prevention. Advancing HIV prevention: new strategies for a changing epidemic—United States, 2003. MMWR 2003;52(15):329–32.
20. Giorgi JV, Lyles RH, Matud JL, et al. Predictive value of immunologic and virulogic markers after long or short duration of HIV-1 infection. J Acquir Immune Defic Syndr 2002;29(4):346–55.
21. DHHS panel on antiretroviral guidelines for adults and adolescents. Guidelines for the use of antiretroviral agents in HIV-1-infected adults and adolescents. Accessible at: http://aidsinfo.nih.gov/ContentFiles/AdultandAdolescentGL.pdf. Accessed January 27, 2008.
22. Friel TJ, Scadden DT. Hematologic manifestations of HIV infection: thrombocytopenia and coagulation abnormalities. Up to Date; June 1, 2007. p. 1–12.
23. Friel TJ, Scadden DT. Hematologic manifestations of HIV infection: anemia. Up to Date; July 26, 2006. p. 1–12.
24. Wyatt CM, Klotman PE. HIV-associated nephropathy in the era of antiretroviral therapy. Am J Med 2007;120(6):488–92.
25. Hoffman RM, Currier JS. Management of antiretroviral treatment-related complications. Infect Dis Clin North Am 2007;21(1):103–32.
26. Jain MK. Drug-induced liver injury associated with HIV medications. Clin Liver Dis 2007;11(3): 615–39.
27. Carpenter CCJ, Flanigan TP, Lederman MM. HIV infection and the acquired immunodeficiency syndrome. In: Andreoli TE, Carpenter CCJ, Griggs RC, et al, editors. Cecil essentials of medicine. 5th edition. Philadelphia: WB Saunders; 2001. p. 841–62.
28. Stringer JR, Bear d CB, Miller RF, et al. A new name (*Pneumocystis jirovecii*) for pneumocystis from humans. Emerging Infect Dis 2003;9(2):276–7.
29. Miller R, Huang L. Pneumocystis jirovecii infection: a review of pneumocystis and the rationale for renaming it. Thorax 2004;59(9):731–3.
30. Spina M, Vaccher E, Carbone A, et al. Neoplastic complications of HIV infection. Ann Oncol 1999; 10(11):1271–86.
31. Di Lorenzo G, Konstantinopoulos PA, Pantanowitz L, et al. Management of AIDS-related Kaposi's sarcoma. Lancet Oncol 2007;8(2):167–76.

32. Maurer TA. Dermatologic manifestations of HIV infection. /2006. Top HIV Med 2005;13(5):149–54.
33. Barr CE, Glick M. Diagnosis and management of oral and cutaneous lesions in HIV-1 disease. Oral Max Fac Surg Clin North Am 1998;10(1):25–44.
34. Neves Ferreira Velho PE, De Souza EM, Cintra ML, et al. Diagnosis of *Bartonella* spp. infection: study of a bacillary angiomatosis case. An Bras Dermatol 2006;81(4):349–53.
35. Schacker T, Hu HL, Koelle DM, et al. Famciclovir for the suppression of symptomatic and asymptomatic herpes simplex virus reactivation in HIV-infected persons. Ann Intern Med 1998;128(1):21–8.
36. Eversole LR. Viral infections of the head and neck among HIV-seropositive patients. Oral Surg Oral Med Oral Pathol 1992;73(2):155–63.
37. Gupta LK, Singhi MK. Tzanck smear: a useful diagnostic tool. Indian J Dermatol Venereol Leprol 2005; 71(4):295–9.
38. Romanowski B, Aoki FY, Martel AY, et al. Efficacy and safety of famciclovir for treating mucocutaneous herpes simplex infection in HIV-infected individuals. AIDS 2000;14(9):1211–7.
39. Palefsky J. Biology of HPV in HIV infection. Adv Dent Res 2006;19(1):99–105.
40. Stuhlberg DL, Galbraith A. Molluscum contagiosum and warts. Am Fam Physician 2003;67:1233–40.
41. Trent JT. Cutaneous manifestations of HIV: a primer. Adv Skin Wound Care 2004;17(3):116–29.
42. Tschachler E, Bergstresser PR, Stingl G. HIV-related skin diseases. Lancet 1996;348(9028): 659–63.
43. Garman ME, Tyring SK. The cutaneous manifestations of HIV infection. Dermatol Clin 2002;20(2). 193–208.
44. Coldiron BM, Bergstresser PR. Prevalence and clinical spectrum of skin disease in patients infected with human immunodeficiency virus. Arch Dermatol 1989;125(3):357–61.
45. Boonchai W, Laohasrisakul R, Manonukul J, et al. Pruritic papular eruption in HIV seropositive patients: a cutaneous marker for immunosuppression. Int J Dermatol 1999;38(5):348–50.
46. Salata RA. Sexually transmitted diseases. In: Andreoli TE, Carpenter CCJ, Griggs RC, et al, editors. Cecil essentials of medicine. 5th edition. Philadelphia: WB Saunders; 2001. p. 832–40.
47. Marrazzo J. Syphilis and other sexually transmitted diseases in HIV infection. Top HIV Med 2007;15(1): 11–6.
48. Center for Disease Control and Prevention. Lymphogranuloma venereum among men who have sex with men—Netherlands, 2003–2004. MMWR Weekly 2004;53(42):985–8.
49. Bartlett JG. Changing trends in bacterial infections: *Staphylococcus aureus*, bacterial pneumonia, *Clostridium difficile*. Top HIV Med 2007;15(3):94–8.
50. Sanchez TH, Brooks JT, Sullivan PS, et al. Bacterial diarrhea in persons with HIV infection, United States, 1992–2002. Clin Infect Dis 2005;41(11): 1621–7.
51. Center for Disease Control and Prevention. Hepatitis C Virus and HIV coinfection. Accessible at: http://www.cdc.gov/idu/hepatitis/hepc_and_hiv_co.pdf; Sep 2002. Accessed February 4, 2008.
52. Bonacini M. Diagnosis and management of cirrhosis in coinfected patients. J Acquir Immune Defic Syndr 2007;45(Suppl 2):s38–46.
53. Kellerman SE, Hanson DL, McNaghten AD, et al. Prevalence of chronic hepatitis B and incidence of acute hepatitis B infection in human immunodeficiency virus-infected subjects. J Infect Dis 2003; 188(4):571–7.
54. Gupta SK, Eustace JA, Winston JA, et al. Guidelines for the management of chronic kidney disease in HIV-infected patients: recommendations of the HIV Medicine Association of the Infectious Diseases Society of America. Clin Infect Dis 2005; 40(11):1559–85.
55. Fine DM. Renal disease and toxicities: issues for HIV care providers. Top HIV Med 2006;14(5):164–9.
56. Spach DH. Selected primary care issues in HIV disease. Top HIV Med 2005;13(4):117–21.
57. Shah SV. Glomerular diseases. In: Andreoli TE, Carpenter CCJ, Griggs RC, et al, editors. Cecil essentials of medicine. 5th edition. Philadelphia: WB Saunders; 2001. p. 253–65.
58. Berhane K, Karim R, Cohen MH, et al. Impact of highly activated antiretroviral therapy on anemia and relationship between anemia and survival in a large cohort of HIV-infected women: women's interagency HIV study. J Acquir Immune Defic Syndr 2004;37(2):1245–52.
59. Adeyemi O. Cardiovascular risk and risk management in HIV-infected patients. Top HIV Med 2007; 15(5):159–62.
60. Friis Moller N, Sabin CA, Weber R, et al. Combination antiretroviral therapy and the risk of myocardial infarction. N Engl J Med 2003;349(21):1993–2003.
61. Balasubramanyam A, Sekhar RV, Jahoor F, et al. Pathophysiology of dyslipidemia and increased cardiovascular risk in HIV lipodystrophy: a model of systemic steatosis. Curr Opin Lipidol 2004; 15(1):59–67.
62. Davaro RE, Thirumalai A. Life-threatening complications of HIV infection. J Intensive Care Med 2007;22(2):73–81.
63. Benson CA, Kaplan JE, Masur H, et al. Treating opportunistic infections among HIV-infected adults and adolescents: recommendations from the CDC, the National Institutes of Health, and the

HIV Medicine Association/Infectious Disease Society of America. Clin Infect Dis 2005;40(Suppl 3). S131–235.
64. Havlir DV, Currier JS. Complications of HIV disease and antiretroviral therapy. Top HIV Med 2006;14(1): 27–35.
65. Currier JS, Havlir DV. Complications of HIV disease and therapy. Top HIV Med 2007;15(2):40–7.
66. Seoane L, Shellito J, Welsh D, et al. Pulmonary hypertension associated with HIV infection. South Med J 2001;94(6):635–9.
67. Mehta NJ, Khan IA, Mehta RN, et al. HIV-related pulmonary hypertension: analytic review of 131 cases. Chest 2000;118(4):1133–41.
68. Brown TT, Cole SR, Li X, et al. Antiretroviral therapy and the prevalence and incidence of diabetes mellitus in the multicenter AIDS Cohort Study. Arch Intern Med 2005;165(10):1179–84.
69. Dube MP. Disorders of glucose metabolism in patients infected with human immunodeficiency virus. Clin Infect Dis 2000;31(6):1467–75.
70. Cohan GR. HIV-associated metabolic and morphologic abnormality syndrome. Postgrad Med 2000; 107(4):141–6.
71. Hadigan C, Meigs JB, Corcoran C, et al. Metabolic abnormalities and cardiovascular disease risk factors in adults with human immunodeficiency virus infection and lipodystrophy. Clin Infect Dis 2001; 32(1):130–9.
72. Glesby MJ. Bone disorders in human immunodeficiency virus infection. Clin Infect Dis 2003; 37(Suppl 2):S91–5.
73. National Institute of Mental Health. Researchers suggest updating criteria for HIV-associated neurocognitive disorders. Available at: http://www.nimh.nih.gov/science-news/2007/researchers-suggest-updating-criteria-for-hiv-associated-neurocognitive-disorders.shtml. Accessed February 23, 2008.
74. Letendre S, Ellis RJ. Neurologic complications of HIV disease and their treatments. Top HIV Med 2006;14(1):21–6.
75. Price RW. AIDS dementia complex. HIV .insite knowledge base chapter June 1998;. Available at: http://hivinsite.ucsf.edu/InSite?page=kb-04-01-03. Accessed February 23, 2008.
76. Letendre S, Ances B, Gibson S, et al. Neurologic complications of HIV disease and their treatment. Top HIV Med 2007;15(2):32–9.
77. Salata RA. Infections of the nervous system. In: Andreoli TE, Carpenter CCJ, Griggs RC, et al, editors. Cecil essentials of medicine. 5th edition. Philadelphia: WB Saunders; 2001. p. 771–81.
78. Zanetti C, Manzano GM, Gabbai AA. The frequency of peripheral neuropathy in a group of HIV-positive patients in Brazil. Arq Neuropsiquiatr 2004;62(2A):253–6.
79. Markarian Y, Wulff EA, Simpson DM. Peripheral neuropathy in HIV disease. In Journal Watch, published in AIDS Clinical Care December 1998;. Available at: http://aids-clinical-care.jwatch.org/cgi/content/full/1998/1201/1. Accessed February 23, 2008.
80. Jabs DA, Green WR, Fox R, et al. Ocular manifestations of acquired immune deficiency syndrome. Ophthalmology 1989;96(7):1092–9.
81. Freeman WR, Lerner CW, Mines JA, et al. A prospective study of the ophthalmologic findings in the acquired immune deficiency syndrome. Am J Ophthalmol 1984;97(2):133–42.
82. Skapik JL, Treisman GJ. HIV, psychiatric comorbidity. Clin Geriatr 2007;15(3):26–36.
83. Tabrizian S, Mittermeier O. HIV and psychiatric disorders. In: Hoffman C, Rockstroh JK, Kamps BS, editors. HIV medicine. 15th edition. Paris: Flying Publisher; 2007. Available at: http://www.hivmedicine.com/hivmedicine2007.pdf; 2007. Accessed February 23, 2008.
84. Ciesla JA, Roberts JE. Meta-analysis of the relationship between HIV infection and risk for depressive disorders. Am J Psychiatry 2001;158(5): 725–30.
85. *Mycobacterium avium* complex (MAC). Project inform pamphlet January 2001. Available at: http://img.thebody.com/legacyAssets/50/20/mac.pdf. Accessed February 17, 2008.
86. Jayasuriya A, Robertson C, Allan PS. Twenty-five years of HIV management. J R Soc Med 2007; 100(8):363–6.
87. Department of Health and Human Services, Office of AIDS Research Advisory Council. Guidelines for the use of antiretroviral agents in HIV-1-infected adults and adolescents. 2007. p. 1–136.
88. Little J, Rhodus NL. HIV and AIDS: update for dentistry. Gen Dent 2007;55(3):184–96.
89. Rana KZ, Dudley MN. Human immunodeficiency virus protease inhibitors. Pharmacotherapy 1999; 19(1):35–59.
90. University of Liverpool HIV drug interaction Web site. Available at: www.hiv-druginteractions.org. Accessed February 26, 2008.
91. Meemken L, Dickinson L. Drug–drug interactions. In: Hoffman C, Rockstroh JK, Kamps BS, editors. HIV medicine. 15th edition. Paris: Flying Publisher; 2007. Available at: http://www.hivmedicine.com/hivmedicine2007.pdf; 2007. Accessed February 23, 2008.
92. Cihlar T. Nucleotide HIV reverse transcriptase inhibitors: tenofovir and beyond. Curr Opin HIV AIDS 2006;1(5):373–9.
93. Lesho EP, Gey DC. Managing issues related to antiretroviral therapy. Am Fam Physician 2003; 68(4):675–86.

94. Hardy H, Skolnik PR. Enfuvirtide, a new fusion inhibitor therapy of human innumodeficiency virus infection. Pharmacotherapy 2004;24(2):198–211.
95. Iwamoto M, Kassahun K, Troyer MD, et al. Lack of a pharmacokinetic effect of raltegravir on midazolam: in vitro/in vivo correlation. J Clin Pharmacol 2008;48(2):209–14.
96. Patton LL. Sensitivity, specificity, and positive predictive value of oral opportunistic infections in adult with HIV/AIDS as markers of immune suppression and viral burden. Oral Surg Oral Med Oral Pathol Oral Radiol Endod 2000;90(2):182–8.
97. Patton LL, McKaig RG, Eron JJ Jr, et al. Oral hairy leukoplakia and oral candidiasis as predictors of HIV viral load. AIDS 1999;13(15):2174–6.
98. Hodgson TA, Greenspan D, Greenspan JS. Oral lesions of HIV disease and HAART in industrialized countries. Adv Dent Res 2006;19(1):57–62.
99. Ramirez-Amador V, Esquivel-Pedraza L, Sierra-Madero J, et al. The changing clinical spectrum of human immunodeficiency virus (HIV)-related oral lesions in 1000 consecutive patients. A 12-year study in a referral center in Mexico. Medicine 2003;82(1):39–50.
100. Patton LL, McKaig R, Strauss R, et al. Changing prevalence of oral manifestations of human immunodeficiency virus in the era of protease inhibitor therapy. Oral Surg Oral Med Oral Pathol Oral Radiol Endod 2000;89(3):299–304.
101. Greenspan D, Gange SJ, Phelan JA, et al. Incidence of oral lesions in HIV-1-infected women: reduction with HAART. J Dent Res 2004;83(2):145–50.
102. Greenspan D, Canchola AJ, MacPhail LA, et al. Effect of highly active antiretroviral therapy on frequency of oral warts. Lancet 2001;357(9266):1411–2.
103. Ramirez-Amador V, Anaya-Saavedra G, Calva JJ, et al. HIV-related oral lesions, demographic factors, clinical staging, and antiretroviral use. Arch Med Res 2006;37(5):646–54.
104. King MD, Reznik DA, O'Daniels CM, et al. Human papillomavirus-associated oral warts among human immunodeficiency virus-seropositive patients in the era of highly active antiretroviral therapy: an emerging infection. Clin Infect Dis 2002;34(5):641–8.
105. Classification and diagnostic criteria for oral lesions in HIV infection. EC-clearinghouse on oral problems related to HIV infection and WHO collaborating centre on oral manifestations of the immunodeficiency virus. J Oral Pathol Med 1993;22(7). 289–91.
106. Patton LL, Phelan JA, Ramos-Gomez FJ, et al. Prevalence and classification of HIV-associated oral lesions. Oral Dis 2002;8(Suppl 2):98–109.
107. Weinert M, Grimes RM, Lynch DP. Oral manifestations of HIV infection. Ann Intern Med 1996;125(6):485–96.
108. Sirois DA. Oral manifestations of HIV disease. Mt Sinai J Med 1998;65(5–6):322–32.
109. Miziara ID, Weber R. Oral candidosis and oral hairy leukoplakia as predictors of HAART failure in Brazilian HIV-infected patients. Oral Dis 2006;12(4):402–7.
110. Ramirez-Amador V, Ponce-de-Leon S, Anaya-Saavedra G, et al. Oral lesions as clinical markers of highly active antiretorviral therapy failure: a nested case–control study in Mexico City. Clin Infect Dis 2007;45(7):925–32.
111. Mercante DE, Leigh JE, Lilly E, et al. Assessment of the association between HIV viral load and CD4 cell count on the occurrence of oropharyngeal candidiasis in HIV-infected patients. J Acquir Immune Defic Syndr 2006;42(5):578–83.
112. Flint SR, Tappuni A, Leigh J, et al. Markers of immunodeficiency and mechanisms of HAART therapy on oral lesions. Adv Dent Res 2006;19(1):146–51.
113. Cassone A, De Bernardis F, Torosantucci A, et al. In vitro and in vivo anticandidal activity of human immunodeficiency virus protease inhibitors. J Infect Dis 1999;180(2):448–53.
114. Cassone A, Tacconelli E, De Bernardis F, et al. Antiretroviral therapy with protease inhibitors has an early, immune reconstitution-independent beneficial effect on candida virulence and oral candidiasis in human immunodeficiency virus-infected subjects. J Infect Dis 2002;185(2):188–95.
115. Greenspan D, Greenspan JS. HIV-related oral disease. Lancet 1996;348(9029):729–33.
116. Reichart PA. Oral manifestations in HIV infection: fungal and bacterial infections, Kaposi's sarcoma. Med Microbiol Immunol 2003;192(3):165–9.
117. Reznik DA. Oral manifestations of HIV disease. Top HIV Med 2006;13(5):143–8.
118. Glick M, Muzyka BC, Lurie D, et al. Oral manifestations associated with HIV-related disease as markers for immune suppression and AIDS. Oral Surg Oral Med Oral Pathol 1994;77(4):344–9.
119. Triantos D, Porter SR, Scully C, et al. Oral hairy leukoplakia: clinicopathologic features, pathogenesis, diagnosis, and clinical significance. Clin Infect Dis 1997;25(6):1392–6.
120. Moura MD, Guimaraes TR, Fonseca LM, et al. A random clinical trial study to assess the efficacy of topical applications of podophyllin resin (25%) versus podophyllin resin (25%) together with acyclovir cream (5%) in the treatment of oral hairy leukoplakia. Oral Surg Oral Med Oral Pathol Oral Radiol Endod 2007;103(1):64–71.
121. Leigh J. Oral warts rise dramatically with use of new agents in HIV. HIV Clin 2000;12(2):7–8.

122. Hagensee ME, Cameron JE, Leigh JE, et al. Human papillomavirus infection and disease in HIV-infected individuals. Am J Med Sci 2004;328(1):57–63.
123. Drake LA, Ceilley RI, Cornelison RL, et al. Guidelines for care for warts: human papillomavirus. J Am Acad Dermatol 1995;32(1):98–103.
124. Baccaglini L, Atkinson JC, Patton LL, et al. Management of oral lesions in HIV-positive patients. Oral Surg Oral Med Oral Pathol Oral Radiol Endod 2007;103(Suppl 1):S50–56.
125. Baccaglini L, Atkinson JC, Patton LL, et al. Management of oral lesions in HIV-positive patients. Oral Surg Oral Med Oral Pathol Oral Radiol Endod 2007;103(Suppl 1):e1–23.
126. Rohrmus B, Thoma-Greber EM, Bogner JR, et al. Outlook in oral and cutaneous Kaposi's sarcoma. Lancet 2000;356(9248):2160.
127. Kerr AR, Ship JA. Management strategies for HIV-associated aphthous stomatitis. Am J Clin Dermatol 2003;4(10):669–80.

Sjögren Syndrome: A Review for the Maxillofacial Surgeon

Rajesh Gutta, BDS, MS[a,*], Landon McLain, DDS, MD[a], Stanley H. McGuff, DDS[b]

KEYWORDS

- Sjögren syndrome • Salivary disease • Parotid swelling
- Keratoconjunctivitis sicca • Dry mouth
- Dry eyes • Xerostomia

Sjögren syndrome is a systemic disease characterized by chronic lymphocytic invasion and eventual destruction of exocrine glandular structures, specifically the lacrimal and salivary glands. The disease, however, is not limited to the head and neck region. It displays a wide array of multisystem abnormalities. Classically, primary Sjögren syndrome is described as a combination of keratoconjunctivitis sicca (KCS) and xerostomia. Secondary Sjögren syndrome is a triad of KCS, xerostomia, and an autoimmune disease, usually rheumatoid arthritis.

Hadden provided the initial descriptions of the condition after noting the relationship between dry mouth and dry eyes with filamentary keratitis. He subsequently coined the term xerostomia to describe dry mouth.[1] In 1892, Mikulicz noted mononuclear infiltration in swollen parotid, submandibular, and lacrimal glands taken from the autopsy of a farmer who died of appendicitis and long had suffered from dry eyes and dry mouth.[1] Thus Mikulicz syndrome was used to describe the swelling of the lacrimal and parotid glands thereafter. The classic term Sjögren syndrome, however, was introduced after the famed Swedish ophthalmologist Henrik Sjögren described the disease in 1933.[1] Patients suspected to have Sjögren syndrome often are referred to an oral and maxillofacial surgeon (OMS) for evaluation and biopsy to rule out Sjögren syndrome. Therefore, a thorough understanding of this disease and its implications is paramount.

EPIDEMIOLOGY AND PATHOPHYSIOLOGY

Approximately 1 to 2 million Americans have Sjögren syndrome, but because of its insidious nature, it is estimated that it is undiagnosed in nearly half of patients who suffer from the disease.[2] The disease is predominantly seen in perimenopausal women. Approximately, 90% to 95% of all known cases are diagnosed in females, usually in the fifth decade.[3] This percentage, however, is slightly lower in secondary Sjögren syndrome. This might indicate a hormonal etiology to this multifactorial disorder. And, nearly 30% of all patients who have rheumatoid arthritis also have Sjögren syndrome. Although not well studied, it is believed that the prevalence is similar among all races and ethnicities. Recent epidemiologic studies have shown nearly identical incidence in China, Finland, Greece, Slovenia, Spain, and the United States.[2]

Although no known chemical or environmental factors are implicated in the pathogenesis of Sjögren syndrome, it is seen more commonly in patients who have sun sensitivity and in drier climates. Sun sensitivity is related directly to the presence of anti-Ro/SSA antibodies, and sicca

---

[a] Department of Oral and Maxillofacial Surgery, MSC 7908, University of Texas Health Science Center, 7703 Floyd Curl Drive, San Antonio, TX 78229, USA
[b] Department of Pathology, MSC 7750, University of Texas Health Science Center, 7703 Floyd Curl Drive, San Antonio, TX 78229, USA
* Corresponding author.
E-mail address: guttar@uthscsa.edu (R. Gutta).

Oral Maxillofacial Surg Clin N Am 20 (2008) 567–575
doi:10.1016/j.coms.2008.06.007
1042-3699/08/$ – see front matter © 2008 Elsevier Inc. All rights reserved.

symptoms are reported more frequently in drier climates, resulting in higher incidence of diagnosis.

Recent studies have elucidated more information in regards to the possible mechanisms that lead to the development of Sjögren syndrome but also have raised more questions on the exact etiology of this disease. Despite multiple theories and associated factors, the exact pathogenesis of this disease is unknown. As commonly noted in autoimmune diseases, multiple infectious etiologies also have been proposed as triggers of Sjögren syndrome. Traditionally, Epstein-Barr virus, and more recently, Coxsackie virus, have been implicated in the priming and maintenance of primary Sjögren syndrome.[4,5] The causal relationship between viruses and their autoimmune association, however, is unclear. It is likely that decreased clearance within glandular cells secondary to chronic sialadenitis may enable the persistence of viruses rather than the opposite. Antihuman T-cell leukemia virus-1 antibody has been reported in association with primary Sjögren syndrome in a patient with chronic sensory neuropathy.[5] Additionally, hepatitis C and HIV viruses have been reported in association with a syndrome in affected patients that is very similar to Sjögren syndrome but lacked the typical autoantibodies associated with the disease. Interestingly, intestinal *Tropheryma whippellii*-associated sicca complex has been reported also, thus expanding the possibilities of potential causes.[6]

Several autoantibodies have been defined and associated with this condition. Even more autoantigens have been associated as possible inciting factors. Anti-SSA/Ro and anti-SSB/La are the most commonly noted and aid in the diagnosis of Sjögren syndrome. Yet, these auto-antibodies are not ubiquitous to the disease and are only a component of the diagnostic criteria, and not definitive. Antimuscarinic receptor antibodies are being implicated more frequently in Sjögren syndrome, as it is thought this antibody blocks autonomic transmission to target salivary and lacrimal glands, thus leading to KCS and xerophthalmia. Unfortunately, marked progress in this arena is slow because of the innate difficulty in identifying these antibodies and the worldwide limitations in technology necessary to perform these studies.

CLINICAL FEATURES
Oral Findings

Saliva is an important participant in many roles of oral function and preservation of health. It offers protection, cleansing, and lubrication of the oral mucosa and defense against caries and periodontal disease, antibacterial function due to the contained lactoferrins, secretory IgA, and peroxidase among others. Digestion also begins in the oral cavity from the enzymes amylase and ptyalin, which are contained in saliva. Xerostomia is the most common oral complaint in patients with Sjögren syndrome. Usually the dental professional is the first to encounter this. There are a multitude of etiologies (chronic or temporary) that might lead to xerostomia, including, but not limited to medications, chronic diseases such as sarcoidosis, HIV, hepatitis C, poorly controlled diabetes, and iatrogenic causes (**Boxes 1** and **2**). The onset may be insidious, and the patient may complain of more vague symptoms like increased fluid intake, difficulty chewing and/or swallowing, sensitivity to acidic foods, and even voice changes. Although there is no set threshold for decreased salivary function, it has been shown that the sensation of oral dryness is not noted until the salivary production drops below one half of normal daily production, which is approximately 1000 to 1500 mL. Salivary flow is diurnal in nature, thus xerostomic symptoms are often worse in the morning, but may fluctuate throughout the day. Rarely will the patient report any feelings of normalcy without consistent fluid intake. Acute xerostomia has been associated with fetor oris, altered taste, and even oral pain. If the diminished salivation persists for an extended period of time, more detrimental changes may begin to occur. Although most patients retain some degree of salivatory capacity, severe cases may not produce any measurable amounts of saliva.

Dental caries will occur more quickly and at differing locations in these patients, sometimes despite excellent oral hygiene. The pattern of decay is often distinctive and displays cavitation at cusp tips of posterior teeth, incisal edges of anterior teeth, and along the cervical neck adjacent to the gingival margin.[7] This upturn in carious decay is related to loss of the salivary buffering capacity, decreased reservoirs of calcium and phosphate that replenish demineralized sites, quantitative reduction in antimicrobial proteins, and reduced mechanical cleansing. These changes lead to increased caries and halitosis because of the overgrowth of odor-causing bacteria. In established cases, the tongue often is depapillated and develops a lobulated surface. Candidal infections are also more common in those affected by the disease. Studies have shown that up to 77% of these patients are *Candida*-positive, compared with a low of 23% in healthy controls. In these patients, an inverse relationship has been noted in the density of *Candida* organisms and stimulated salivary flow rates.[8] Interestingly, periodontal disease has not been shown to be more severe in Sjögren syndrome. In fact, numerous studies

> **Box 1**
> **Drugs commonly associated with dry mouth**
>
> Antianxiety
>   Alprazolam
>
> Antihypertensive
>   Clonidine
>   Methyldopa
>
> Antidepressant
>   Amitriptyline
>   Citalopram
>   Doxepin
>   Fluoxetine
>   Imipramine
>   Nefozodone
>   Nortriptyline
>   Paroxetine
>   Venlafaxine
>
> Antihistamine
>   Cetirizine
>   Chlorpheniramine
>   Diphenhydramine
>   Hydroxyzine
>   Loratadine
>   Perchlorperazine
>   Promethazine
>
> Antipsychotic
>   Chlorpromazine
>   Clozapine
>   Fluphenazine
>   Haloperidol
>   Loxapine
>   Molindone
>   Olanzapine
>   Quetiapine
>   Risperidone
>   Thioridazine
>   Thiothixene
>   Trifluoperazine
>   Ziprasidone
>
> Anti-Parkinson's
>   Benztropine
>   Selegiline
>   Trihexyphenidyl
>
> Antiacne
>   Isotretinoin
>
> Decongestant
>   Pseudoephedrine
>
> Bronchodilator
>   Ipratropium
>   Albuterol
>
> Muscle relaxant
>   Cyclobenzaprine
>
> *Data from* Wu AJ, Daniels TE. The dry mouth: a dental perspective on Sjögren's. In: Wallace DJ, Bromet EJ, Grayzel A, et al, editors. The new Sjogrne's syndrome handbook, 3rd edition. New York: Oxford University Press; 2005.

have found no difference in periodontal disease among patients who have Sjögren syndrome and the general population.[7] This perplexing finding is possibly due to the fact that patients who have Sjögren syndrome often have increased awareness to the benefits of strict hygiene. Oral function also is diminished because of the hyposalivation, and this may lead to speech difficulty, dysphagia, and difficulty retaining removable prostheses, particularly lower complete dentures. Speech impairment might be related to oral dryness and the tongue sticking to the palate. Salivary gland enlargement is seen in about one third of patients. This is usually symmetric and gradual in onset, although it may fluctuate in severity over a period of weeks to months.

Ophthalmologic Findings

Xerophthalmia is the most dominant feature of Sjögren syndrome. Termed keratoconjunctivitis sicca, the dry-eyed patient may experience foreign body sensation in the eyes, burning, photophobia, ocular fatigue, decreased visual acuity, and even periods of paradoxical hyperlacrimation.[3] Tear film is a layered structure, and in Sjögren syndrome, the base layer (adsorbed mucin layer) is deficient, which leads to diminished wetting of the cornea, cleansing, and lubrication of the ocular surface. Destruction of the corneal and bulbar conjuctival epithelium often may develop, leading to clinical findings such as distorted light reflex,

> **Box 2**
> **Various causes of dry mouth**
>
> Temporary dry mouth
>   Short-term drug use
>   Virus infections (eg, mumps)
>   Dehydration
>   Psychogenic conditions
>
> Chronic dry mouth
>   Chronic drug usage (**Box 1**)
>   Chronic diseases
>   Sjögren syndrome
>   Sarcoidosis
>   HIV or hepatitis C infection
>   Depression
>   Diabetes mellitus
>   Amyloidosis
>   Central nervous system disorders
>   Absent or malformed glands (rarely)
>   Head and neck radiation
>   Graft-versus-host disease
>
> *Data from* Wu AJ, Daniels TE. The dry mouth: a dental perspective on Sjögren's. In: Wallace DJ, Bromet EJ, Grayzel A, et al, editors. The new Sjögren's syndrome handbook, 3rd edition. New York: Oxford University Press; 2005.

filamentary keratitis, meibomian gland dysfunction, and enlarged lacrimal glands. Xerophthalmia could be multifactorial in nature similar to xerostomia. Some of these factors may include contact lens irritation, use of cosmetics, allergic or infective conjunctivitis, and blepharitis. It is very important to assess the patient's ability to produce irritant or emotional tears. A lack of stimulated tear production is a good indicator of severe lacrimal gland involvement.

OTHER HEAD AND NECK MANIFESTATIONS

Multiple other head and neck structures may be involved in Sjögren syndrome and are of particular importance to the OMS. An evaluation of these structures and elicitation of associated symptoms should be part of the routine head and neck evaluation in these patients.

Ear, Nose, and Throat

Nasal secretions also may be decreased, and this could lead to an inflammatory response consisting of atrophic rhinitis, foul-smelling crusting, intermittent epistaxis, and even septal perforation. Patients additionally may complain of anosmia and sense of fullness in the nose. Paranasal sinuses can be involved by inflammatory obstruction of the ostea, leading to obstructive and/or infective sinusitis. Also included in this obstructive process is the eustachian tube dysfunction, which may lead to tinnitus, otalgia, and conductive hearing loss.

Larynx

Laryngeal involvement in Sjögren syndrome typically is characterized by intermittent coughing and hoarseness. This is noted more commonly in patients who use their voice more frequently, such as singers and announcers. Thickening of the laryngeal secretions also is noted and may lead to chronic laryngitis.

Thyroid

Nearly 50% of Sjögren syndrome patients have autoimmune thyroid disease, making it the most common organ-specific manifestation outside of the exocrine glands. Hypothyroidism is the most common form and has an increased association with Sjögren syndrome patients who suffer from primary biliary cirrhosis.

SYSTEMIC MANIFESTATIONS
Gastrointestinal

Dysphagia is a frequent complaint in Sjögren syndrome and often is related to decreased lubrication and hydration of the food bolus as it passes through the esophagus. This also may be caused by esophageal dysmotility that is seen in up to one third of patients who have Sjögren syndrome, however. Gastro–esophageal reflux from diminished esophageal muscle tone and even dyspepsia related to atrophic gastritis from destruction of the exocrine glands of the stomach wall additionally have been associated with Sjögren syndrome. Pernicious anemia can develop because of the hindered absorption of cyanocobolamin (vitamin B12) in these patients. Pancreatic insufficiency with diarrhea and steatorrhea can be seen, as well as acute pancreatitis. Of note, nearly 25% of patients who have Sjögren syndrome might have elevated amylase levels related to salivary gland destruction rather that pancreatitis.

There is a very high correlation between primary biliary cirrhosis and Sjögren syndrome.[9] Primary biliary cirrhosis is caused by autoimmune inflammation and destruction of the small to medium bile ducts of the liver. As a result, bile salts build up in the liver, leading to hepatic inflammation and eventually cirrhosis. This impairment leads to the usual sequelae of liver disease including pruritus, jaundice, malabsorption, coagulopathy, varices, and eventual hepatic failure. Unfortunately, there is no known cure for primary biliary cirrhosis other than orthotopic liver transplantation; although treatment with ursodeoxycholic acid may delay the progression of the disease. Chronic active hepatitis also has been associated with Sjögren syndrome and can lead to cirrhotic liver disease. Chronic active hepatitis, however, is treatable with steroids or other immunosuppressive drugs, notably azathioprine.

Connective Tissue Disorders

Rheumatoid arthritis (RA) is the most common rheumatologic disease and is the most commonly associated autoimmune disorder seen with Sjögren syndrome. RA is characterized by autoimmune-mediated inflammation of the joint synovium, characteristically the proximal interphalangeal and metacarpophalangeal joints. The shoulders, hips and knees often are involved symmetrically. RA is associated with early morning stiffness and fatigue, as well as subcutaneous nodules around pressure points of the extremities. Diagnosis of RA is based on clinical, radiologic, and laboratory evidence. The diagnosis of RA or prior history of RA in a patient who has Sjögren syndrome implies secondary Sjögren syndrome. These patients have a highly variable onset. In addition, the condition is generally milder in form, and there is less association with lymphoma than primary Sjögren syndrome. Notably, the primary form of the disease also can be associated with other autoimmune diseases and remain primary in nature, but those diseases are limited to Hashimoto's thyroiditis, Raynaud's phenomenon, and antiphospholipid antibody syndrome. Systemic lupus erythematosus, scleroderma, polymyositis, dermatomyositis, and a range of other vasculitides have been associated with Sjögren syndrome. The interplay among these diseases and the relative effect on one another are unclear, however, and remain an integral part of ongoing research about Sjögren syndrome.

Neurologic

Up to 20% of the patients with Sjögren syndrome have some form of associated neurologic disease, usually a peripheral neuropathy or carpal tunnel syndrome. Recent literature, however, supports an increasing association with central nervous system deficits such as optic neuropathy, seizures, cognitive dysfunction, and a syndrome mimicking multiple sclerosis.[10] As many as 80% of these patients also will display depression disorder or symptoms associated with depression.

Pulmonary

Pulmonary manifestations of Sjögren syndrome display various features, categorized into four broad patterns. These are: diffuse interstitial disease, small airway disease, desiccation of the tracheobronchial tree, and large airway obstruction.[11] The most common CT findings are ground glass attenuation, followed by multiple subpleural nodules and cystic airspaces. Rarely, pulmonary hypertension may develop. Pulmonary findings also might be the first indicator of malignant lymphoma development.[12,13]

Hematology

Patients who have Sjögren syndrome are at a 44-fold greater risk for developing a malignant lymphoma, and the total prevalence is estimated to be around 4%. Lymphomas arising in these patients are usually low-grade non-Hodgkin's type, usually found in the mucosa-associated lymphoid tissue (MALT) of the intestinal tract. The bone marrow rarely is affected, as these lesions usually are confined to salivary glands, lymph nodes, and the stomach. The low-grade lymphomas affecting the exocrine glands are usually left untreated, as the survival rates are identical to treated groups. In the small subset of patients who develop high-grade lymphoma, however, combination chemotherapy is required. It remains associated with poor outcome, however. Predictors of lymphoma development are low complement levels, serum cryoglobulins, and the presence purpura. Fortunately, the life expectancy of patients who have Sjögren syndrome is normal, excluding the patients who develop lymphoma.[12]

DIAGNOSIS

The current standards for diagnosis are the revised European–American criteria introduced in 2002 (**Box 3**).[14] Earlier, the diagnosis of Sjögren syndrome was less stringent and often one of subjectivity, without any ability to formulate clinical trials or strict epidemiologic research.

The diagnosis of primary Sjögren syndrome requires four of the six criteria, including either a positive lip biopsy or positive anti- SSA/Ro or anti-SSB/La. Secondary Sjögren syndrome requires an established connective tissue disease and at least one sicca symptom plus two out of three objective tests for either xerophthalmia or xerostomia. Note that Sjögren syndrome also can be diagnosed in the absence of sicca symptoms if three out of four objective tests are positive.

> **Box 3**
> **Revised American–European criteria for classification of Sjögren syndrome**
>
> Ocular symptoms (1 of 3)
>
> > Dry eyes for longer than 3 months
> > Sensation of a foreign body in the eye
> > Use of artificial tears more than three times a day
>
> Oral symptoms (1 of 3)
>
> > Dry mouth for longer than 3 months
> > Swollen salivary glands
> > Need liquids to swallow
>
> Ocular tests (1 of 2)
>
> > Unanesthetized Schirmer's test (less than 5 mm in 5 minutes)
> > Vital dye staining
>
> Positive lip biopsy (focus score more than .25 mm²)
>
> Oral test (1 of 3)
>
> > Unstimulated salivary flow (less than 0.1 mL/min)
> > Abnormal parotid sialography
> > Abnormal salivary scintigraphy
>
> Positive anti-SSA and/or SSB
>
> *Data from* Vitali C, Bombardier S, Jonsson R, et al. Classification criteria for Sjögren's syndrome: a revised version of the European criteria proposed by the American European group. Ann Rheum Dis 2002; 61:554–8.

OBJECTIVE TESTS
Schirmer Test

The Schirmer test is objectively used to measure tear secretion. The test is performed by placing a porous filter strip in the inferior fornix of each unanesthetized eye for 10 minutes. A healthy eye should wet more than 15 mm of the standard filter strip in 5 minutes. A more reliable assessment, however, is made by staining the cornea with 1% rose Bengal dye and examining with a slit lamp to show punctate or filamentary keratitis if the cornea is dry.

Sialometry

This test can be used as a diagnostic tool mainly in two ways: collection of whole saliva (ie, combined secretions of all salivary glands) and collection of glandular saliva (ie, gland specific saliva). Collection of whole saliva is the method most often used, because it is very easy to perform, taking only a few minutes, without the need for a collecting device. Glandular saliva usually is collected directly from the glands (parotid, submandibular and sublingual).[15] The assessment should be performed in such a way to minimize the fluctuations related to a circadian rhythm of salivary secretion and composition. Salivary flow also can be measured by comparing unstimulated saliva with stimulated salivary flow.

Sialography

This method has been used for many years as a means to assess the salivary component of Sjögren syndrome. Typical sialographic findings in Sjögren syndrome are dilatations of the ducts (sialodochiectasis), duct strictures, and punctate collections of extravasated contrast medium (sialectasis). When interpreting the significance of punctate sialectasis, one should remember that this is a radiographic image affected by the technique. This has been called pseudosialectasis when contrast medium is forced through the weakened ducts.[16]

Scintigraphy

The oral component of Sjögren syndrome also may be evaluated by salivary gland scintigraphy. This is a noninvasive nuclear medicine technique to assess the salivary glands. A radionuclide, pertechnetium m^{99}, is infused intravenously, and the images of the salivary glands are captured after 1 hour. The uptake of the radionuclide by the glands is observed as well as the amount of saliva containing the radionuclide. Although the test is highly sensitive for Sjögren syndrome, it has a low specificity.

Biopsy

Of importance to the OMS is the labial minor salivary gland biopsy, first introduced by Calman and Reifman in 1966.[17] The oral labial minor salivary gland biopsy provides a means of assessing the salivary component of Sjögren syndrome. A positive biopsy is utilized as one of the major diagnostic criteria for this disease. Salivary glands involved by this condition show a focal lymphocytic pattern of infiltration, in which there are multiple interstitial aggregate foci of inflammatory cells. The infiltrate should consist predominantly of lymphocytes (**Figs. 1–3**). An aggregate focus is defined as a collection of greater than 50 inflammatory cells.[18] There may be admixed plasma cells and histiocytes, but these cells should not comprise a significant portion of the infiltrate. Granulomatous

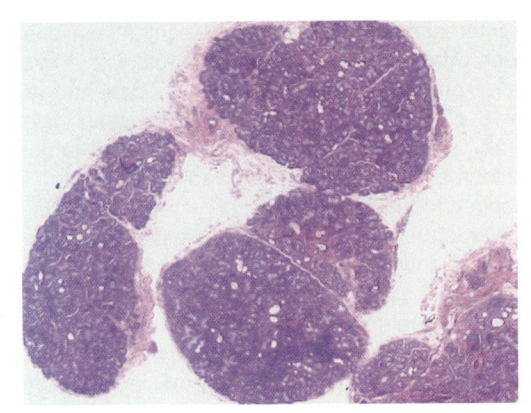

Fig. 1. Minor salivary glands exhibiting a focal lymphocytic pattern of inflammatory cell infiltration (original magnification 1.6×).

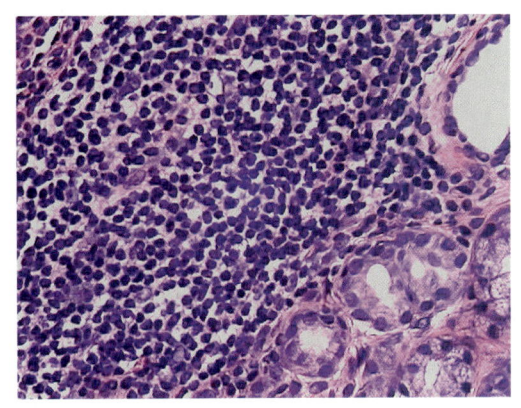

Fig. 3. Section showing a dense aggregate of lymphocytes with adjacent intact salivary gland parenchyma (original magnification 25×).

inflammation should not be present. The adjacent salivary gland parenchyma is usually intact, without acinar atrophy, fibrosis, ductal ectasia, inspissated secretions, or acute inflammation. The presence of such regressive/degenerative parenchymal changes is considered to be nonspecific and is not characteristic of an autoimmune exocrinopathy.[19]

The Sjögren syndrome focus score is a semiquantitative method of grading the degree of salivary gland inflammatory infiltration. Histomorphometric analysis is utilized by the pathologist to quantitate the area of salivary gland parenchyma in square millimeters. The number of lymphocytic aggregates is counted, and a focus score is calculated utilizing the following formula:

$$\frac{\text{Number of Lymphocytic Aggregates} \times 4}{\text{Area of Salivary Gland Parenchyma}} = \text{Focus Score}$$

The focus score represents the number of lymphocytic aggregates per 4 mm^2 of salivary gland tissue. Therefore, an absolute minimum of 4 mm^2 of salivary gland tissue is required to calculate the focus score. Generally, harvesting 5 to 10 minor salivary glands should be quantitatively sufficient.

A focus score of 1 or greater (greater than one lymphocytic aggregate per 4 mm^2 of salivary gland tissue) is considered supportive of the diagnosis of Sjögren syndrome. The focus score can range from 0 to 12, with a focus score of 12 representing diffuse glandular effacement by the lymphocytic infiltrate. The presence of a dense effacing infiltrate should raise concern for possible progression to lymphoma.

The oral labial minor salivary gland biopsy is a valuable diagnostic tool, especially in patients who present with inconclusive clinical findings.[20] A positive Sjögren syndrome focus score is not diagnostic of Sjögren syndrome by itself, but the results of the biopsy must be correlated with each of the other diagnostic criteria in order to establish an accurate diagnosis. The minor salivary gland biopsy is also helpful in excluding other conditions, such as sarcoidosis, which may be associated with a sicca syndrome. Biopsy of the parotid and lacrimal glands also has been utilized for assessing Sjögren syndrome.[20,21] Some authors recommend biopsy of the parotid tail over labial biopsy. The lymphocytic infiltrate occurs earlier and more severely in the parotid gland than in minor glands. The parotid biopsy requires less regimented histopathologic grading.[22]

TREATMENT

Although Sjögren syndrome is unlikely to be primarily managed by the OMS, a thorough knowledge of the tenants of treatment is important. Xerostomia is the hallmark of the disease process and the most likely component to be encountered

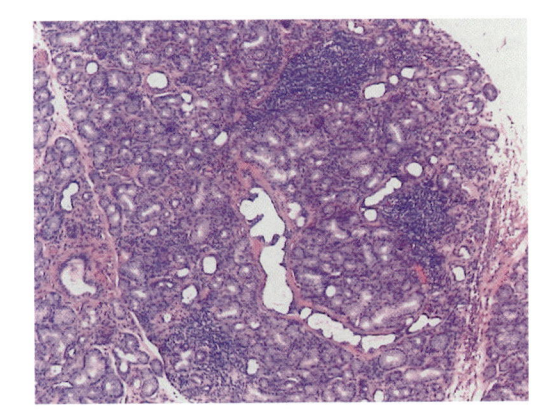

Fig. 2. Minor salivary glands with multiple lymphocytic aggregate foci (original magnification 4×).

and treated by the OMS. Certainly, impeccable oral hygiene is vital because of the diminished anticariogenic properties of salivary flow, and the avoidance of refined carbohydrates. Ideal treatment should address xerostomia, prevention of oral complications, stimulation of salivary flow, and repair of inflamed salivary glands. Currently, there is no panacea for patients who have Sjögren syndrome.

Adequate hydration remains the simplest yet most effective means to treat xerostomia. Frequent small sips of water not only rehydrate the oral cavity but also cleanse and reduce microbial load. Avoidance of dehydration is paramount to maintain baseline salivary flow. Caffeinated sodas should be avoided because of the diuretic effect of caffeine and the acidity of the soda. Fluoride carriers and remineralization solutions may be necessary for caries control. The use of nighttime humidifiers is a consideration that will minimize oral drying during sleep, as this is the diurnal nadir of salivary flow.

Several modes of salivary stimulation are available. Ranging from topical to systemic, these therapies are based upon some remaining secretory capacity of the salivary glands. The disadvantage of all these therapies is their transient nature, although symptomatic relief may persist beyond the period of increased salivation and is likely related to the obtundant effects of saliva on the oral mucosa.[23]

Local therapies include sugar-free gums, candies, or lozenges as stimulants to gustatory and masticatory salivary flow. Xylitol is an acceptable artificial sweetener and has been shown to reduce caries. Clinical trials have supported the use of anhydrous crystalline maltose lozenges as an effective means to treat xerostomia.[24]

Oral pilocarpine 5 mg three to four times daily also has been recommended. The use of this parasympathomimetic has been around for over 100 years and has been shown in several clinical trials to be an effective means to stimulate salivary flow. There is no tolerance associated, and adverse reactions including sweating, flushing, and frequent urination are rare. This drug, however, is contraindicated in acute narrow-angle glaucoma, uncontrolled asthma, and acute iritis. Other effective agents include:

> Cevimeline, which may have a longer duration of action than pilocarpine, but similar pharmacologic profile
> Bromhexine
> Interferon-alpha in indictable or lozenge form, which has shown increased salivation and decreased salivary gland inflammation
> Infliximab, a tumor necrosis factor α blocker[2]

Interestingly, favorable early results have been seen with tibolone, a synthetic steroid with androgenic properties, when used to treat patients who have Sjögren syndrome. Tibolone, when given orally at a dosage of 2.5 mg/d, has been shown to increase oral, ocular, and vaginal lubrication in postmenopausal women.[25]

Xerophthalmia is also a key target of anti-Sjögren syndrome therapy and often is addressed by the ophthalmologist. Local therapy includes mainly nonpreservative-containing artificial tears in the form of eye drops, gels, or ointments. Topical steroids are advocated by some, in addition to warm ocular compresses and massage aimed at reducing meibomian inflammation. Temporary or permanent punctal occlusion may benefit those who have severe ocular symptoms.[26] In addition, systemic administration of androgens methyl-testosterone or mesterolone and cyclosporine has been linked with beneficial effects on lacrimal and meibomian function.[1] Some authors even have suggested transplantation of minor sublingual salivary glands.[26]

For the 6% to 10% of patients who may progress into lymphoma, a complete workup to assess other locations and staging is recommended. Any parotid focus of lymphoma is typically treatable with radiotherapy and any change in size, color, or architecture of the involved parotid gland mandates repeat biopsy.

FUTURE DIRECTIONS

Because most of the current therapy for Sjögren syndrome is mostly symptomatic, there remains a dearth of treatment directed at the exact etiology behind the disease. Future therapy likely will be directed at more tissue-specific receptors, resulting in less side effects. In patients who have little to no remaining exocrine function, tissue-specific transplantation or biocompatible artificial lacrimal or salivary glands may be feasible.[2] There has even been promising work in local gene transfer of interleukin-10 by means of an adenovirus in a mouse model. The possibility of human success with gene transfer remains hopeful.[27]

REFERENCES

1. Tabbara KF, Vera-Cristo CL. Sjögren syndrome. Curr Opin Ophthalomol 2000;11(6):449–54.
2. Wallace DJ. Who develops Sjögren's syndrome. In: Wallace DJ, Bromet EJ, Grayzel A, et al, editors. The new Sjögren's syndrome handbook. 3rd edition. New York: Oxford University Press; 2005. p. 10–2.
3. Lash AA. Sjögren's syndrome: pathogenesis, diagnosis, and treatment. Nurse Pract 2001;26(8):50, 53–8.

4. Fox RI, Pearson G, Vaughan JH. Detection of Epstein-Barr virus-associated antigens and DNA in salivary gland biopsies from patients with Sjögren's syndrome. J Immunol 1986;137(10):3162–8.
5. Hansen A, Lipsky PE, Dorner T. New concepts in the pathogenesis of Sjögren syndrome: many questions, fewer answers. Curr Opin Rheumatol 2003;15(5):563–70.
6. Bosman C, Boldrini R, Borsetti G, et al. Sicca symptoms associated with *Trophermyma whippleii* intestinal infection. J Clin Microbiol 2002;40(8):3104–6.
7. Wu AJ, Daniels TE. The dry mouth: a dental perspective on Sjögren's. In: Wallace DJ, Bromet EJ, Grayzel A, et al, editors. The new Sjögren's syndrome handbook. 3rd edition. New York: Oxford University Press; 2005. p. 58–67.
8. Radfar L, Shea Y, Fischer SH, et al. Fungal load and candidiasis in Sjögren's syndrome. Oral Surg Oral Med Oral Pathol Oral Radiol Endod 2003;96(3):283–7.
9. Mandel L, Dehlinger N. Primary biliary cirrhosis and Sjögren's syndrome: case report. J Oral Maxillofac Surg 2003;61(11):1358–61.
10. Delalande S, de Seze J, Fauchais AL, et al. Neurologic manifestations in primary Sjögren syndrome: a study of 82 patients. Medicine 2004;83(5):280–91.
11. Constantopoulos SH, Papadimitriou CS, Moutsopoulos HM. Respiratory manifestations in primary Sjögren's syndrome: a clinical, functional, and histologic study. Chest 1985;88(2):226–9.
12. Koyama M, Johkoh T, Honda O, et al. Pulmonary involvement in primary Sjögren's syndrome: spectrum of pulmonary abnormalities and computed tomography findings in 60 patients. J Thorac Imaging 2001;16(4):290–6.
13. Levy RA, Vilela VS, Abreu MM. Useful studies: blood tests, imaging, biopsies, and beyond. In: Wallace DJ, Bromet EJ, Grayzel A, et al, editors. The new Sjögren's syndrome handbook. 3rd edition. New York: Oxford University Press; 2005. p. 97–105.
14. Vitali C, Bombardier S, Jonsson R, et al. Classification criteria for Sjögren's syndrome: a revised version of the European criteria proposed by the American European group. Ann Rheum Dis 2002;61(6):554–8.
15. Kalk WW, Vissink A, Spijkervet FK, et al. Sialometry and sialochemistry: diagnostic tools for Sjögren's syndrome. Ann Rheum Dis 2001;60(12):1110–6.
16. Daniels TE, Benn DK. Is sialography effective in diagnosing the salivary component of Sjögren's syndrome? Adv Dent Res 1996;10(1):25–8.
17. Calman HI, Reifman S. Sjögren's syndrome: report of a case. Oral Surg Oral Med Oral Pathol 1966;21(2):158–62.
18. Chisholm DM, Mason DK. Labial salivary gland biopsy in Sjögren's disease. J Clin Pathol 1968;21(5):656–60.
19. Daniels TE. Labial salivary gland biopsy in Sjögren's syndrome: assessment as a diagnostic criterion in 362 suspected cases. Arthritis Rheum 1984;27(2):147–56.
20. Lee M, Rutka JA, Slomovic AR, et al. Establishing guidelines for the role of minor salivary gland biopsy in clinical practice for Sjögren's syndrome. J Rheumatol 1998;25(2):247–53.
21. Pijpe J, Kalk WW, van der Wal JE, et al. Parotid gland biopsy compared with labial biopsy in the diagnosis of patients with primary Sjögren's syndrome. Rheumatology 2007;46(2):335–41.
22. Marx RE, Stern D. Oral and maxillofacial pathology: a rationale for diagnosis and treatment. Hanover Park, IL: Quintessence Publishing Co; 2003. p. 497–526.
23. Al-Hashimi I. The management of Sjögren's syndrome in dental practice. J Am Dent Assoc 2001;132(10):1409–17.
24. Brennan MT, Shariff G, Lockhart PB, et al. Treatment of xerostomia: a systematic review of therapeutic trials. Dent Clin North Am 2002;46(4):847–56.
25. Sartore A, Grimaldi E, Guaschino S. The treatment of Sjögren's syndrome with tibolone: a case report. Am J Obstet Gynecol 2003;189(3):894.
26. Murube J, Murube E. Treatment of dry eye by blocking the lacrimal canaliculi. Surv Ophthalmol 1996;40(6):463–80.
27. Hansen A, Lipsky PE, Dorner T. Immunopathogenesis of primary Sjögren's syndrome: implications for disease management and therapy. Curr Opin Rheum 2005;17(5):558–65.

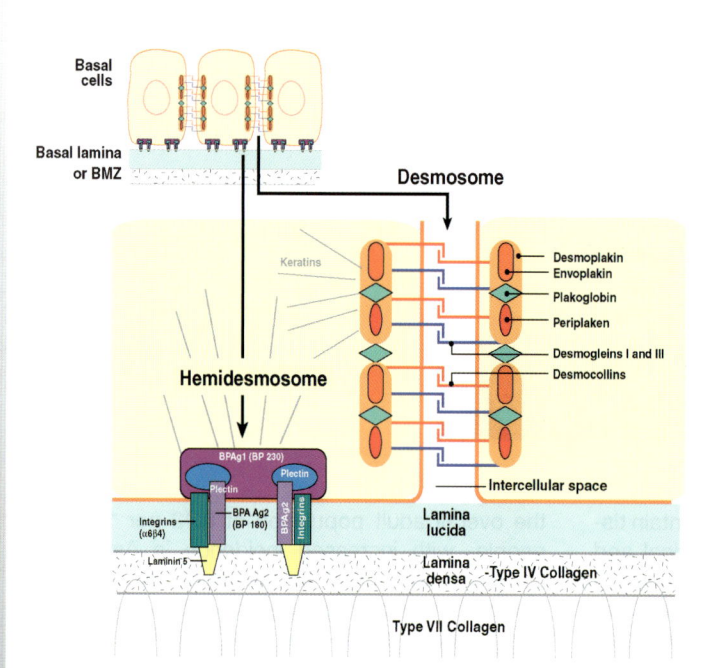

Fig. 1. Anatomic and molecular basis of bullous dermatoses.

patients have high serum titers of antidesmoglein 3 antibodies and low or no titers of antidesmoglein 1 antibodies. The function of desmoglein 1 in the skin is preserved, preventing the development of cutaneous lesions, but the impaired adhesive function of desmoglein 3 produces acantholysis in the oral cavity. Most patients who have PV develop cutaneous lesions. The clinical picture of mucocutaneous PV emerges when cutaneous lesions appear as antibodies to both desmoglein 1 and 3 develop. Clinical phenotypes thus are determined by the relative amounts of antibodies against desmoglein 1 and 3.

A subset of pemphigus patients only produces desmoglein 1 antibodies, a condition known as pemphigus foliaceus. These patients do not have mucosal involvement.

Clinical Presentation

Figs. 2, 3, and 4 depict the delicate superficial blisters and chronic ulcerations of the skin and mucosa that are the hallmark of PV. Pisanti and colleagues found that the oral cavity was the sole initial site of PV lesions in 56% of the cases, and that 88% of patients had primary lesions in the mouth alone or in combination with other sites.[5] Sirois reported survey results of 99 patients who had PV and found that 81% had oral lesions first.[16]

Table 1	
Autoimmune bullous dermatoses and antigens targeted by autoantibodies	
Autoimmune Bullous Dermatoses	**Antigen**
Mucosal dominant pemphigus vulgaris (PV)	Desmoglein 3
Mucocutaneous PV	Desmoglein 3, desmoglein 1, and possibly desmoglein 4
Paraneoplastic pemphigus	Desmoglein 3, desmoglein 1, and plakin proteins
Pemphigus foliaceus	Desmoglein 1
IgA pemphigus	Desmocolin
Bullous pemphigoid	BP 180 and BP 230
Lichen planus pemphigoides	BP 180
Epidermolysis bullosa acquisita	Type 7 collagen
Erythema multiforme	Desmoplakins
Dermatitis herpetiformis	Tissue transglutaminase

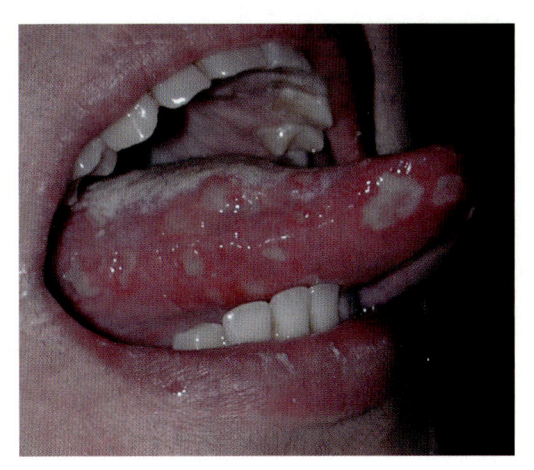

Fig. 2. Painful pemphigus vulgaris tongue lesions.

The lesions begin as short-lived vesicles or blisters that rapidly rupture because of their suprabasilar position. Vesicles or even bullae will be seen more commonly on the skin because of the increased thickness of skin epithelium and a greater keratin layer as compared with mucosa. The oral lesions are particularly painful, and oral and skin lesions can become secondarily infected. All the mucosal surfaces can become involved, including oral, pharyngeal, laryngeal, ocular, nasal, upper respiratory, and anogenital. Ocular lesions can result in severe corneal desquamation and symblepharon between bulbar and palpebral conjunctivae, which can lead to functional blindness. Tissue fragility is common, and oral superficial tissue sloughing and ulceration can occur with common frictional maneuvers such as tooth brushing, removable prosthetic appliance wear, or tissue manipulation. Nikolsky sign classically is described as the extension of a skin blister when lateral pressure is applied to peri-lesional skin. It

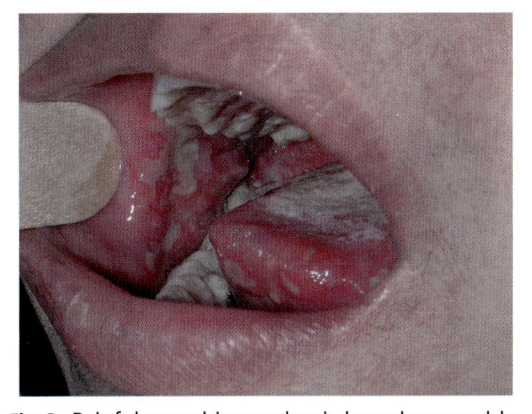

Fig. 3. Painful pemphigus vulgaris buccal mucosal lesions from the same patient.

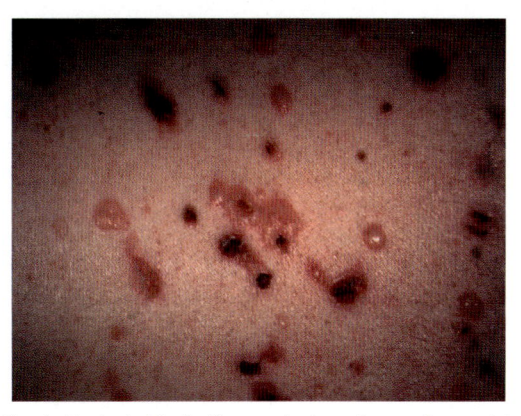

Fig. 4. Typical skin bullae and ulcerations of pemphigus vulgaris.

was coined Nikolsky sign after Pyotr Vasilyewich Nikolsky (1858 to 1940), a Russian dermatologist who studied at the University of Kiev and first described the phenomenon in 1896. This test is difficult to reproduce in the oral cavity, because blisters and vesicles are extremely short-lived. A positive Nikolsky sign in the oral cavity usually is applied when tissue ulceration or blistering is noted after applying mucosal pressure by blowing air or using a blunt instrument or finger. Nikolsky sign is not specific for PV, however, because it can be provoked in other diseases such as PNP, epidermolysis bullosa, oral lichen planus, mucous membrane pemphigoid, linear IgA disease, lupus erythematosus, dermatomyositis, chronic erythema multiforme, or graft-versus-host disease.[17]

Diagnostic Work-Up

Definitive diagnosis of PV requires biopsy of the oral mucosa or skin that includes clinically normal tissue. The preferred biopsy site is considered oral mucosa, because the diagnostic suprabasilar separation and acantholysis are seen best in such tissues. The ulcerated tissues should be avoided when selecting the biopsy site, because it may not show the roof of the vesicle, or the tissues may be obscured by secondary inflammation and necrosis. Obtaining two biopsy specimens or dividing a single biopsy specimen into two representative specimens is ideal. One specimen is submitted in 10% neutral-buffered formalin for hematoxylin and eosin (H and E) staining, and the other submitted in Michel's medium for direct immunofluorescence (DIF) studies. This medium prevents tissue degradation without damaging the immunoreactants such as immunoglobulins, complement, and fibrin. Various sections then are incubated with fluorescein-labeled antibodies directed against different human immunoglobulins, complement, fibrin, and fibrinogen. When the slides are examined under the microscope, DIF typically demonstrates homogenous epithelial cell surface staining with IgG.[18] DIF is costly and is not required in unequivocal cases but will confirm or rule out the diagnosis when there is doubt. Tissues placed in formalin cannot be used for DIF.

Indirect immunofluorescence (IIF) may be performed to assess the titer of circulating autoantibodies, and it is thought to be an index of disease severity against which to adjust treatment dosage. Assessing the titer of circulating antibodies is costly, however, and is not as accurate as the patient's observed clinical disease severity.[8]

A more sensitive and recent technique for determining circulating antibodies is ELISA. This technique can detect circulating antibodies to desmoglein 1 or 3, and the titers directly correlate with disease activity. Because of its specificity, ELISA can help differentiate between patients who have pemphigus foliaceus and those who have PV.[14]

Histopathology

The characteristic histologic features of PV observed using a standard H and E stain include intraepithelial clefts, acantholysis (separation of the epithelial cells), and a dense mononuclear lymphocytic infiltration (**Fig. 5**). In **Fig. 6**, DIF staining reveals the characteristic spider web distribution of autoantibody between the epithelial cells.

Treatment

Patients who present initially with PV frequently are dehydrated, in pain, and possibly suffering from secondary infection. Hospital admission may be necessary to provide fluid resuscitation, pain control, and antibiotic administration while

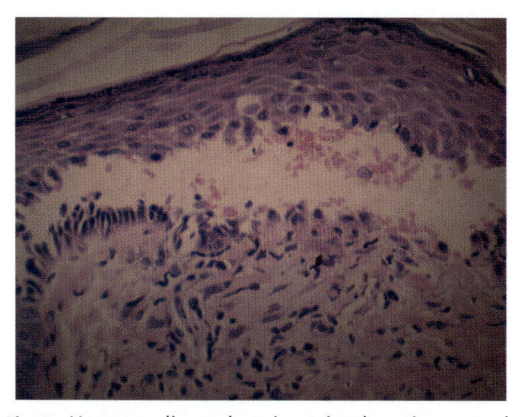

Fig. 5. Hematoxylin and eosin stained section revealing suprabasilar separation, mononuclear infiltrate, and acantholysis.

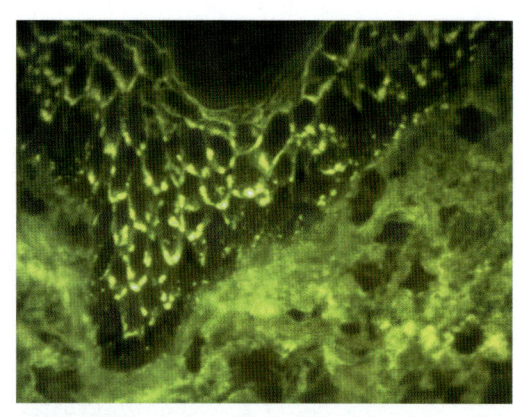

Fig. 6. Direct immunofluorescence staining (IgG) showing pemphigus vulgaris antigen distribution in the spaces between squamous epithelial cells. Specimen obtained from intraoral peri-lesional biopsy specimen with intact mucosa.

preparing for biopsy. Biopsy and diagnosis should be performed prior to starting corticosteroid therapy. If corticosteroid therapy is initiated, and the biopsy specimen is nondiagnostic, subsequent biopsies will have an altered tissue response, obscuring diagnosis and complicating treatment.

Corticosteroid therapy became the mainstay therapy for patients with PV around 1950; before that, PV was almost invariably fatal (usually from septicemia) within 5 years. Lever's classic 1965 monograph, *Pemphigus and Pemphigoid*, summarizes the dismal prognosis of his patients treated between 1937 and 1949. Of 33 patients, 30 died within 5 years, and an additional patient died within 6 years.[19] The two survivors received large doses of adrenal cortical extracts and therefore probably received significant doses of glucocorticoids.

Prednisone dramatically changed the prognosis for patients with PV. Prednisone quickly suppresses blistering and dramatically decreases mortality from disease. Patients tend to relapse when prednisone is tapered, however, and long-term steroid therapy can produce severe complications such as osteoporosis, osteonecrosis, cataracts, hyperglycemia, weight gain, opportunistic infections, and hypothalamic-pituitary-adrenal axis suppression.[20] In fact, Rosenberg's review in 1976 showed more deaths from corticosteroid adverse effects than from uncontrolled pemphigus.[21]

The problems with prednisone therapy for patients who had PV led to an active search for adjuvant treatment protocols that would have a steroid-sparing effect. These agents, along with earlier diagnosis and treatment and better medical treatment of glucocorticoid therapy complications, have helped decrease the mortality from PV to fewer than 10%.[22]

The mainstay adjuvant immunosuppressive drug therapy for PV over the last 20 years has been cyclophosphamide or azathioprine.[23–25] Both drugs can cause thrombocytopenia, leukopenia, and anemia. Also, chronic immunosuppression with these drugs increases the risk of neoplasia. Azathioprine additionally can cause hepatotoxicity, requiring monitoring of liver function tests. Cyclophosphamide can cause sterility, hemorrhagic cystitis, urinary bladder fibrosis, congestive heart failure, and hemorrhagic myocarditis.

After establishing adjuvant immunosuppressive treatment with cyclophosphamide or azathioprine, plasmapheresis can be helpful in controlling persistent disease.[26–28] Plasmapheresis removes autoantibodies from the blood, with a direct effect on the disease process.

Two of the new medications being used for PV are mycophenolate (CellCept) and rituximab (Rituxan). Mycophenolate most often is used in combination with prednisone and cyclosporine to prevent rejection of renal allogeneic transplants.[29] Mycophenolic acid, the active metabolite, suppresses B- and T-cell proliferation through its inhibition of inosine monphosphate dehydrogenase, an essential enzyme in the pathway of de novo guanine nucleotide synthesis. Adverse effects of mycophenolate are mainly gastrointestinal (diarrhea, dyspepsia, abdominal pain, or nausea) and myelosuppression.[29] At this time, mycophenolate is a good choice to use for a patient with PV receiving prednisone who requires adjuvant therapy but does not respond to, or cannot tolerate azathioprine.[30]

Enk and Knop presented 12 patients with PV who initially were treated with prednisone (2 mg/kg daily) and azathioprine (1.5 to 2 mg/kg daily).[31] These patients initially improved but relapsed when prednisone was tapered. The azathioprine was discontinued, and the patients subsequently received combination therapy with mycophenolate (1 g twice daily) and prednisolone (2 mg/kg daily). Eleven of the 12 patients responded to therapy and showed no relapse of their disease even after tapering of the steroid dose to 2.5 mg/day by 9 months. One patient did not respond. During the 9- to 12-month follow-up, none of the 11 patients showed reappearance of pemphigus lesions.

Rituximab is another important addition to the armamentarium of therapy for PV. It is a monoclonal antibody directed against the CD20 antigen of B lymphocytes and has been effective in various autoimmune diseases.[32–38] Joly and colleagues[39] recently studied 21 patients with pemphigus whose disease had not responded to, or they could not tolerate, prednisone. They received four weekly infusions of rituximab, and 18 of 21 patients had a complete remission at 3 months.

There are several other adjuvant therapies that have been described but have not found widespread use in the United States. These include dapsone,[40,41] intramuscular gold,[42,43] intravenous immunoglobulin,[44,45] cyclosporine,[46,47] extracorporeal photopheresis,[48,49] and tetracycline with niacinamide.[50]

PARANEOPLASTIC PEMPHIGUS
Epidemiology

The term PNP was first suggested by Anhalt and colleagues in 1990 after describing five patients with underlying neoplasm in whom painful mucosal ulcerations and polymorphous skin lesions developed, usually with progression to blistering eruptions on the trunk and extremities.[51] PNP most commonly is associated with B-cell lymphoproliferative disorders. In a review of 18 patients fulfilling the diagnostic criteria for PNP, 77.7% of patients had a lymphoid neoplasm.[52] Hodgkin's lymphoma, chronic lymphocytic leukemia, Castleman's disease, sarcomas, thymomas, and Waldernstrom's macroglobuninemia make up the most common malignancies seen in association with PNP.[53] Most patients who have PNP range in age from 45 to 70 years, but cases have been reported as young as 7 years old.[53] There appears to be a slight male predilection.[53]

Pathophysiology

The pathogenesis of PNP involves the humoral and cellular immune systems.[54] Three theories that link PNP to neoplasia have been developed. First, neoplasias involving the immune system, such as thymomas, may cause deregulation by altering signal pathways such as overproduction of interleukins.[53] Second, carcinomas may produce antigenic components that interact with the cell surface of epithelial cells and lead to an autoimmune response. In fact, it has been shown that some lymphomas can atypically express desmosomes.[53] Third, the primary paraneoplastic process can be viewed as a lichenoid reaction in which the necrotic keratinocytes drive the humoral response.[53]

Clinical Presentation

Oral lesions are seen in almost all cases of PNP and often times can be the first symptom of the disease process.[53] Oral lesions associated with PNP are often severe, diffuse, persistent erosions extending to all regions of the oral cavity, including posterior extension to the hypopharynx and esophagus.[52,53] In addition, oral ulcerations often extend outward onto the lip, approaching the vermillion border.[53] In up to 50% of patients, oral manifestations of PNP are present prior to the diagnosis of a neoplasm and can be the first sign of disease in nearly 25% of cases.[52] In some cases, however, erosive lesions can arise up to 16 years after the diagnosis of a malignancy and even have arisen following the remission of the cancer.[53] Skin lesions on the other hand tend to be polymorphous and can mimic several dermatologic conditions. Flaccid or tense blisters with or without erosions are the most common skin findings.[53] Surprisingly, the skin of the face typically is spared. Ocular involvement with PNP is common and can be devastating. Bilateral conjunctival ulcerations are common and can be seen in up to 72.2% of patients, leading to pseudomembranous conjunctivitis, symblepharon, and loss of vision.[52,53] Most patients also develop respiratory problems that are a complication of PNP or its treatment. Confounding this problem is the direct effect on the respiratory system that leads to bronchiolitis obliterans, which eventually leads to a fatal respiratory failure.[53–55]

Diagnostic Work-Up

The diagnostic criteria for PNP include the following:[53,56,57]

1. Polymorphous eruptions involving skin and mucosa
2. Histopathology demonstrating intraepidermal acantholysis and dyskeratosis along with basal layer vacuolar changes
3. Intraepidermal and/or basement membrane zone deposition of IgG and C3 with direct immunofluorescence
4. Serum autoantibodies to multiple epithelia (simple, columnar, and transitional)
5. Unique immunoprecipitation complex of 250, 230, 210, and 190 Kd antigens

These above criteria have been revised by Camisa and Helm and contain major and minor criteria.[53] Major criteria include:

Polymorphous mucocutaneous eruption
Concurrent internal neoplasia
Specific serum immunoprecipitation pattern

Minor criteria include:

Histologic evidence of acantholysis
DIF showing intercellular and basement membrane staining

IIF staining with rat bladder (transitional epithelium)

Diagnostic workup of patients who have PNP and no associated malignancy should have a directed work-up aimed at the most common associated malignancies. This work-up should include a CT of the chest/abdomen/pelvis, complete blood cell count (CBC) with differential, serum protein electrophoresis and diagnostic biopsies as indicated.[53]

Histopathology

In addition to the acantholysis seen in pemphigus, PNP includes necrosis of individual keratinocytes and vacuolar interface changes.[52] DIF will show deposition of IgG, with or without C3 on the cell surface, and a characteristic combination of both granular–linear complements deposition along the basement membrane and in the epithelial intercellular spaces.[52] In contrast, the reaction seen in PV is intercellular only. Indirect immunofluorescence has a similar pattern to PV, in that both will contain high titers of autoantibodies to the intercellular substance of human epidermis (stratified squamous epithelium). The autoantibodies seen with PNP, however, will bind to simple, columnar, and transitional epithelium.[52,54] Urinary epithelium usually is chosen based on its high density of desmosomes.[56] In addition, the pattern of immunoprecipitation seen in PNP is unique and is the most reliable technique for confirmation of diagnosis.[53] Autoantibodies against desmoplakin II (210Kd) and peri-plakin (190 Kd) are the most specific markers for PNP.[53,58]

Treatment

Treatment of patients who have PNP remains similar to the treatment of PV in addition to the treatment of the patient's malignancy. Resection of benign tumors in certain cases has been shown to improve clinical symptoms and decrease autoantibody titers.[53] Correlation between tumor burden and PNP activity, however, generally is lacking. In fact, treatment of malignant neoplasms is not commonly associated with improvement in clinical symptoms of PNP.[53] Lesions associated with PNP are persistent and resistant to therapy.[56] The mortality rate for PNP is 75% to 80%, compared with 10% for PV.[56] Despite traditional and modern advancements in chemotherapy, most patients who have PNP die from septicemia, pneumonia, respiratory failure, or the neoplasm itself.[52]

SUMMARY

The history, epidemiology, pathophysiology, clinical presentation, diagnostic work-up, histopathology, and treatment of PV and PNP have been presented. These life-threatening, autoimmune, mucocutaneous bullous conditions may be encountered first by oral health providers and, therefore, deserve keen understanding and attention by the oral and maxillofacial surgeon. Great diagnostic and management strides have been made, but morbidity and life quality issues remain a reality for these chronically ill patients.

REFERENCES

1. Huber O. Structure and function of desmosomal proteins and their role in development and disease. Cell Mol Life Sci 2003;60(9):1872–90.
2. Kowalczyk AP, Bornslaeger EA, Norvell SM, et al. Desmosomes: intercellular adhesive junctions specialized for attachment of intermediate filaments. Int Rev Cytol 1999;185:237–302.
3. Garrod DR, Merritt AJ, Nie Z. Desmosomal adhesion: structural basis, molecular mechanism, and regulation [review]. Mol Membr Biol 2002;19(2):81–94.
4. Chidgey M. Desmosomes and disease: an update. Histol Histopathol 2002;17(4):1179–92.
5. Pisanti S, Sharav Y, Kaufman E, et al. Pemphigus vulgaris: incidence in Jews of different ethnic groups, according to age, sex, and initial lesion. Oral Surg Oral Med Oral Pathol 1974;38(3):382–7.
6. Simon DG, Krutchkoff D, Kaslow RA, et al. Pemphigus in Hartford County, Connecticut, from 1972 to 1977. Arch Dermatol 1980;116(9):1035–7.
7. Ahmed AR. Clinical features of pemphigus. Clin Dermatol 1983;1(2):13–21.
8. Marx RE, Stern D. Oral and maxillofacial pathology: a rationale for diagnosis and treatment. Carol Stream (IL): Quintessence Publishing Co, Inc; 2003.
9. Tsunoda K, Ota T, Suzuki H, et al. Pathogenic autoantibody production requires loss of tolerance against desmoglein 3 in both T- and B-cells in experimental pemphigus vulgaris. Eur J Immunol 2002;32(3):627–33.
10. Amagai M, Tsunoda K, Suzuki H, et al. Use of autoantigen-knockout mice in developing an active autoimmune disease model for pemphigus. J Clin Invest 2000;105(5):625–31.
11. Brenner S, Bialy-Golan A, Ruocco V. Drug-induced pemphigus. Clin Dermatol 1998;16(3):393–7.
12. Ruocco V, Brenner S, Lombardi ML. A case of diet-related pemphigus. Dermatology 1996;192(4):373–4.
13. Brenner S, Tur E, Shapiro J, et al. Pemphigus vulgaris: environmental factors. Occupational, behavioral, medical, and qualitative food frequency questionnaire. [erratum appears in Int J Dermatol 2003 Sep;42(9):760 Note: Silva MR [corrected to Ramos-e-Silva M]]. Int J Dermatol 2001;40(9):562–9.
14. Amagai M, Tsunoda K, Zillikens D, et al. The clinical phenotype of pemphigus is defined by the antidesmoglein autoantibody profile. J Am Acad Dermatol 1999;40(2 Pt 1):167–70.
15. Harman KE, Seed PT, Gratian MJ, et al. The severity of cutaneous and oral pemphigus is related to desmoglein 1 and 3 antibody levels. [see comment]. Br J Dermatol 2001;144(4):775–80.
16. Sirois DA, Fatahzadeh M, Roth R, et al. Diagnostic patterns and delays in pemphigus vulgaris: experience with 99 patients. Arch Dermatol 2000;136(12):1569–70.
17. Salopek TG. Nikolsky's sign: is it dry or is it wet? Br J Dermatol 1997;136(5):762–7.
18. Ettlin DA. Pemphigus. Dent Clin North Am 2005;49(1):107–25.
19. Lever W. Pemphigus and pemphigoid. 1st edition. Springfield (IL): Charles C Thomas Publishers; 1965.
20. Williams LC, Nesbitt LT Jr. Update on systemic glucocorticosteroids in dermatology. Dermatol Clin 2001;19(1):63–77.
21. Rosenberg FR, Sanders S, Nelson CT. Pemphigus: a 20-year review of 107 patients treated with corticosteroids. Arch Dermatol 1976;112(7):962–70.
22. Bystryn JC, Steinman NM. The adjuvant therapy of pemphigus. An update. [see comment]. Arch Dermatol 1996;132(2):203–12.
23. Fellner MJ, Katz JM, McCabe JB. Successful use of cyclophosphamide and prednisone for initial treatment of pemphigus vulgaris. Arch Dermatol 1978;114(6):889–94.
24. Ahmed AR, Hombal S. Use of cyclophosphamide in azathioprine failures in pemphigus. J Am Acad Dermatol 1987;17(3):437–42.
25. Aberer W, Wolff-Schreiner EC, Stingl G, et al. Azathioprine in the treatment of pemphigus vulgaris. A long-term follow-up. J Am Acad Dermatol 1987;16(3 Pt 1):527–33.
26. Mazzi G, Raineri A, Zanolli FA, et al. Plasmapheresis therapy in pemphigus vulgaris and bullous pemphigoid. Transfus Apher Sci 2003;28(1):13–8.
27. Roujeau JC, Andre C, Joneau Fabre M, et al. Plasma exchange in pemphigus. Uncontrolled study of ten patients. Arch Dermatol 1983;119(3):215–21.
28. Blaszczyk M, Chorzelski TP, Jablonska S, et al. Indications for future studies on the treatment of pemphigus with plasmapheresis. Arch Dermatol 1989;125(6):843–4.
29. Hood KA, Zarembski DG. Mycophenolate mofetil: a unique immunosuppressive agent. Am J Health Syst Pharm 1997;54(3):285–94.
30. Stanley JR. Therapy of pemphigus vulgaris. Arch Dermatol 1999;135(1):76–8.

31. Enk AH, Knop J. Mycophenolate is effective in the treatment of pemphigus vulgaris. [see comment]. Arch Dermatol 1999;135(1):54–6.
32. Kazkaz H, Isenberg D. Anti B-cell therapy (rituximab) in the treatment of autoimmune diseases. Curr Opin Pharmacol 2004;4(4):398–402.
33. Stasi R, Stipa E, Forte V, et al. Variable patterns of response to rituximab treatment in adults with chronic idiopathic thrombocytopenic purpura. [comment]. Blood 2002;99(10):3872–3.
34. Narat S, Gandla J, Hoffbrand AV, et al. Rituximab in the treatment of refractory autoimmune cytopenias in adults. Haematologica 2005;90(9):1273–4.
35. Zaja F, De Vita S, Russo D, et al. Rituximab for the treatment of type II mixed cryoglobulinemia. Arthritis Rheum 2002;46(8):2252–4 [author reply 2254–5].
36. Specks U, Fervenza FC, McDonald TJ, et al. Response of Wegener's granulomatosis to anti-CD20 chimeric monoclonal antibody therapy. Arthritis Rheum 2001;44(12):2836–40.
37. Levine TD. Rituximab in the treatment of dermatomyositis: an open-label pilot study. Arthritis Rheum 2005;52(2):601–7.
38. Arzoo K, Sadeghi S, Liebman HA. Treatment of refractory antibody-mediated autoimmune disorders with an anti-CD20 monoclonal antibody (rituximab). [see comment]. Ann Rheum Dis 2002;61(10):922–4.
39. Joly P, Mouquet H, Roujeau J-C, et al. A single cycle of rituximab for the treatment of severe pemphigus. [see comment]. N Engl J Med 2007;357(6):545–52.
40. Haim S, Friedman-Birnbaum R. Dapsone in the treatment of pemphigus vulgaris. Dermatologica 1978;156(2):120–3.
41. Piamphongsant T. Pemphigus controlled by dapsone. Br J Dermatol 1976;94(6):681–6.
42. Penneys NS, Eaglstein WH, Frost P. Management of pemphigus with gold compounds: a long-term follow-up report. Arch Dermatol 1976;112(2):185–7.
43. Pandya AG, Dyke C. Treatment of pemphigus with gold. Arch Dermatol 1998;134(9):1104–7.
44. Colonna L, Cianchini G, Frezzolini A, et al. Intravenous immunoglobulins for pemphigus vulgaris: adjuvant or first-choice therapy? Br J Dermatol 1998;138(6):1102–3.
45. Sami N, Qureshi A, Ruocco E, et al. Corticosteroid-sparing effect of intravenous immunoglobulin therapy in patients with pemphigus vulgaris. Arch Dermatol 2002;138(9):1158–62.
46. Barthelemy H, Frappaz A, Cambazard F, et al. Treatment of nine cases of pemphigus vulgaris with cyclosporine. J Am Acad Dermatol 1988;18(6):1262–6.
47. Lapidoth M, David M, Ben-Amitai D, et al. The efficacy of combined treatment with prednisone and cyclosporine in patients with pemphigus: preliminary study. J Am Acad Dermatol 1994;30(5 Pt 1):752–7.
48. Liang G, Nahass G, Kerdel FA. Pemphigus vulgaris treated with photopheresis. J Am Acad Dermatol 1992;26(5 Pt 1):779–80.
49. Rook AH, Jegasothy BV, Heald P, et al. Extracorporeal photochemotherapy for drug-resistant pemphigus vulgaris. Ann Intern Med 1990;112(4):303–5.
50. Chaffins ML, Collison D, Fivenson DP. Treatment of pemphigus and linear IgA dermatosis with nicotinamide and tetracycline: a review of 13 cases. J Am Acad Dermatol 1993;28(6):998–1000.
51. Anhalt GJ, Kim SC, Stanley JR, et al. Paraneoplastic pemphigus. An autoimmune mucocutaneous disease associated with neoplasia. N Engl J Med 1990;323(25):1729–35.
52. Sklavounou A, Laskaris G. Paraneoplastic pemphigus: a review. Oral Oncol 1998;34(6):437–40.
53. Kimyai-Asadi A, Jih MH. Paraneoplastic pemphigus. Int J Dermatol 2001;40(6):367–72.
54. Nguyen VT, Ndoye A, Bassler KD, et al. Classification, clinical manifestations, and immunopathological mechanisms of the epithelial variant of paraneoplastic autoimmune multiorgan syndrome: a reappraisal of paraneoplastic pemphigus. Arch Dermatol 2001;137(2):193–206.
55. Nousari HC, Deterding R, Wojtczack H, et al. The mechanism of respiratory failure in paraneoplastic pemphigus. [see comment]. N Engl J Med 1999;340(18):1406–10.
56. Favia GF, Di Alberti L, Piattelli A. Paraneoplastic pemphigus: a report of two cases. Oral Oncol 1998;34(6):571–5.
57. Ostezan LB, Fabre VC, Caughman SW, et al. Paraneoplastic pemphigus in the absence of a known neoplasm. J Am Acad Dermatol 1995;33(2 Pt 1):312–5.
58. Joly P, Richard C, Gilbert D, et al. Sensitivity and specificity of clinical, histologic, and immunologic features in the diagnosis of paraneoplastic pemphigus. J Am Acad Dermatol 2000;43(4):619–26.

Systemic Lymphoproliferative Diseases

Aaron Liddell, DMD, Sidney L. Bourgeois, Jr., DDS*

KEYWORDS
- Lymphoma • Lymphoproliferative disorders • Neoplasms

As the practice of medicine becomes increasingly compartmentalized, oral and maxillofacial surgeons are finding themselves integral in what has become a multi-disciplinary approach to treating lymphoproliferative disorders. Roles vary from initial diagnosis and staging to treatment, maintenance, and surveillance. Nevertheless, the need to understand the myriad of disorders with head and neck sequelae is increasingly important in day-to-day practice. Among these illnesses lies the broad disease entity of lymphoma, which, in many instances manifests with head and neck abnormalities. This article focuses on lymphoma and subclasses that the oral and maxillofacial surgeon may encounter in practice. It elucidates a brief historical review of lymphoma, including a basic review of classification schemes. Additionally, it will give a general overview of the pathology, pathophysiology, and current treatment modalities with specific attention paid to the head and neck manifestations and complications.

BASIC PATHOPHYSIOLOGY

The intricate process of hematopoiesis has been described classically as cell growth originating from tissues of lymphoid or myeloid origins. This compartmentalization is generally theoretic, and there is significant interplay between lymphoid and myeloid tissues, both in normal physiology and pathophysiology. Any aberrancy in the maturation of cells from primordial, pluripotential stem cells along their specific pathways, to committed stem cells, and finally mature, differentiated cells may lead to malignant lymphoproliferation.[1–3] This abnormal lymphocytic differentiation may be of multiple etiologies. Frequently, inborn errors associated with genetic diseases contribute to genomic instability with a predilection toward abnormal lymphopoiesis, as frequently is seen with Trisomy 21 (childhood leukemia). Additionally, viruses increasingly are being implicated in the etiology of leukemia and lymphoma. Epstein Barr virus (EBV) is associated with Burkitt's lymphoma (BL) and HL and human T-cell lymphotropic virus 1 (HTLV-1), which is associated with T-cell leukemias. The role of these viruses in malignant cellular transformation seems to be amplified in the setting of immunodeficiency specifically involving suppression within the T-cell lineage (HIV/AIDS).[1–3]

Chromosomal translocations associated with oncogenes are associated most frequently with lymphoproliferative disorders. The dynamic nature of the human leukocyte antigen/major histocompatibility complex (HLA/MHC) makes leukocytes especially prone to genetic alterations during normal immunoglobulin and T-cell receptor selection. It is during these genetic rearrangements that aberrant splicing of immunoglobulin or T-cell antigen receptor (TCR) sequences adjacent to proto-oncogenes occurs, enabling activation and expression, or inhibition and suppression, of many cell cycle regulators, enabling uncontrolled lymphoproliferation.[1,3]

Finally, environmental factors that induce chronic inflammation have been associated with abnormal lymphopoiesis and ultimately malignancy. Long-term sequelae associated with chemotherapy and radiation therapy have been

---

Department of Oral and Maxillofacial Surgery, University of Texas Health Science Center, 7703 Floyd Curl Drive, San Antonio, TX 78229, USA
* Corresponding author.
E-mail address: bourgeois@uthscsa.edu (S.L. Bourgeois).

implicated in genomic instability and cellular transformation, with an endpoint of lymphoproliferative disease and hematologic malignancy.[1]

Hematologic malignancies often are compartmentalized within two large diagnostic entities, namely the leukemias and lymphomas. The distinction between leukemia (classically atypical bone marrow proliferation with peripheral blood involvement) and lymphoma (classically distinct neoplastic lymphoid tissue masses) is, in many instances, arbitrary, as both disease entities may present, or evolve, to include manifestations within the spectrum of their counterpart's disease processes. That being said, the terms generally are used to describe the global distribution of neoplastic cells as being either predominantly within the bone marrow and peripheral blood, or as single or multiple well-defined tissue masses.[2,3]

Lymphoma has been classified broadly into two distinct diagnostic entities, namely Hodgkin's lymphoma (HL) and non-Hodgkin's lymphomas (NHL). These two diagnostic entities are defined based on specific clinical, histologic, and immunophenotypic behaviors, and treatment modalities. There have been numerous classification systems used to describe lymphomas. This is frequently a point of confusion for practitioner and patient alike. Of the many classification schemes used, the World Health Organization's (WHO) classification of lymphoma is the most clear, up-to-date, and frequently cited in the literature. This WHO classification scheme defines individual disease entities based on phenotype, genotype, morphology, and clinical characteristics.[4–6]

MEDICAL EVALUATION

Medical evaluation of suspected lymphomas of all kinds begins with a thorough history and physical examination with particular attention to constitutional symptoms. Radiological evaluation includes plain film chest radiography and CT scans of head and neck (**Fig. 1**), chest, abdomen, and pelvis. Additional imaging modalities, including bone and positron emission tomography (PET) scans (**Fig. 2**), may be used as adjunctive diagnostic aids in the initial evaluation.[3,7–9] Hematologic studies including complete blood cell count (CBC) with differential, liver function tests, Chem 20, lactate dehydrogenase (LDH), and erythrocyte sedimentation rate are essential. Bone marrow biopsy is integral in initial staging of the disease and should be included in the preliminary work-up to determine the extent of disease. Any head and neck mucosal lesion should be biopsied with the specimens sent for histopathologic and immunohistochemical staining. If possible, specimens should be submitted for frozen-section examination, with additional tissue submitted for permanent histopathologic diagnosis, immunohistochemical, and flow cytometric studies. Neck masses may be biopsied directly or assessed cytologically with the aid of fine needle aspiration. If cervical lymph node biopsy is undertaken, the goal should be to acquire the node with an intact capsule. PET scanning has seen an emergence into many treatment algorithms, both in the assessment of response to therapy, and in prediction of relapse risk. It seems destined to become an integral tool in the work-up, assessment, and surveillance.[9]

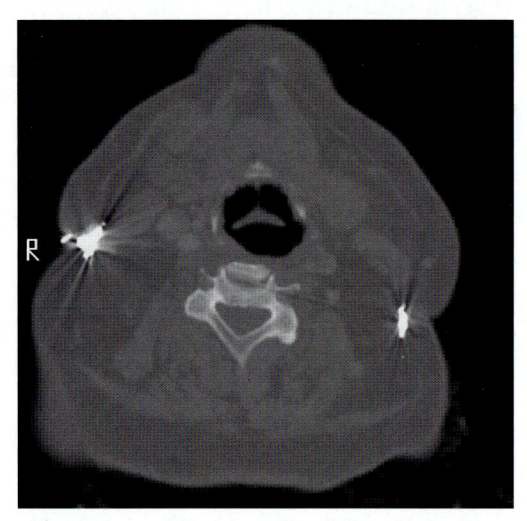

Fig. 1. CT scan—diffuse large B-cell lymphoma.

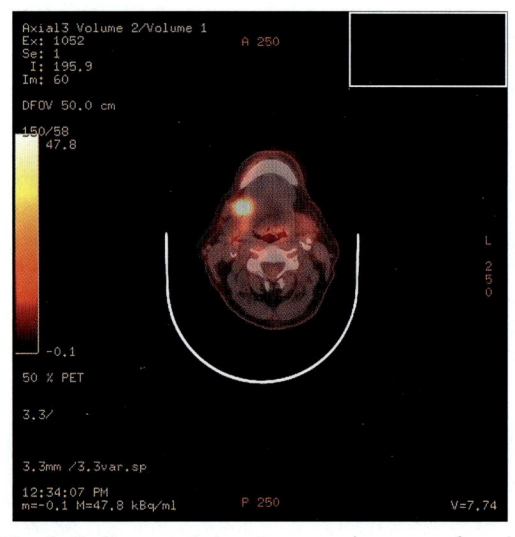

Fig. 2. Positron emission tomography scan of neck lesion.

HODGKIN'S LYMPHOMA

Hodgkin's lymphoma (HL) is named after British physician Thomas Hodgkin who first described the entity in 1832. Based on the WHO classification, HL can be divided into what are now two separate entities. The first is classic HL (CHL), which include in order of frequency nodular sclerosing (cNSHL, 60% to 80%), mixed cellularity (cMCHL, 15% to 30%), lymphocyte-rich (cLRHL, 6%), and lymphocyte-depleted (cLDHL, approximately 1%). and the other is a separate entity, nodular lymphocyte-predominant HL (NLPHL, 4% to 5%).[5] CHLs, with its variants, account for approximately 95% of Hodgkin's lymphomas, with the remaining 5% attributed to NLPHL.[2,3,7] HL classically has been described as having a bimodal distribution of incidence, with the first peek frequently seen in the 15- to 34-year-old age group, with an additional peak around the age of 65.[1–3,7,10] There are approximately 8000 cases diagnosed annually in the United States, of which there is a slight male predilection (1.4:1). The age-adjusted incidence in the United States is approximately 3 cases per 100,000 population.[11] Remarkably, with modern therapeutic intervention, the 5-year survival of patients with HL is approximately 80%.[12,13]

HL is a peculiar lymphoproliferative disorder in that Reed-Sternberg (RS) cells (**Fig. 3**), the pathognomonic neoplastic cell, classically constitute less than 5% of the total cell population within the tumor mass.[2,3] The bulk of the mass consists of a mixed stroma of inflammatory cells, including predominantly T lymphocytes (Tc), eosinophils, plasma cells, neutrophils, and histiocytes.[7,10] This reactive, inflammatory background is important from the standpoint of proper classification and staging, as it has been noted that there is a correlation between this reactive stroma and the cellular morphology of the neoplastic cells.

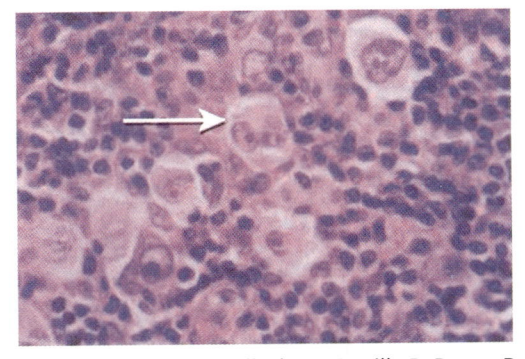

Fig. 3. Reed Sternberg cells. (*From* Neville B, Damm D, Allen C, et al. Hematologic disorders. In: Oral and maxillofacial pathology, 2nd edition. Philadelphia: W.B. Saunders; 2002. p. 517; with permission.)

Regardless of class or prevalence, however, the definitive diagnosis of HL depends upon identification of RS cells in a proper inflammatory background.[1]

Historically, there has been debate pertaining to the etiology of RS cells. Evidence now suggests that these cells are predominantly of B-cell (Bc) lineage, with less than 2% being derived from Tc.[1–3,5] RS cells are giant cells, frequently five to six times the size of normal lymphocytes (approximately 15 μm).[1,2] They are typically bi- or multinucleated, with prominent nucleoli, surrounded by a clear zone, giving them the characteristic appearance of owl eyes. There are multiple variants to the classic RS cell, which are defined morphologically. These include the Hodgkin's cell (mononuclear), lacunar cell (multilobed, copious cytoplasm), and lymphocytic and histiocytic (L&H) cells (multilobed, convoluted nuclei, also referred to as popcorn cells based on cytologic morphology). Quantitative presence of these cells within the various HLs has been shown to correlate with tumor aggressiveness.[1,2,7]

Although all HLs are defined histologically by the RS cell or its variants, there is immunophenotypic variation between the CHLs and NLPHL, leading to the WHO division of these two disease entities.[5,6] CHLs typically express CD15, CD30, and CD20 (approximately 25%), and are CD3 and CD45 negative. NLPHL, on the other hand, expresses CD45, in addition to CD19, CD20, CD22, and CD79A, but specifically lacks CD15 and CD30. In addition, in the inflammatory stroma, Bc predominates, in contrast to CHL, where Tc is the predominant lymphocyte.[4]

Presentation of HL may be either in the occult form, often initially thought to be of infectious etiology, or in the overt form, with numerous symptoms. The importance of a systematic, thorough head and neck examination cannot be overemphasized. The typical presentation of HL is a young adult with asymptomatic cervical or supraclavicular lymphadenopathy.[2,3,7] Less frequently, nodes of the axilla, mediastinum, abdomen, or pelvis initially are involved.[7] In addition to persistently enlarging nodal regions, there may be report of weight loss, night sweats, generalized pruritus, or fatigue. Fevers may be cyclical, in the classic Pel-Ebstein pattern (high fever for 1 to 2 weeks with defervescent period of 1 to 2 weeks), or not present at all.[14] Pain is not associated with HL frequently, although in as many as 10% of patients, pain in the region of the lymphoma can be elicited by even scant alcohol consumption.[8]

Oral involvement has been described in HL but is infrequent. When present, lesions of the oral cavity often represent undiagnosed primary sites, or may indicate worsening of systemic disease, as opposed to isolated primary lesions, which are cited infrequently in the literature.[10,15–19] Although lesions may present in any region of the oral cavity, they most frequently involve the maxillary or mandibular buccal vestibule or alveolar ridge.[16–18] Isolated involvement of the dorsal tongue and bony involvement of both the maxilla and mandible also have been described.[10,15,19,20] Oral lesions are minimally tender to palpation, often indurated, discrete masses with raised, rolled margins and central ulceration with or without necrotic debris.[10,16–19] Other findings may include pathologic fracture, regional anesthesia, failure of extraction sockets to heal, or tooth mobility.[17] These lesions may be accompanied by underlying bony involvement and lymphadenopathy.[16,20] When lymphadenopathy is present, clinical examination findings will vary, based on extent of disease. Although initially mobile, with progression, lymph nodes become matted and fixed to surrounding soft tissues, and, if untreated, atypical lymphocytes frequently spread to involve the spleen or extralymphatic tissues.[7]

From the standpoint of prognosis and treatment, staging is paramount, in terms of directing therapy toward the least toxic, most efficacious treatment. Staging historically followed the four-stage system established at the Ann Arbor conference of 1974.[21,22] In 1988, however, the Cotswold's Staging Classification revised the Ann Arbor System, and it frequently is used today to predict prognosis and drive therapy.[7,8] This system uses four stages with subclasses within Stage 3 (**Box 1**).[7,8,21]

Recently, joint efforts have contributed to a prognostic index (International Prognostic Index) based on seven factors: serum albumin, gender, Hgb, age, stage (Ann Arbor), peripheral leukocytosis, and presence of lymphocytopenia.[23–25] For most early stages (2/2), combination therapy, including field radiation and chemotherapy, generally has replaced mantle field radiation as a single treatment modality. The radiation field involves the nodes of the neck, axilla, and lungs, and is between 40 and 45 Gy for cervical HL lesions. The mandibular architecture below the lingula also is included.[2,12] Historically, MOPP (mechlorethamine, vincristine, procarbazine, prednisone) was used as a multidrug, chemotherapeutic approach given over 6 to 12 months; however, long-term adverse effects (leukemia/myelodysplasia, sterility) have made this regimen unfavorable in many instances.[12,26] Currently, ABVD (doxorubicin, bleomycin, vinblastine, dacarbazine), which has a smaller adverse effect profile, is the chemotherapy regimen being used. ABVD, in combination with radiation therapy, has been shown to be superior to alternating MOPP/ABVD pulses or MOPP alone.[12,13,26] More advanced stage disease (3/4) generally is treated with multidrug chemotherapy alone, which typically consists of ABVD for 6 to 8 months.[27]

Patients who have early stage disease and a favorable response to early treatment have as high as a 90% 10-year survival rate, while patients who have stage 3/4 disease have a 55% to 75% 10-year survival rate.[12,13] Unfortunately, for those patients who have an unfavorable response to early treatment modalities, the prognosis is poor. Modern research increasingly shows that stem cell transplantation salvage treatment has the best prognosis, yielding event-free survival rates as high as 56%, superior to salvage chemotherapy, which has only a 10% to 37% survival rate.[26] With continued development, PET scans will be a great adjuvant in assessing treatment response and surveillance of both early and advanced disease.[28]

Box 1
Cotswold's staging system

Stage 1—involvement of a single lymph node region (or lymphoid structure [ie, thymus, spleen, or Waldeyer's ring)

Stage 2—involvement of more than 2 lymph node regions on the same side of the diaphragm (the mediastinum is a single site, hilar lymph nodes lateralized; the number of anatomic sites is indicated by subscript)

Stage 3—involvement of lymph node structures on both sides of the diaphragm

Stage 3_1—with or without splenic, hilar, celiac, or portal nodes (upper abdomen)

Stage 3_2—with para-aortic, iliac, mesenteric nodes (lower abdomen)

Stage 4—involvement of extranodal site(s) beyond that designated E

* Individual stages are augmented by modifying features designated A, B, X, or E. A indicates a paucity of systemic symptoms. B indicates constitutional symptoms such as fever, night sweats, and unexplained weight loss of at least 10% total body weight. X is used to indicate bulky disease, including greater than one third widening of the mediastinum or greater than 10 cm diameter nodal mass. E represents involvement of a single, contiguous extranodal site.

Adapted from Warburton G, Childs RC, Charles M, et al. Hodgkin's lymphoma: a case report involving the mandible. J Oral Maxillofac Surg 2003;61(12): 1492–6; with permission.

NON-HODGKIN'S LYMPHOMA

NHL consists of a wide, complex, spectrum of disorders of lymphoreticular histogenesis.[1,2] NHL can be separated into Bc lymphomas (**Figs. 4 and 5**) or Tc lymphomas.[4,5] There is significantly more diversity among NHLs when compared with HL. NHLs frequently have worse prognoses as compared with HLs.[2] Greater than 60,000 cases of NHL are diagnosed annually in the United States alone, constituting approximately 3% of all newly diagnosed malignancies. There is a slight predilection toward males without a true racial predilection before the age of 50. After 50 years of age, Caucasians have a slightly higher incidence. Unlike the bimodal distribution of HL, the incidence of NHL progressively increases with age, with the median age of onset being 55.[11] Although more frequently seen in adults, NHL is not uncommon in children. NHL represents the third most common cancer in children.[29] As previously mentioned, there appears to be an increased incidence of NHL in the setting of immunosuppression and autoimmune diseases.[3,30–32] Viruses (EBV) increasingly are associated with many of the NHLs.[33]

Numerous classification schemes have been used over time to define individual disease entities. The earliest classification scheme was based on tumor morphology (Rappaport), differentiating follicular versus diffuse growth patterns.[34] With the development of immunophenotypic testing assays, the Lukes-Collins classification was created, which used immunologic markers (Bc/Tc) to differentiate specific disease entities.[35] With increasing disparity and confusion among various classification protocols, the "Working Formulation for Clinical Use" was created, which grouped lymphomas into low-, intermediate-, and high-grade categories, at the same time using differentiation and tumor morphology from other classification systems.[36] When immunohistochemical markers became critical to the diagnosis of NHL, the Revised European American Classification of Lymphoid Neoplasms (REAL) was developed. The REAL Classification System was revised by the REAL/WHO Classification System (**Box 2**), which is used most frequently today.[4,5] With the development of novel diagnostic testing assays and recognition of new NHL subclasses, the REAL/WHO classification system is dynamic, with frequent modifications and revisions.

Not unlike HL, most NHL pathogenesis lies within the lymph node, with proliferation forming masses consisting of abnormal lymphocytes (**Fig. 6**). Of the NHLs, it is estimated that upwards of 85% of American and European diagnoses are of Bc lineage, the remaining being of histiocyte or Tc derivation.[3] Within tumor masses, there are varying levels of cellular differentiation, which is used to designate tumor grade. Low-grade tumors consist of well-differentiated, small lymphocytes, and high-grade tumors consist of poorly differentiated cells.[2] Lymphomas may have either follicular growth patterns (representing germinal center architecture), or they may be diffuse with no germinal center semblance, the former being more common when abnormal cells are of Bc lineage. There is frequently effacement and destruction of lymph node architecture when located anatomically within the lymph node chain.[1] When extralymphatic NHL exists, the malignant cells tend to invade adjacent soft tissues with extensive infiltration. Regardless of growth pattern, NHLs tend to grow in broad, infiltrative sheets with uniform cytologic architecture.[2]

Of the numerous NHLs that have been classified, there are varieties with higher prevalence in the general population and more frequent oro–facial manifestations. These include diffuse large B-cell lymphoma (30% to 40% of all NHLs), small (peripheral) B-cell lymphomas (low-grade), mucosa-associated lymphatic tissue (MALT) lymphoma, follicular lymphoma, mantle cell lymphoma,[11] BL, and nasal T/NK-cell lymphoma.[2,3]

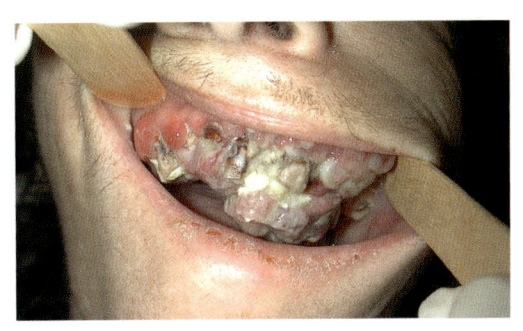

Fig. 5. Diffuse large B-cell lymphoma of the maxilla.

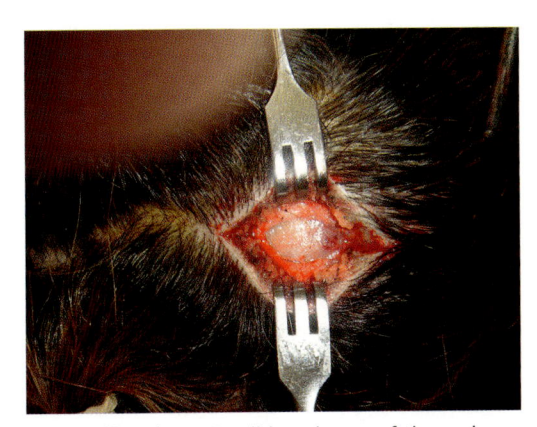

Fig. 4. Diffuse large B-cell lymphoma of the scalp.

> **Box 2**
> **Revised European American Lymphoma/World Health Organization Classification**
>
> Precursor B-cell neoplasm
>   Precursor B-lymphoblastic leukemia/lymphoma
>   Precursor B-cell acute lymphoblastic leukemia
>
> Mature (peripheral) B-cell neoplasm
>   B-cell chronic lymphocytic leukemia/small lymphocytic lymphoma
>   B-cell prolymphocytic leukemia
>   Lymphoplasmacytic lymphoma
>   Splenic marginal zone B-cell lymphoma (plus or minus villous lymphocytes)
>   Hairy cell leukemia
>   Plasma cell myeloma/plasmacytoma
>   Extranodal marginal zone B-cell lymphoma of mucosa-associated lymphoid tissue type
>   Nodal marginal zone lymphoma (plus or minus monocytoid B-cells)
>   Follicular lymphoma
>   Mantle cell lymphoma
>   Diffuse large cell B-cell lymphoma
>   Mediastinal large B-cell lymphoma
>   Primary effusion lymphoma
>   BL/Burkitt's cell leukemia
>
> T-cell and natural killer cell neoplasms
>   Precursor T-cell Neoplasm
>   Precursor T-lymphoblastic lymphoma/leukemia
>   Precursor T-cell acute lymphoblastic leukemia
>
> Mature (peripheral) T-cell and NK-cell neoplasms
>   T-cell prolymphocytic leukemia
>   T-cell granular lymphocytic leukemia
>   Aggressive NK-cell leukemia
>   Adult T-cell lymphoma/leukemia (HTLV 1+)
>   Extranodal NK/T-cell lymphoma, nasal type
>   Enteropathy-type T-cell lymphoma
>   Hepatosplenic gamma-delta T-cell lymphoma
>   Subcutaneous panniculitis-like T-cell lymphoma
>   Mycosis fungoides/Sezary syndrome
>   Anaplastic large cell lymphoma, T/null-cell, primary cutaneous type
>   Peripheral T-cell lymphoma, not otherwise characterized
>   Angioimmunoblastic T-cell lymphoma
>   Anaplastic large cell lymphoma, T/null-cell, primary systemic type
>
> Hodgkin's lymphoma
>   Nodular lymphocyte predominant HL
>   Classical HL
>   Nodular sclerosis HL
>   Lymphocyte-rich classical HL
>   Mixed cellularity HL
>   Lymphocyte depletion HL

The clinical presentation of NHLs can be broad and multifocal. They may represent widespread systemic involvement or a solitary, primary lesion. Initial presentation is usually nodal; however up to 24% of NHL presents with extranodal manifestations. Patients classically present with a slowly enlarging, nontender mass, frequently involving the cervical, thoracic, axillary, or inguinal nodes.[37] As with HL, nodes are freely mobile initially; however with disease progression, lesions infiltrate the surrounding tissues, leading to matted, fixed nodes.[2]

Oro–facial manifestations may include unexplained tooth mobility, odontalgia, cranial nerve paresthesias, gingival swelling, bony expansion of the maxilla or mandible, mucosal swelling, and mucosal ulceration.[38,39] Intraoral lesions are described as having a boggy consistency with overlying erythema, which may be accompanied by overlying or peri-lesional telangiectasia.[40] Radiographic signs of osseous involvement may vary from extensive, ill-defined ragged changes that mimic chronic osteomyelitis to no changes at all. Untreated intraosseous lesions almost always undergo expansile changes with subsequent

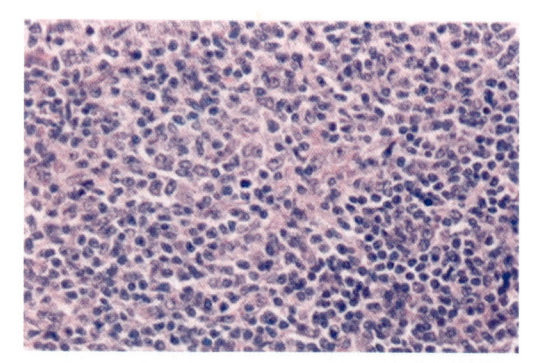

Fig. 6. Non-Hodgkin's lymphoma. (*From* Neville B, Damm D, Allen C, et al. Hematologic disorders. In: Oral and maxillofacial pathology, 2nd edition. Philadelphia: W.B. Saunders; 2002. p. 521; with permission.)

cortical perforation and invasion of the adjacent soft tissues.[2]

Treatment of NHL, like HL, typically involves chemotherapy, radiation therapy, or a combination of both.[37] In the assessment of NHL, the international prognostic index becomes critical in tailoring treatment to each individual patient. For decades, the treatment of NHL has involved use of CHOP (cyclophosphamide, doxorubicin, vincristine, and prednisone) at various intervals and various dosing intensities.[41] Research is ongoing for more efficacious, less toxic options. At present, Rituximab (a chimeric anti-CD20 IgG1 monoclonal antibody) in addition to ACVBP (doxorubicin, cyclophosphamide, vindesine, bleomycin, and prednisone) at varying intensities and with different treatment intervals is being used. The combination of Rituximab and ACVBP is yielding better results than standard CHOP therapy.[42,43] Radiotherapy is tailored to the individual based on stage and disease bulk. The efficacy of autologous stem cell transplantation both in patients with relapse and at initial diagnosis has yielded favorable results and likely will play a larger role in NHL treatment in the future.[41]

BURKITT'S LYMPHOMA

BL is of particular interest because of the frequency of head and neck manifestations that may present at any stage during the disease process. BL is a high-grade, rapidly proliferating NHL with aggressive tendencies and an astonishing doubling time of 24 hours. BL has been described as consisting of three subclasses, namely endemic (African), sporadic (United States), and HIV-associated, which may declare with vastly different initial and long-term presentations.[44] Endemic BL (eBL) is traditionally a malignancy of African children, with the mean age of onset between 4 and 7 years.[45] There is a predilection toward development of tumors of the jaws (maxilla more than mandible), although this association is age-dependent, with an inverse relationship between jaw tumors and age.[2] Sporadic BL (sBL) tends to present in a slightly older population when compared with the endemic form, with a mean age of onset of approximately 11 years.[46] Initial complaints are predominantly abdominal—abdominal pain, nausea, constipation and vomiting.[47] There are less frequent maxillofacial manifestations, although Waldeyer's ring may be involved.[46] HIV-associated BL (hBL) classically presents in young adults and frequently includes involvement of the bone marrow and lymphatic chains. Presentation of BL varies based on the type and location. Complaints may include abdominal pain, nausea, constipation and vomiting, weight loss, fevers, and general malaise. Oro–facial complaints may include atypical, severe odontalgia, tooth mobility, bony expansion, soft tissue masses, or unexplained craniofacial neuropathy.[48,49]

Etiology of BL classically has been described as being associated with the genetic translocation t(8:14), which approximates the c-myc oncogene of chromosome 8 next to either a variable heavy or light chain immunoglobulin sequence (there are other translocations, always involving the 8 chromosome).[45] This translocation activates c-myc and ensuing cell cycle abnormalities leading to abnormal lymphoproliferation.[1] EBV infection has been found to be intimately associated with BL: sBL 15% to 30% EBV+, eBL nearly 100% EBV+, hBL up to 60% EBV+.[45]

Histologically, BL presents with uniform sheets of lymphocytes (Bc) with basophilic manifestations of high mitotic activity.[2,45,46] There is frequent, marked apoptosis present, secondary to outgrowth of perfusion capabilities relative to the doubling time of this neoplasm. Because of the apoptotic potential, there is typically an influx of reactive macrophages that ingest the cellular debris of apoptosis. These macrophages tend to have less stain uptake, and therefore create the classic starry sky appearance histologically (Fig. 7) as they are distributed in this generally basophilic sea of lymphocytes.[45]

Treatment of BL varies based on specific disease type, with eBL displaying marked sensitivity to chemotherapy, while sBL and hBL are less sensitive and have traditionally worse prognoses.[44] Generally, limited-duration, high-intensity

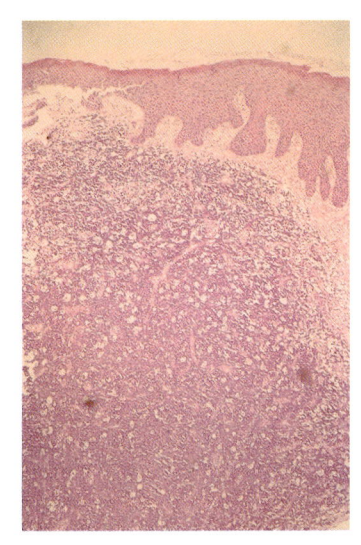

Fig. 7. Burkitt's lymphoma.

chemotherapy with or without CNS prophylaxis has produced excellent survival in the pediatric population, with 5-year survival as high as 90% with localized disease.[50] Adults tend to have less favorable prognoses, with overall survival rates between 50% and 70%. The CODOX-M/IVAC (alternating cycles of cyclophosphamide, vincristine, doxorubicin, methotrexate/ifosfamide, etoposide, high-dose cytarabine) protocol, Rituximab, and hyper-CVAD (hyperfractionated cyclophosphamide, vincristine, doxorubicin, dexamethasone) with intrathecal prophylaxis have yielded encouraging long-term survival with improving adverse effect profiles.[44,51,52]

NASAL T/NK-CELL LYMPHOMA (ANGIOCENTRIC LYMPHOMA)

Known by many different names (midline lethal granuloma syndrome, midline malignant reticulosis, idiopathic midline destructive disease), nasal T/NK-cell lymphoma is not encountered frequently, but which has impressive in oro/nasopharyngeal manifestations. It now is understood that this entity is usually a malignancy of the sino-nasal tract, usually of T, or NK cell lineage.[53,54] These lymphomas are rare in Western populations, with a predilection for Asian and South American populations.[3,53] Lesions tend to involve Waldeyer's ring, sino–nasal soft and hard tissues.[55] There is a strong association with EBV, with nearly 100% of nasal T/NK- cell lymphomas testing positive for EBV using in situ hybridization (EBER ½).[54,56] Classically, this lesion presents in the Asian male as a persistent ulcerative or necrotic lesion in the naso/oropharyngeal mucosa.[53] Palatal swelling with accompanying orbital edema is frequently present.[54] When clinical suspicion suggests lymphoma, tissue samples should be taken and submitted for inmunohistochemical studies (ideally unfixed, fresh tissue), and complete medical evaluation as previously described is undertaken.[53] Histologically, these lesions are characterized by atypical cellular polymorphism surrounding frank ulceration and often extensive necrosis. There is a predilection toward angio-invasion with perivascular infiltrate, although this is not necessarily diagnostic, and may not be present in as many as 40% to 50% of cases.[54] When the lesion is localized to the nasopharynx/oral cavity, treatment is usually local radiation involving all tumor sites and any immediately contiguous regions. With more disseminated disease, combination therapy is employed, which includes multidrug chemotherapy, CHOP, and ACVBP, in addition to preliminary success with purine and pyrimidine analogs, gemcitabine, pentostatin, and field radiation therapy of varying intensities based on tumor characteristics.[53,57]

The prognosis of nasal T/NK-cell lymphoma has been poor, with a 5-year disease-free survival of approximately 25%.[58] Despite therapy, relapse remains frequent, and many of these lymphomas are chemotherapy-resistant. Expression of p53 tumor suppressor protein often is seen in poorly responsive cases and heralds a poor prognosis.[53]

EXTRANODAL MARGINAL ZONE B-CELL /MUCOSA-ASSOCIATED LYMPHATIC TISSUE LYMPHOMA

MALT first was described as a distinct entity in 1994 in the REAL classification, and subsequently included in the WHO classification of lymphoma, extranodal marginal zone Bc lymphoma. MALT lymphoma displays frequent head and neck manifestations.[4–6,58–65] This subtype of lymphoma is by no means rare, accounting for approximately 7% to 8% of all NHLs.[59] MALT is most common in the gastrointestinal (GI) tract, but also is seen frequently in the head and neck region, including salivary glands, ocular adnexae, and thyroid.[59,60] The lesions are composed of mature B-cells, which are CD5- and CD10-negative.[61] There are two types of MALTs that have been described. The native type frequently is found in the GI tract (Peyer's patches), whereas the acquired type can be found in sites of chronic inflammation from various stimuli, including autoimmune (Sjogren's syndrome, Hashimoto's thyroiditis) and infectious (*Helicobacter pylori*, hepatitis C virus) disorders.[61–63] In the presence of chronic lymphoreactive proliferation, pathologic clones may develop and progressively replace normal lymphocytes, leading to MALT lymphoma.[61,62]

This disease entity is particularly common Sjogren's syndrome, or in the context of myoepithelial sialadinitis (MESA). It is the most common lymphoma of the salivary gland.[54,61–64] The maxillary sinus, hard palate, and nasal cavity also may be involved.[65] MALT lymphomas present in the head and neck region as extranodal infiltrates that occupy the salivary glands (particularly parotid).[2,59–65] This infiltration results in nonpainful, nonulcerated enlargement of the oral soft tissues.[2]

Staging is accomplished using the Ann Arbor Staging System. Most patients who have nongastric lymphoma present with advanced stage disease (Ann Arbor 3/4). Because of the indolent nature of the disease, however, prognosis remains good.[60–62] The International Prognostic Index has been used in terms of outcome prediction and prognosis and in guiding treatment algorithms.[23,61] There are no set algorithms for treating

MALT lymphoma; consequently, treatment usually is tailored to individuals based on location and extent of lesion. Treatment consists of chemotherapy, radiation therapy, surgical excision, or any combination of these modalities.[2,60,66] This treatment consists of chemotherapy, multicycle CHOP or CNOP (cyclophosphamide, mitoxantrone, vincristine, prednisolone), radiation therapy, surgical excision, or any combination of these modalities.[2,60,66,67] The addition of Rituximab to existing chemotherapy protocols also has shown early promising results.[58,67]

COMPLICATIONS OF TREATMENT

Complications of treatment of lymphomas may include pan-cytopenia; isolated neutropenia; infection with or reactivation of varicella, herpes simplex, hepatitis B and C, cytomegalovirus, and candidiasis; mucositis; and osteoradionecrosis. Rituxamab-related complications are listed in **Box 3**.

Box 3
Rituxamab-related complications

Hypoxia
Pulmonary infiltrates
Adult respiratory distress syndrome
Myocardial infarction
Ventricular fibrillation
Cardiogenic shock
Acute renal failure associated with tumor lysis syndrome
Fatal mucositis
Progressive multifocal leukoencephalopathy
Nausea
Pruritus
Angioedema
Asthenia
Hypotension
Headache
Bronchospasm
Rhinitis
Urticaria
Vomiting
Myalgia
Dizziness,
Hypertension

A review of current literature reveals that fully or partially absorbed antifungals (clotrimazole, fluconazole, ketoconazole) may be more efficacious than topical agents (nystatin) from the standpoint of preventing and treating candidiasis.[68] Development of mucositis is common in the context of chemotherapy and radiation therapy. Signs and symptoms include dysphagia, odynophagia, and severe oral pain, which may be accompanied by increased salivary outflow. With all of the data currently available, there is no consensus on the management or prevention of chemo/radiation-induced mucositis. Drugs such as amifositine, benzydamine, and calcium phosphate, and more holistic approaches using ice-chips, honey, and Chinese medicine have shown efficacy and potential to minimize the severity of mucositis.[69] Anecdotal recommendations include systemic antibiotics or topical analgesics. Ultimately, a tincture of time is the best remedy, as these lesions generally will resolve with discontinuation of chemotherapy or radiation therapy. Radiation therapy also can lead to osteoradionecrosis (ORN). The treatment of ORN is controversial and beyond the scope of this issue.

SUMMARY

With advancements in diagnosis and treatment for lymphoma, it is important that physicians be up to date in the management of these lymphoproliferative disorders, their associated complications, and the complications of treatment. The importance of a thorough examination of the oro–facial complex and neck on all patients cannot be overemphasized. Oral and maxillofacial surgeons continue to make significant contributions in what has become a multidisciplinary approach to managing lymphoproliferative disease.

REFERENCES

1. Aster JC. Diseases of white blood cells, lymph nodes, spleen and thymus. In: Kumar V, Abbas A, Fausto N, editors. Robbins and cotran: pathologic basis of disease. 7th Edition. Philadelphia: Elsevier; 2005. p. 661–709.
2. Marx R, Stern D. Neoplasms of the immune system: lymphomas, leukemias, and langerhans cell histiocytosis. In: Marx R, Stern D, editors. Oral and maxillofacial pathology: a rationale for diagnosis and treatment. Chicago: Quintessence; 2003. p. 829–75.
3. Neville B, Damm D, Allen C, et al. Hematologic disorders. In: Oral and maxillofacial pathology. 2nd edition. Philadelphia: W.B Saunders; 2002. p. 497–531.
4. Harris NL, Jaffe ES, Stein H, et al. A revised European-American classification of lymphoid

neoplasms: a proposal from the international lymphoma study group. Blood 1994;84(5):1361–92.
5. Jaffe ES, Harris NL, Stein H, et al. World Health Organization classification of tumors of hematopoietic and lymphoid tissues. Lyon, France: IARC Press; 2001.
6. Cogliatti SB, Schmid U. Who is WHO and what was REAL? Swiss Med Wkly 2002;132(43–44):607–17.
7. Warburton G, Childs RC, Charles M, et al. Hodgkin's lymphoma: a case report involving the mandible. J Oral Maxillofac Surg 2003;61(12):1492–6.
8. Lister TA, Crowther D, Sutcliffe SB, et al. Report of a committee convened to discuss the evaluation and staging of patients with Hodgkin's disease: Cotswolds meeting. J Clin Oncol 1989;7(11):1630–6.
9. Haioun C, Itti E, Rahmouni A, et al. [18F]Fluoro-2-deoxy-D-glucose positron emission tomography (FDG-PET) in aggressive lymphoma: an early prognostic tool for predicting patient outcome. Blood 2005;106(4):1376–81.
10. Cohen MA, Bender S, Struthers PJ. Hodgkin's disease of the jaws: review of the literature and report of a case. Oral Surg Oral Med Oral Pathol 1984; 57(4):413–7.
11. Hodgkin's and non-Hodgkin's lymphoma. Available at: www.seer.cancer.gov. Accessed February 19, 2008.
12. Engert A, Franklin J, Eich HT, et al. Two cycles of doxorubicin, bleomycin, vinblastine, and dacarbazine plus extended-field radiotherapy is superior to radiotherapy alone in early favorable Hodgkin's lymphoma: final results of the GHSG HD7 trial. J Clin Oncol 2007;25(23):3495–502.
13. Rueda Dominguez A, Marquez A, Guma J, et al. Treatment of stage I and II Hodgkin's lymphoma with ABVD chemotherapy: results after 7 years of a prospective study. Ann Oncol 2004;15(12):1798–804.
14. Good GR, DiNubile MJ. Images in clinical medicine: cyclic fever in Hodgkin's disease (Pel-Ebstein fever). N Engl J Med 1995;332(7):436.
15. Ishimaru T, Hayatsu Y, Ueyama Y, et al. Hodgkin's lymphoma of the mandibular condyle: report of a case. J Oral Maxillofac Surg 2005;63(1):144–7.
16. Mathews FR, Appleton SS, Wear DJ. Intraoral Hodgkin's disease. J Oral Maxillofac Surg 1989;47(5): 502–4.
17. Bathard-Smith PJ, Coonar HS, Markus AF. Hodgkin's disease presenting intraorally. Br J Oral Surg 1978; 16(1):64–9.
18. Peters RA, Beltaos E, Greenlaw RG, et al. Intraoral extranodal Hodgkin's disease. J Oral Surg 1977; 35(4):311–2.
19. Kinnman J, Shin HI, Wetteland P. Hodgkin's disease of the tongue: report of a case in a Korean male. Laryngoscope 1969;79(3):446–57.
20. Jamshed A, Allard WF, Mourad WA, et al. Primary Hodgkin's disease of the mandible: a case report and review of the literature. Oral Surg Oral Med Oral Pathol Oral Radiol Endod 1997;83(6):680–4.
21. Carbone PP, Kaplan HS, Musshoff K, et al. Report of the committee on Hodgkin's disease staging classification. Cancer Res 1971;31(11):1860–1.
22. Rosenberg SA, Boiron M, DeVita V, et al. Report of the committee on Hodgkin's disease staging procedures. Canc Res 1971;31(11):1862–3.
23. Hasenclever D, Diehl V. A prognostic score for advanced Hodgkin's disease. N Engl J Med 1998; 339(21):1506–14.
24. Sehn LH. Optimal use of prognostic factors in non-Hodgkin lymphoma. Hematology Am soc Hematol Educ Program 2006;1:295–302.
25. Armitage JO. Staging non-Hodgkin lymphoma. CA Cancer J Clin 2005;55(6):368–76.
26. Byrne BJ, Gockerman JP. Salvage therapy in Hodgkin's lymphoma. Oncologist 2007;12(2):156–67.
27. Canellos GP, Anderson JR, Propert KJ, et al. Chemotherapy of advanced Hodgkin's disease with MOPP, ABVD, or MOPP alternating with ABVD. N Engl J Med 1992;327(21):1478–84.
28. Gallamini A, Rigacci L, Merli F, et al. The predictive value of positron emission tomography scanning performed after two courses of standard therapy on treatment outcome in advanced stage Hodgkin's disease. Haematologica 2006;91(4):475–81.
29. Percy CL, Smith MA, Linet M, et al. Lymphomas and reticuloendothelial neoplasms. SEER Program. In: Ries LA, Smith MA, Gurney JG, et al, editors. Cancer incidence and survival among children and adolescents: United States SEER program 1975–1995. Bethesda: National Cancer Institute; 1999. p. 35–50. NIH Pub. No. 99-4649.
30. Mandel L, Surattanont F, Dourmas M. T-cell lymphoma in the parotid region after cardiac transplant: case report. J Oral Maxillofac Surg 2001;59(6): 673–7.
31. Ugboko VI, Oginni FO, Adelusola KA, et al. Orofacial non-Hodgkin's lymphoma in Nigerians. J Oral Maxillofac Surg 2004;62(11):1347–50.
32. Zintzaras E, Voulgarelis M, Moutsopoulos HM. The risk of lymphoma development in autoimmune diseases: a meta-analysis. Arch Intern Med 2005; 165(20):2337–44.
33. Rezk SA, Weiss LM. Epstein-Barr virus-associated lymphoproliferative disorders. Hum Pathol 2007; 38(9):1293–304.
34. Hicks EB, Rappaport H, Winter WJ. Follicular lymphoma: a re-evaluation of its position in the scheme of malignant lymphoma based on a survey of 253 cases. Cancer 1956;9(4):792–821.
35. Lukes RJ, Collins RD. Immunologic characterization of human malignant lymphomas. Cancer 1974; 34(4Supp):1488–503.
36. National Cancer Institute-sponsored study of classifications of non-Hodgkin's lymphomas: summary and

37. Pazoki A, Jansisyanont P, Ord RA. Primary non-Hodgkin's lymphoma of the jaws: report of 4 cases and review of the literature. J Oral Maxillofac Surg 2003;61(1):112–7.
38. Eisenbud L, Scuibba J, Babia M, et al. Oral presentations in non-Hodgkin's lymphoma: a review of thirty-one cases. Part II: fourteen cases arising in bone. Oral Surg Oral Med Oral Pathol 1984;57(3):272–80.
39. Gusenbauer AW, Katsikeris NF, Brown A. Primary lymphoma of the mandible: report of a case. J Oral Maxillofsac Surg 1990;48(4):409–15.
40. Eisenbud L, Scuibba J, Babia M, et al. Oral presentations in non-Hodgkin's lymphoma. Part I: data analysis. Oral Surg Oral Med Oral Pathol 1983;56(2):151–6.
41. Gisselbrecht C, Mounier N. Managing large cell lymphoma. iv. Ann Oncol 2006;17(Suppl 4):8–11.
42. Mounier N, Briere J, Gisselbrecht C, et al. Rituximab plus CHOP (R-CHOP) in the treatment of elderly patients with diffuse large B-cell lymphoma (DLBCL) overcomes BCL-2 chemotherapy resistance. Blood 2003;101(11):4279–84.
43. Reyes F, Lepage E, Ganem G, et al. ACVPB versus CHOP plus radiotherapy for localized aggressive lymphoma. N Engl J Med 2005;352(12):1197–205.
44. Ferry JA. Burkitt's lymphoma: clinicopathologic features and differential diagnosis. Oncologist 2006;11(4):375–83.
45. Jaffe E, Harris N, Stein H, et al. Pathology and genetics of tumors of hematopoietic and lymphoid tissues. Washington, DC: IARC Press; 2001. p. 181–4.
46. Landesberg R, Yee H, Datikashvili M, et al. Unilateral mandibular lip anesthesia as the sole presenting symptom of Burkitt's lymphoma: case report and review of literature. J Oral Maxillofac Surg 2001;59(3):322–6.
47. Gupta H, Davidoff AM, Pui CH, et al. Clinical implications and surgical management of intussusception in pediatric patients with Burkitt lymphoma. J Pediatr Surg 2007;42(6):998–1001.
48. Nissenbaum M, Kaban LB, Troulis MJ. Toothache, paresthesia, and Horner syndrome: an unusual presentation of disseminated Burkitt's lymphoma. J Oral Maxillofac Surg 2007;65(7):1395–401.
49. Durmus E, Oz G, Guler N, et al. Intraosseous mandibular lesion. J Oral Maxillofac Surg 2003;61(2):246–9.
50. Cairo MS, Sposto R, Perkins SL, et al. Burkitt's and Burkitt-like lymphoma in children and adolescents: a review of the children's cancer group experience. Br J Haematol 2003;120(4):660–70.
51. Thomas DA, Faderl S, O'Brien S, et al. Chemoimmunotherapy with hyper-CVAD plus rituximab for the treatment of adult Burkitt and Burkitt-like lymphoma or acute lymphoblastic leukemia. Cancer 2006;106(7):1569–80.
52. Mead GM, Sydes MR, Walewski J, et al. An international evaluation of CODOX-M and CODOX-M alternating with IVAC in adult Burkitt's lymphoma: results of United Kingdom lymphoma group LY06 study. Ann Oncol 2002;13(8):1264–74.
53. Tsang WM, Tong AC, Lam KY, et al. Nasal T/NK cell lymphoma: report of 3 cases involving the palate. J Oral Maxillofac Surg 2000;58(11):1323–7.
54. Jaffe ES. Lymphoid lesions of the head and neck: a model of lymphocyte homing and lymphomagenesis. Mod Pathol 2002;15(3):255–63.
55. Yamanaka N, Harabuchi Y, Sambe S, et al. Non-Hodgkin's lymphoma of Waldeyer's ring and nasal cavity: clinical and immunologic aspects. Cancer 1985;56(4):768–76.
56. Chan JF, Yip TT, Tsang WY, et al. Detection of Epstein-Barr viral RNA in malignant lymphomas of the upper aerodigestive tract. Am J Surg Pathol 1994;18(9):938–46.
57. Greer JP. Therapy of peripheral T/NK neoplasms. Hematology Am Soc Hematol Educ Program 2006;1:331–7.
58. Cheung MM, Chan JK, Lau WH, et al. Primary non-Hodgkin's lymphoma of the nose and nasopharynx: clinical features, immunophenotype, and treatment outcome in 112 patients. J Clin Oncol 1998;16(1):70–7.
59. Zucca E, Conconi A, Pedrinis E, et al. Nongastric marginal zone B-cell lymphoma of mucosa-associated lymphoid tissue. Blood 2003;101(7):2489–95.
60. Papaxoinis G, Fountzilas G, Rontogianni D, et al. Low-grade mucosa-associated lymphoid tissue lymphoma: a retrospective analysis of 97 patients by the Hellenic cooperative oncology group (HeCOG). Available at: http://annonc.oxfordjournals.org/cgi/content/full/mdm529v1?maxtoshow=&;HITS=10&hits=10&RESULTFORMAT=1&title=Low-grade+mucosaassociated+lymphoid+tissue+lymphoma&andorexacttitle=and&andorexacttitleabs=and&andorexactfulltext=and&searchid=1&FIRSTINDEX=0&sortspec=relevance&resourcetype=HWCIT. Accessed February 18, 2008.
61. Cavalli F, Isaacson PG, Gascoyne RD, et al. MALT lymphomas. Hematology Am Soc Hematol Educ Program 2001;241–58.
62. Cohen SM, Petryk M, Varma M, et al. Non-Hodgkin's lymphoma of mucosa-associated lymphoid tissue. Oncologist 2006;11(10):1100–17.
63. Ando M, Matsuzaki M, Murofushi T. Mucosa-associated lymphoid tissue lymphoma presented as diffuse swelling of the parotid gland. Am J Otol 2005;26(4):285–8.
64. Ellis GL. Lymphoid lesions of salivary glands: malignant and benign. Med Oral Patol Oral Cir Bucal 2007;12(7):E479–85.
65. Tauber S, Nerlich A, Lang S. MALT lymphoma of the paranasal sinuses and the hard palate: report of two cases and review of the literature. Eur Arch Otorhinolaryngol 2006;263(1):19–22.

66. Oh SY, Kwon HC, Kim WS, et al. Nongastric marginal zone B-cell lymphoma: a prognostic model from a retrospective multicenter study. Cancer Lett 2007;258(1):90–7.
67. Raderer M, Wohrer S, Streubel B, et al. Activity of rituximab plus cyclophosphamide, doxorubicin/mitoxantrone, vincristine, and prednisone in patients with relapsed MALT lymphoma. Oncology 2005;70(6):411–7.
68. Worthington HV, Clarkson JE, Eden OB. Interventions for treating oral candidiasis for patients with cancer receiving treatment. Cochrane Database Syst Rev 2007;(2):CD001972.
69. Worthington HV, Clarkson JE, Eden OB. Interventions for preventing oral mucositis for patients with cancer receiving treatment. Cochrane Database Syst Rev 2007;(4):CD000978.

The Leukemias

Vernon P. Burke, DMD, MD, James M. Startzell, DMD, MS*

KEYWORDS
- Leukemia • Oral effects • Oral surgery
- Oral and maxillofacial surgery • Oral mucosa disorders
- Management

Leukemia is a disease of mesenchymal origin in which there is an abnormal proliferation or an increased lifespan of myeloid or lymphoid cells. In the not so distant past these diseases were a death sentence, but in the past 40 years the medical community has made great strides in their treatment. Complete cure of or long periods of remission in many of these diseases is now possible. As technology for surface markers and cytogenetics has developed, so has the understanding of these diseases. Leukemia affects people throughout the lifespan and may present in many different forms. Leukemia can present in an indolent or alarmingly rapid way so only astute observation and a high level of suspicion can insure timely detection of the disorder.

Pathologic changes may occur within the oral cavity early in the course of the disease or may be induced in oral tissues secondary to treatment or as delayed sequelae of the disorder. An oral and maxillofacial surgeon (OMS) may be consulted for interpretation of oral lesions before a definitive diagnosis is made or after diagnosis for treatment of dentoalveolar disease or management of symptoms related to leukemia or its treatment. An in-depth discussion of each leukemia type, its diagnosis, and treatments is beyond the scope of this article. Instead, a brief overview of the types of leukemia and the common oral implications and treatments of the oral manifestations of these diseases are presented.

NORMAL DEVELOPMENT OF WHITE BLOOD CELLS

All blood cells are believed to develop from a common pluripotent stem cell. This stem cell can differentiate into a myeloid precursor or a lymphoid precursor. In an oversimplified description, myeloid cells are those formed in the bone marrow and lymphoid cells are those formed in the lymphatic tissue. The common lymphoid precursor then gives rise to plasma (B cells), T cells, or natural killer (NK) cells. Likewise, the common myeloid precursor gives rise to erythrocytes, polymorphonuclear lymphocytes, macrophages/monocytes, platelets, eosinophils, and basophils. The four major types of leukemia are classified based on the primary cell line of origin, lymphoid or myeloid, and are further divided according to the usual onset and progression of the disease, acute or chronic. There are other less common forms of leukemia and related syndromes.

THE LYMPHOID LEUKEMIAS

It is widely accepted that lymphoid leukemias are a result of a single progenitor cell mutation. The implication is that all resultant cells resemble the progenitor or, in other words, the daughter cells are true clones of the progenitor. The relationship between these neoplasms and the lymphomas of lymphoid cell origin is unclear and is beyond the depth of this review (see the article by Liddell and Bourgeois elsewhere in this issue). The two most important categories for discussion in this article are acute lymphoblastic leukemia (ALL) and chronic lymphoblastic leukemia (CLL).

Acute Lymphocytic Leukemia

Acute lymphocytic leukemia, acute lymphoblastic leukemia, and acute lymphoid leukemia are synonymous terms, all abbreviated ALL. There is broad array of ALL types. The majority are B-cell ALLs, representing approximately 85% of all ALLs. This

---

Department of Oral and Maxillofacial Surgery, University of Texas Health Science Center, Mail Code 7961, 7703 Floyd Curl Drive, San Antonio, TX 78229-3900, USA
* Corresponding author.
E-mail address: startzell@uthscsa.edu (J.M. Startzell).

is a disease of early childhood with a peak incidence at 4 years old. Following in occurrence are the T-cell ALLs and then the rare NK-cell leukemias. T-cell ALL is found more typically in adolescents and the NK-cell ALLs are more common in adults.[1]

Manifestations

The typical presentation can be nonspecific and confusing for unsuspecting practitioners. Patients often present with systemic signs of infection, fatigue, fever, pallor, and bleeding that are spontaneous or difficult to stop. Complete blood count often shows peripheral cytopenia. The white blood cell count cannot be relied on to diagnose the disease because there can be leukocytosis, leucopenia, or a normal leukocyte count. Patients also may present with symptomatic nodes or extranodal involvement of the central nervous system or testicles, hepatomegaly, or splenomegaly. Bone marrow biopsy usually is required for diagnosis and exact classification of the type of ALL.

The most common oral manifestation is spontaneous gingival bleeding (especially if platelet counts are below 10,000 to 20,000/mm^3).[2] Patients also may experience candidiasis, gingival hypertrophy/inflammation, neutropenic ulceration of the oral mucosa, herpetic infections that do not obey normal confinement to the keratinized mucosa, and rarely chloroma. Another manifestation is an infiltration of leukemic cells in one area of the oral mucosa. Numb chin syndrome also is reported as an initial and late presentation of ALL.[3] Unexplained paresthesia never should be minimized, especially in patients who have prior malignancy.[3]

Treatment and prognosis

The treatment of ALL is highly variable depending on the type of ALL. In childhood ALLs the typical format is

1. Induction—to reduce the number of blasts
2. Consolidation—to further reduce leukemic blasts
3. Interim maintenance—to allow normal bone marrow to recover
4. Delayed intensification—to address resistant leukemic cells
5. Maintenance—to extend disease remission. Oral, intravenous, or intrathecal drug regimen may be employed.

The medications used in treatment are multiple and can include those causing pancytopenia, immune dysregulation, and xerostomia, all of which are of interest to an OMS.

One of the great successes in modern medicine has been overcoming the once dismal prognosis of leukemia, and ALL is one of the leukemias where the greatest successes have been achieved. This is especially true in the childhood ALLs, in that as many as 85% may have complete remission and be considered cured. In adults, this number is closer to 50%. Unfortunately, there remain variants within ALL that have a poorer prognosis. Examples include ALLs with the t(9;22) translocation, certain cytogenetic abnormalities, extremely high white counts at presentation, or central nervous system involvement.[4] Of particular interest to OMSs managing patients under treatment of ALL is a tendency for children to become hypoglycemic easily during episodes of fasting. This tendency correlates somewhat with the age of a child, with younger children more prone to hypoglycemia. Halonen and colleagues[5] found that 19 of 35 children treated with 6-mercaptopurine and methotrexate became hypoglycemic during overnight fasting. Six of the patients became hypoglycemic in less than 13 hours, and 13 of the 19 hypoglycemic children became symptomatic. The implication of this data is that in planning surgery in children who are under treatment of ALL, monitoring of blood sugar may be in order.

Chronic Lymphocytic Leukemia

In the Western hemisphere, CLL is the most common form of leukemia.[4] Rare in the Asian countries, CLL is found to affect mostly older individuals yet can be seen in early middle age. Like ALL, B-cell phenotype predominates, representing approximately 95% of cases. The cause of CLL is uncertain with the exception of increased occurrence among those individuals exposed to Agent Orange in Vietnam. One theory of pathogenesis holds that cells in CLL are especially long lived, avoiding the usual pathways for apoptosis.

Manifestations

CLL can manifest at different levels of disease advancement and severity. Often the disease is an incidental finding on routine CBC in completely asymptomatic individuals or is discovered after investigation of enlarged lymphocytic or extralymphatic organs. The disease occurs along a spectrum, in some cases including cells with marker characteristics and histology essentially identical to small lymphocytic lymphoma. B symptoms may be present, which include intermittent fever over 38°C, drenching sweats, occurrence most often at night, and unintentional weight loss greater than or equal to 10% of body weight in 6 months or less.[1] Similar to ALL, patients who have CLL may present with fatigue, frequent infections, bleeding tendencies, and lymphadenopathy.

The diagnosis is suspected with a sustained lymphocytosis greater than 5×10^9/L consisting of monoclonal plasma cells expressing CD5 antigen. Classically the peripheral blood examination reveals smudge cells, which are friable white blood cells damaged during slide preparation. The bone marrow biopsy is confirmatory when it shows infiltration of the bone marrow with the same plasma cells seen in peripheral blood.[1,4] Practitioners should be acutely aware that persons suffering from CLL have a tendency to concurrently suffer from autoimmune complications, which include autoimmune hemolytic anemia and autoimmune thrombocytopenia. For poorly understood reasons, patients suffering from CLL also frequently present with hypogammaglobulinemia. These latter three conditions can be of great concern to OMSs asked to consult on patients who have CLL.

Oral manifestations are similar to those of ALL. There may be petechial hemorrhage resulting from thrombocytopenia, gingival bleeding, chloroma, or opportunistic infection, such as candidiasis. Also, Anhalt and colleagues[6] described a variant of pemphigus, which they termed, *paraneoplastic pemphigus*, seen in patients who have underlying neoplasms (see the article by Edgin, Pratt, and Grimwood elsewhere in this issue). This form starts in the oral cavity and progresses to involve the skin of the trunk and extremities. The lesions are characterized by "cutaneous blisters, a positive Nikolsky's sign, and epidermal and esophageal acantholysis."[6]

Treatment and prognosis

The B-cell CLL lymphoid leukemias are categorized by staging systems, such as the Rai (**Table 1**), which consider the combination of lymphocytosis plus alterations in other cell counts or involvement of other organ systems. Additional staging systems include the Binet and the International Workshop on Chronic Lymphocytic Leukemia, which attempts to combine the Binet and Rai staging systems.[4] The stage suggests prognosis and treatment protocols. Age and health of patients also are factors in deciding treatment options. Treatment may be withheld in asymptomatic patients who have low-risk disease. If treatment is deemed necessary, younger healthier patients may be offered more aggressive treatment than older sicker patients. Pharmacologic treatment may consist of single-agent intravenous fludarabine or oral chlorambucil. Other strategies call for multidrug protocols similar to those traditionally used for lymphomas, such as cyclophosphamide, vincristine, and prednisone or cyclophosphamide, doxorubicin, vincristine, and prednisone. There also is a place for bone marrow transplantation (BMT) in this disease, again depending on age and health status of patients. Radiation may be used on the spleen and occasionally splenectomy is performed.[1,4]

Autoimmune hemolytic anemia, autoimmune thrombocytopenia, and hypogammaglobulinemia are treated independently of CLL. These conditions should be corrected as best as possible before any necessary surgical treatments are performed on these patients. Tight coordination with oncologists is best in these situations.

THE MYELOID LEUKEMIAS

As discussed previously, myeloid leukemias represent an interruption in the normal production of cells in the myeloid line. The precursor cells are responsible for the eventual development of erythrocytes, granulocytes, and platelets. Typically, in myeloid leukemias there is a somatic gene mutation that results in the loss of control at one level

Table 1
Rai's chronic lymphoblastic leukemia staging system

Stage	Absolute Lymphocytosis	Lymph Nodes	Blood or Organ Involvement	Prognosis in Years
0	>15,000/mm^3	—	—	12–15
I	+	Enlarged	—	5–11
II	+	With or without	Enlarged liver or spleen	4–9
III	+	With or without	Anemia with or without enlarged liver or spleen	1–3.5
IV	+	With or without	Thrombocytopenia with or without enlarged liver or spleen	1–3.5

of production. This loss of control then leads to increased, decreased, or normal levels of production of that line and disturbed production of other cell lines resulting from crowding or inhibitory suppression in the bone marrow. Not only can quantitative disturbances be seen but also qualitative disturbance, in that the function of cells can be affected. Myeloid leukemias are clinically similar in their common infiltration of the bone marrow and often low numbers of blasts found in peripheral blood. Frequently, there are decreased blood counts of specific cell lines found on peripheral smear and evidence of poor function of the cells present.[4,7] Like other malignancies, these diseases can transform over time into more aggressive forms of leukemia.[8]

Acute Myelogenous Leukemia

Acute myelogenous leukemia (AML) has been classified in many ways, which can add confusion when trying to understand this group of diseases. The French-American-British (FAB) classification was first proposed in 1976 and includes eight categories, designated M0 to M7, based on morphology and cytochemistry. In an attempt to increase the value of the classification system in determining treatment, prognosis, and research, the World Health Organization (WHO) created a new classification system based on morphology, molecular, and clinical features. In addition to molecular classification, chromosomal analysis and immunophenotyping often are used to aid in the classification of the disease. **Table 2** lists the FAB classification and **Table 3** the WHO classification.[60]

Table 2
FAB classification of acute lymphoblastic leukemia

M0	Minimally differentiated leukemia
M1	Myeloblastic leukemia without maturation
M2	Myeloblastic leukemia with maturation
M3	Hypergranular promyelocytic leukemia
M4Eo	Variant: increase in abnormal marrow eosinophils
M4	Myelomonocytic leukemia
M5	Monocytic leukemia
M6	Erythroleukemia (Di Guglielmo disease)
M7	Megakaryoblastic leukemia

Data from Armitage JO, Longo DL. Malignancies of lymphoid cells. In: Braunwald E, Hauser SL, Fauci AS, et al, editors. Harrison's principles of internal medicine, 15th edition. New York: McGraw-Hill; 2001. p. 715–26.

The incidence of AML is 2.3 per 100,000 people. The incidence increases with age and is more common in men than woman. Several factors are involved in the disease, including heredity, environmental exposure, drugs and radiation. Fanconi's anemia; Down, Klinefelter's, and Patau's syndromes; and neurofibromatosis all lend a predisposition to certain AMLs. Occupational exposure to benzene and petroleum also are linked to AML. Chemotherapy agents, usually alkylating agents, such as busulfan, cisplatin, carboplatin, chlorambucil, and cyclophosphamide, used to treat other cancers are associated with an increase in AML. The role of radiation used to treat malignancy and its relation to development of AML is controversial, although exposure to atomic blast radiation has been established as a cause of AML with increased likelihood proportional on exposure level.[4,7]

Manifestations

The disease presentation can vary somewhat depending on the subtype of AML but typically is diagnosed weeks to months after the onset of symptoms. The most common presenting complaint is fatigue. Weight loss and anorexia are common presenting symptoms followed by fever and problems with coagulation, such as bleeding or easy bruising. On physical examination, clinicians are likely to see hepatosplenomegaly, fever, mild lymphadenopathy, evidence of coagulopathy, and infection. Sternal pain also may be present. Particularly striking in this group of diseases is the finding of a bleeding diathesis especially from the linings of body cavities. This is true especially in the M3 subtype, acute promyelocytic leukemia, in which affected leukemic cells release procoagulant factors and fibrinolytic factors. Practitioners should be on the lookout for disseminated intravascular coagulation in patients who have M3 type AML.[4,7,8]

Patients who have AML can present with leukocyte counts in excess of 100,000/μL but more frequently have counts less than 5000/μL. Thrombocytopenia is a common feature in AML with approximately 75% of patients presenting with platelets less than 100,000/μL and as many as 25% with less than 25,000/μL. These low platelet counts place patients at increased risk for spontaneous bleeding. Hemorrhage, decreased production, and poor survival leads to a frequent finding of decreased erythrocytes in a typically normocytic normochromic anemia.[4,7] Microscopic examination of the peripheral blood also may demonstrate Auer rods. These are aggregates of granules from within the leukemic cells. They are seen as groups of rod-shaped red inclusions in

Table 3
World Health Organization classification of acute lymphoblastic leukemia

I. AMLs
  a. AMLs with recurrent cytogenetic translocations
  b. AML with t(8;21) (q22;q22), AML1(CBF-alpha)/ETO
  c. Acute promyelocytic leukemia (AML with t(15;17) (q22;q11-12) and variants, PML/RAR-alpha)
  d. AML with abnormal bone marrow eosinophils (inv(16) (p13q22) or t(16;16) (p13;q11), CBF-alpha/MYH11X)
  e. AML with 11q23 (MLL) abnormalities

II. AML with multilineage dysplasia
  a. With prior MDS
  b. Without prior MDS

III. AML and MDS, therapy related
  a. Alkylating agent related
  b. Epipodophyllotoxin related (some may be lymphoid)
  c. Other types

IV. AML not otherwise categorized
  a. AML minimally differentiated
  b. AML without maturation
  c. AML with maturation
  d. Acute myelomonocytic leukemia
  e. Acute monocytic leukemia
  f. Acute erythroid leukemia
  g. Acute megakaryocytic leukemia
  h. Acute basophilic leukemia
  i. Acute panmyelosis with myelofibrosis
  j. Acute biphenotypic leukemias

Data from Harris NL, Jaffe ES, Diebold J, et al. World Health Organization classification of neoplastic diseases of the hematopoietic and lymphoid tissues: report of the clinical advisory committee meeting-Airlie House, Virginia, November 1997. J Clin Oncol 1999;17(12):3835–49; with permission.

the cytoplasm. This finding not only can help with diagnosis of AML but also may help in prognostic evaluation.[8]

Oral manifestations are more common in some of the subsets of AML. Although rare, chloroma may be a presenting feature of AML and invariably progresses into systemic disease. Infiltration of the gingiva, seen as gingival hyperplasia, is more common in the M4 and M5 forms of the disease that represent AMLs with monocytic differentiation. Monocytes have a tendency to infiltrate out into tissue as a part of their normal behavior. **Fig. 1** is a clinical photograph of a patient who had known AML who developed a tongue infiltrated with AML cells. Such infiltration may not have the characteristic marginal definition of a mass. This lesion, shown here shortly after biopsy, presented as a diffuse erythematous firm enlargement of the tongue without discrete margins. Similar to the previously described lymphoid leukemias, opportunistic bacterial infection or exaggerated viral infections may be recognized in the setting of immunodeficient states. Gingival bleeding is a frequent finding. Sweet's syndrome, or acute febrile neutrophilic dermatosis, is an ulcerative condition seen in the mouth in AML. Sweet's syndrome may be confused with Behçet's or aphthous ulcers.[9]

Treatment and prognosis
There are several different strategies for treating AML. Typically AML is treated with a combination of an anthrocycline and the antimetabolite, cytosine arabinoside (Ara-C). Therapy with these two agents is described numerically: anthrocycline

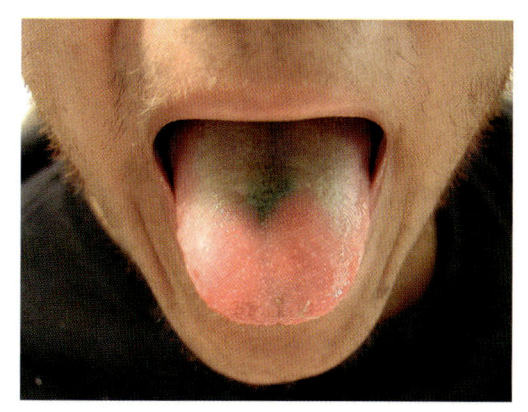

Fig. 1. Tongue infiltration by AML.

+ Ara-C. A popular and effective combination is the 3 + 7 regimen in which patients receive 3 days of idarubicin or daunorubicin and 7 days of Ara-C. This induction type of therapy produces clinical remission in 60% to 70% of patients.[4] The main causes of failure to obtain a clinical remission are death before remission and failure to achieve bone marrow hypoplasia. After induction therapy, treatment can progress to the typical maintenance therapy or, otherwise, to consolidation or intensification therapy. There is a wide range of opinions on therapy lengths and strategies, a topic too in depth for the purposes of this article.[4]

Prognosis of treatment is judged with several variables that include the age of patients, presence of certain karyotypes associated with better or worse prognosis, and performance status of patients at the time of induction. Unfortunately, the success of treatment of AML has not achieved the same success as that of childhood ALL. According to Hoffman and colleagues, only 20% of persons treated for AML with a standard therapy or its variants achieve a long-term survival without disease.[4]

Chronic Myelogenous Leukemia

Chronic myelogenous leukemia (CML) is an exciting topic in the hematologic malignancies because so much is known about the disease. CML is diagnosed by the identification of a reciprocal translocation of chromosomes 9 and 22. The region from chromosome 22 is called the breakpoint cluster region (BCR) and the region from chromosome 9 is the Abelson murine leukemia locus (ABL). This translocation leads to the disease in that the product of this fusion is a tyrosine kinase (TK) capable of constitutive autophosphorylation. This TK activation leads to subsequent enhanced cell division and evasion of apoptosis of mature myeloid cells that are clonal in nature.[8]

Manifestations

Typically a disease seen in older patients, occurrence of CML increases with age. It is rarely seen in children and, if found, carries a poor prognosis. Patients often are asymptomatic at the time of diagnosis and the disease is found incidentally on examination of blood. If patients have a complaint at the time of diagnosis it is likely to be fatigue followed by anorexia or weight loss.

In untreated CML there generally are three phases of the disease. The initial or chronic stage typically lasts 5 to 6 years. In the chronic phase, the peripheral blood reveals elevated counts of platelets and elevated white blood cell counts. Mature granulocytes among metamyelocytes and myelocytes often are seen. Bone marrow shows near 100% cellularity compared with the usual 50%. Extramedullary hematopoeisis occurs, resulting most commonly in splenomegaly and possible hepatomegaly and lymphadenopathy. The second stage, the accelerated stage, is characterized by increasing anemia, basophilia, and thrombocytopenia. Invariably CML progresses to the third stage, blast crisis. Blast crisis is marked by a transition from a chronic leukemia to an acute leukemia. Histologic examination reveals blasts of several lineages, thrombocytopenia, and anemia not explained by other causes (hemorrhage or chemotherapy). Blast crisis leads to rapid deterioration in patient health and eventual death.[4,7,8]

Oral manifestations of CML are the result of immunocompromise and thrombocytopenia. Petechiae, mucosal bleeding, and acute periodontitis may be witnessed. Overgrowth of oral flora may present as candidiasis.

Treatment and prognosis

Historically CML was treated with interferon-α with a success rate of approximately 20% measured by cytogenetic remission.[4] Hydroxyurea and busulfan also are used as oral chemotherapeutic agents that provide patients with hematologic remission for a limited time. Neither drug prevents the inevitable blast crisis. The use of these drugs diminished after the development of imatinib mesylate (Gleevec). As discussed previously, the causative problem in CML seems to be the production of a constitutively activated TK.

Imatinib mesylate (400 mg daily) acts by inhibiting the TK in its inactive form by binding to the ATP binding site.[10] Doses of 600 to 800 mg may be used in adults during accelerated phase or blast crisis. Patients who begin their treatment in the chronic phase receive the most benefit. According to Kantarjian and colleagues, more than 90% have a hematologic response and more than 60% have a cytogenetic response.[11] The response is far worse for those patients who begin treatment in the accelerated or blast phase. Monitoring of disease is important in CML despite optimism with imatinib mesylate.[12,13] There are reports of developed resistance to imatinib mesylate resulting from overexpression of the BCR-ABL gene or genetic alteration.[10,13]

There has been a decrease in the use of stem cell transplantation (SCT) in the treatment of CML since the release of imatinib mesylate, yet it remains the only therapy that is potentially curative. In younger patients using allogenic graft from an HLA-matched sibling or in HLA-matched unrelated donors, the long-term success can be as high as 85% and 70%, respectively. The major incidence of mortality is during preparation for and at the time of transplantation. Because mortality increases substantially at increased age there has been reluctance to offer SCT to older patients.[4,7,14]

MYELODYSPLASTIC SYNDROMES

Myelodysplastic syndromes (MDS) are a group of disorders affecting the myeloid cell lineage. These disorders are characterized by clonal expansion of a myeloid progenitor that maintains its ability to produce mature cells. The control mechanisms for coordinated cellular production are disrupted. Two main classification systems exist for MDS. In the traditional FAB system it is separated into five categories. Recently WHO amended this classification system into four categories. For the purposes of this article, the overarching characteristics of the syndromes, the usual treatments, and implications for OMSs are discussed.

Certain populations are at increased risk for MDS. Persons who have Down syndrome or Fanconi's anemia not uncommonly develop MDS. Exposure to radiation is a known causative factor in MDS as is previous treatment with alkylating agents and DNA topoisomerase inhibitors. This is a devastating late complication of life-saving treatment with these medications that develops 5 to 7 years after treatment with alkylating agents and only 2 years after DNA topoisomerase inhibitors.[4,7,8,14]

Manifestations

Like CML, MDS is a disease with increasing frequency as patients age. Rarely it is seen before age 50, with a mean onset age of 68.[7] The disease has an insidious onset and is found incidentally in nearly half of cases. If symptomatic, patients often complain of increasing fatigue and shortness of breath. Pallor is seen on clinical examination and it is not unusual to note fever or weight loss. These symptoms coincide with the degree of cytopenia, especially anemia. Sweet's syndrome also may be noted.[9]

On peripheral blood examination, anemia is the predominate feature. Red blood cells and platelets often are large, which makes it important to exclude the macrocytic anemias during the differential diagnosis process. Approximately half of all patients who have MDS have thrombocytopenia. Neutrophils have decreased numbers of granules and may contain Döhle bodies (round inclusions in the cytoplasm of neutrophils often seen in cancer). Polymorphonuclear lymphocytes s often are hyposegmented and the total white count usually is normal or low. Bone marrow examination relies on an evaluation of the morphology of the cells present and the percentages of certain cells in the marrow, such as myeloblasts, karyotyping, and cytogenetics. Often multiple bone marrow aspirates and biopsies are required over time to determine the specific type of MDS and rule out other disease entities.[4,7,8,14]

Oral manifestations often are a result of the qualitative and quantitative defect in platelets. Petechiae and gingival bleeding frequently are seen. The oral manifestations of Sweet's syndrome are a rare but recognized entity associated with MDS.[8]

Treatment and Prognosis

The success of treatment of MDS varies widely and therapy lacks standardization. The advanced age and poor performance status of typical patients diagnosed with MDS are contributing factors in the difficulty treating MDS. Treatment strategies range from supportive to intensive therapies. These myriad strategies hint at the limited understanding and lack of a definitive treatment of MDS.

Supportive care is of critical importance to patients suffering from MDS. In anemia, supportive care includes blood transfusion when necessary, possible use of erythropoietin, and, if indicated, iron therapy. Thrombocytopenia often is untreated unless platelet counts are low. The logic behind this is the real risk for alloimmunization and the subsequent inability to use platelet transfusion later. Irradiated blood products often are used to help diminish this problem. Because the quality of the circulating platelets is poor, even if the count is normal, patients may exhibit bleeding diathesis.

Depending on the subtype of MDS, there may be a grim prognosis of just a few months or, in another subtype, patients may survive with supportive therapy for years. The International Prognostic Scoring System predicts prognosis of MDS.[15] This system creates a score based on blast percentage, cytopenia, presence of an abnormal karyotype, and cytogenetics. The higher the score the lower the prognosis measured in years. The likelihood of progression to AML also is listed in this system. In patients who have MDS, about one third die as a result of transformation to AML. This subtype of AML carries a poor prognosis. Approximately 20% die of an infection related to immunosuppression. Others die as a result of bone marrow failure.[14,15]

TREATMENT OF ORAL MANIFESTATIONS

In leukemia there are oral manifestations of the disease and there are manifestations related to treatment. **Table 4** lists constitutional symptoms,

Table 4
Common leukemia complaints and examination findings

Constitutional	General Physical Examination Findings	Oral Examination Findings
Malaise	Bruising	Pallor
Fatigue	Epistaxis	Gingival bleeding
Anorexia	Lymphadenopathy	Mucosal petechiae
Weight loss	Organomegaly	Gingivo-periodontitis
Low-grade fever	Organ infiltration	Gingival hyperplasia
Night sweats	Bacterial or viral infections	Tissue mass or enlargement
Bleeding without obvious cause	—	Mucosal ulceration
—	—	Candidal erythema or plaques
—	—	Xerostomia

general physical examination findings, and oral findings found commonly among the leukemias. There might be overlap between those conditions that are seen as a result of the disease and those arising as a result of treatment. Each must be considered in its relevance to patient care and the determination of which steps should be taken in the treatment provided by an OMS. Oral candidiasis is a good example in that the immunodeficiency of leukemia or the immunodeficiency of the chemotherapeutic agents can contribute to this condition. Patients being conditioned for BMT or who have received BMT may have the additional problems of xerostomia and the unfortunate shift to more cariogenic oral bacteria.[16] Xerostomia is common in those receiving chemotherapy and contributes to the problems (discussed later).

For the sake of organization and usefulness to readers, each entity is described and the treatments outlined. This not meant as an all-inclusive treatment protocol but rather as an outline and a list of conditions that merit further reading. OMSs should remember to encourage good oral hygiene as a cornerstone to the prevention of some of the conditions that follow.[17,18]

Candidiasis

Oral candidiasis or thrush, as it sometimes is called, is a disease caused by the growth of a fungus, most commonly *Candida albicans*, that is characterized by white wipeable material on an erythematous oral mucosal base. The presence of Candida species is frequent in healthy controls and increases with age most often without formation of lesions. The lesions associated with Candida in its milder forms is nonpainful but in severe cases can be painful. Dysphagia also can result from Candida infection. There is concern in immunosuppressed patients for progression of oral Candidal infection to systemic infection, which can be a devastating and fatal complication. Although not as commonly, *Aspergillosis* is implicated in morbid and fatal infections in immunocompromised patients and should be treated in a matter similar to Candida.[19,20] Many studies have been performed in an attempt to establish oral fungal infection as a cause of the high incidence of systemic fungal infections seen in immunosuppressed patients and those receiving BMT. At this time it is unknown how often oral fungus is the source of systemic fungal infection in these patients and if prophylaxis decreases mortality.[20–28]

Treatment of oral candidiasis has been performed with nystatin,[25] clotrimazole[21,22,29] itraconazole, ketaconazole, fluconazole, miconazole, amphotericin B, and even chlorhexidine. A Cochrane review noted that the medications absorbed from the gastrointestinal tract partially or completely are more efficacious than those medications that are not. These medications include the partially absorbed clotrimazole and miconazole and the completely absorbed fluconazole, itraconazole, and ketaconazole. The Cochrane review found that nystatin lacked benefit and amphotericin B had only a small benefit in treating oral candidiasis.[27,30]

Oral Herpes

Oral herpes in the setting of leukemia treatment is grouped commonly with mucositis. Because it is a discrete etiologic agent, herpes simplex virus (HSV-1) is discussed separately. HSV-1 is common in the healthy population and typically presents with somewhat painful ulcers and cosmetic problems. In immunocompromised patients and undergoing chemotherapy and BMT, HSV-1 infection can cause devastating ulcers affecting a patient's ability to eat and occasionally transitions into a systemic infection. These ulcers provide an avenue for virus and bacteria to cause a systemic superinfection. The lesions found in immunocompromised patients do not obey the normal boundaries of HSV-1 infection and often are found throughout the mouth. It even is suggested in the literature that HSV-1 may be a contributing factor in acute necrotizing ulcerative gingivitis found in patients undergoing treatment of leukemia.[31] It has been long established that prophylactic treatment of HSV-1 with acyclovir in leukemic patients under chemotherapeutic treatment decreases the amount of oral manifestations associated with HSV-1[31-41] and increases survival in patients who have BMT.[42,43] Following the all too common archetype, resistance to acyclovir is reported in the literature.[44-46] For these resistant cases, cidofovir has been advocated as a successful alternative.[45,47]

Typically, patients are treated prophylactically after initiation of chemotherapy if they are known to be HSV-1 infected. Prophylactic treatment is highly efficacious in BMT patients and usual dosing is acyclovir (200 mg 5 times a day). Reactivation of HSV-1 in this population is treated in a stepwise fashion depending on severity, from 800 mg twice a day to initiation of intravenous acyclovir (5–10 mg/kg every 8 hours).[48] Typical treatment courses range from 5 to 10 days. Topical acyclovir should be avoided because of its lack of efficacy.

GRAFT-VERSUS-HOST DISEASE

In the setting of SCT in the treatment of leukemia, graft-versus-host disease (GVHD) is not uncommon. GVHD is a potential complication anytime immunocompetent transplantation of T lymphocytes takes place into an immunocompromised host. Acute and chronic forms exist, with the acute form occurring in the first 100 days after transplantation. The T lymphocytes attack the recipient's cells, which result in the manifestations of the disease with involvement mainly of the liver, skin, gastrointestinal tract, and eyes. Weight loss is common, as are lichenoid mucositis, xerostomia, and esophageal strictures.[49,50] Most importantly, GVHD can cause a severe immunosuppression that can be fatal.

Prevention of GVHD is important in the acute phase and usually entails the use of drugs, such as cyclosporine, tacrulimus, methotrexate, or corticosteroids, and most patients experience at least a mild form of GVHD immediately post graft. In the case of increased severity of acute GVHD, treatment includes monoclonal antibodies, increased corticosteroids,[14] and antithymocyte globulin.[51,52] Chronic GVHD frequently is found in older patients and in those who have acute GVHD. Treatment is similar to acute GVHD in the use of steroids and cyclosporine but thalidomide also may be added. It has been reported in the pediatric population that deoxycoformycin (Pentostatin), a purine nucleoside analog, also may help in the treatment of chronic GVHD.[53]

Oral findings in GVHD can be difficult to differentiate from other entities. They often present as shallow ulcerations on the lips and mucosa, which may mimic HSV-1 or aphthae. GVHD also occasionally presents as a white lesion, which can be confused with a lichenoid reaction, Candida, or squamous cell carcinoma. It is recommended lesions in patients after grafting be tested for fungus and viral cultures performed before assuming a diagnosis of GVHD.[50] It is most prudent to biopsy the lesion to confirm the diagnosis as reports of second malignancy are present in the literature.[49] Treatment of the oral manifestations of GVHD is accomplished primarily by treatment of the underlying GVHD. Sialogogues are in order for xerostomia and saline or bicarbonate rinses may provide patients relief of related symptoms. Pain management is of particular importance and OMSs should work diligently to provide topical, systemic or a combination of both analgesics to provide patients with the most comfort possible.

MUCOSITIS

Mucositis is common in the persons being treated for hematologic malignancy.[54] It has been reported to occur in 75% of this population and can at times limit the continuation of therapy. Because of the break in physical barrier to infection that comes with mucositis, the mouth can become a source for systemic infection. Several reports in the medical literature point to cases of bacteremia with organisms commonly associated with the normal oral flora.[55,56] Acute periodontal disease also should be watched for and treated with appropriate antibacterial regimens and dental treatment regimens indicated to eliminate this as a source. Patients can find the pain of mucositis overwhelming and the delivery of proper nutrition can become a problem as a result. The etiology of mucositis is multifactoral and can vary widely from patient to patient and with medication regimens. In general mucositis is worse in days immediately after administration of chemotherapeutic agents and is made worse by the addition of radiation.[57]

Basic oral hygiene is the cornerstone to the prevention and treatment of mucositis.[17,18] The pretreatment stomatologic evaluation of patients slated for chemotherapy can eliminate factors that may contribute to the development of mucositis.[58] Meeting with a dentist or dental specialist also can provide the opportunity for reinforcement of oral hygiene principles. Successful strategies for prevention and treatment of mucositis remain elusive. Many agents and interventions are advocated, but few are shown effective in clinical trials.[59] In their review of the literature, the Cochrane group found only ice chips, Chinese herbal preparations, and amifistone displayed evidence these interventions may benefit patients. Of the three, amifistone showed the greatest benefit, but most studies were conducted in patients who had solid tumors and not leukemia.[59] It should be emphasized that practitioners should treat pain and discomfort in the oral region. Frequently used, but with unknown benefit, are saline and bicarbonate rinses. Additionally, many preparations are available to practitioners that have topical anesthetic and barrier properties (coating rinses). Although strong data are lacking on products, such as oral sucralfate and combination rinses, if pain relief and increased ability to tolerate oral intake is gained there may be a subjective benefit.

SURGICAL MANAGEMENT OF LEUKEMIC PATIENTS

Any of the pathologic conditions commonly managed by an OMS may occur in patients who have leukemia. These include mucosal disorders requiring biopsy or supportive care, dental or gingivoperiodontal disease, soft tissue or bony trauma, mucosal pathology, tumors, or developmental disorders. The primary threats to patients who have leukemia and who require the services of a dentist or OMS are failure of a practitioner to recognize that a patient has the disease, to biopsy lesions suggestive of leukemia, or to account for anemia, thrombocytopenia, or immunodeficiency in developing management plans for the presenting disorder.

REFERENCES

1. Armitage JO, Longo DL. Malignancies of lymphoid cells. In: Braunwald E, Hauser SL, Fauci AS, et al, editors. Harrison's: principles of internal medicine. 15th edition. New York: McGraw-Hill; 2001. p. 715–26.
2. Neville BW, Damm DD, Allen CM, et al. Oral & maxillofacial pathology. 2nd edition. Philidelphia: W.B. Saunders; 2002. p. 510–2.
3. Hiraki A, Nakamura S, Abe K, et al. Numb chin syndrome as an initial symptom of acute lymphocytic leukemia: report of three cases. Oral Surg Oral Med Oral Pathol Oral Radiol Endod 1997;83(5): 555–61.
4. Estey EH, Kantarjian HM. Hematologic malignancies. In: Hoffman R, Benz EJ, Shattil SJ, et al, editors. Hoffman: hematology: basic principles and practice. 4th edition. Philadelphia: Elsevier; 2005. Available at: http://www.mdconsult.com.libproxy.uthscsa.edu/das/book/body/93451089-4/0/1267/0.html; 2005. Accessed April 29, 2008.
5. Halonen P, Salo MK, Mäkipernaa A. Fasting hypoglycemia is common during maintenance therapy for childhood acute lymphoblastic leukemia. J Pediatr 2001;138(3):428–31.
6. Anhalt GJ, Kim SC, Stanley JR. Paraneoplastic pemphigus: an autoimmune mucocutaneous disease associated with neoplasia. N Engl J Med 1990; 323(25):1729–35.
7. Wetzler M, Byrd J, Bloomfield C. Acute and chronic myeloid leukemias. In: Braunwald E, Hauser SL, Fauci AS, et al, editors. Harrison's: principles of internal medicine. 15th edition. New York: McGraw-Hill; 2001. p. 706–14.
8. Astor J. Diseases of white blood cells, lymph nodes, spleen, and thymus. In: Kumar V, Abbas AK, Fausto N, editors. Pathologic basis of disease. 7th edition. Philadelphia: Elsevier; 2005. p. 661–710.
9. Femiano F, Gombos F, Scully C. Sweet's syndrome: recurrent oral ulceration, pyrexia, thrombophlebitis, and cutaneous lesions. Oral Surg Oral Med Oral Pathol Oral Radiol Endod 2003;95(3): 324–7.
10. Nardi V, Azam M, Daley GQ. Mechanisms and implications of imatinib resistance mutations in BCR-ABL. Curr Opin Hematol 2004;11(1):35–43.
11. Kantarjian H, Sawyers C, Hochhaus A, et al. Hematologic and cytogenetic response to imitanib mesylate in chronic myelogenous leukemia. N Engl J Med 2002;346(9):645–52.
12. Goldman J. Monitoring minimal residual disease in BCR-ABL-positivie chronic myeloid leukemia in the imatinib era. Curr Opin Hematol 2005;12(1): 33–9.
13. Morimoto A, Ogami A, Chiyonobu T, et al. Early blast transformation following complete cytogenetic response in a pediatric chronic myeloid leukemia patient treated with imatinib mesylate. J Pediatr Hematol Oncol 2004;26(5):320–2.
14. Kantarjian H, Faderi S. Acute lymphoid leukemias in adults. In: Abeloff MD, Armitage JO, Niederhuber JE, et al, editors. Clinical oncology. 3rd edition. Elsevier; 2004. Available at: http://www.mdconsult.com.libproxy.uthscsa.edu/das/book/body/93451089-4/0/1241/0.html; 2004. Accessed April 29, 2008.
15. Greenberg P, Cox C, LeBeau MM, et al. International scoring system for evaluating prognosis in myelodysplastic syndromes. Blood 1997;89(6): 2079–88.

16. Dens F, Boogaerts M, Boute P, et al. Caries-related salivary microorganisms and salivary flow rate in bone marrow recipients. Oral Surg Oral Med Oral Pathol Oral Radiol Endod 1996;81(1):38–43.
17. McGuire DB, Yeager KA, Dudley WN, et al. Acute oral pain and mucositis in bone marrow transplant and leukemia patients: data from a pilot study. Cancer Nurs 1998;21(6):385–93.
18. Yeager KA, Webster J, Crain M, et al. Implementation of an oral care standard for leukemia and transplantation patients. Cancer Nurs 2000;23(1):40–8.
19. Myoken Y, Sugata T, Myoken Y, et al. Antifungal susceptibility of aspergillus species isolated from invasive oral infection in neutropenic patients with hematologic malignancies. Oral Surg Oral Med Oral Pathol Oral Radiol Endod 1999;87(2):174–9.
20. Sugata T, Myoken Y, Kyo T, et al. Oral aspergillosis in compromised patients. Oral Surg Oral Med Oral Pathol Oral Radiol Endod 1996;81(6):632–3.
21. Cuttner J, Troy KM, Funaro L, et al. Clotrimazole treatment for prevention of oral candidiasis in patients with acute leukemia undergoing chemotherapy: results of a double blind study. Am J Med 1986;81(5):771–4.
22. Owens NJ, Nightingale CH, Schweizer RT, et al. Prophylaxis of oral candidiasis with clotrimazole troches. Arch Intern Med 1984;144(2):290–3.
23. Williams C, Whitehouse JM, Lister TA, et al. Oral candidial prophylaxis in patients undergoing chemotherapy for acute leukemia. Med Pediatr Oncol 1977;3(3):275–80.
24. Gafter-Gvili A, Fraser A, Paul M, et al. Antibiotic prophylaxis for bacterial infections in afebrile neutropenic patients following chemotherapy. Cochrane Database Syst Rev 2005;19(4):CD004386.
25. Gotzche PC, Johansen HK. Nystatin prophylaxis and treatment in severely immunodepressed patients. Cochrane Database Syst Rev 2002;(2):CD002033.
26. Epstein JB, Ransier A, Lunn R, et al. Prophylaxis of candidiasis in patients with leukemia and bone marrow transplants. Oral Surg Oral Med Oral Pathol Oral Radiol Endod 1996;81(3):291–6.
27. Clarkson JE, Worthington HV, Eden OB. Interventions for preventing oral candidiasis for patients with cancer receiving treatment. Cochrane Database Syst Rev 2007;(1):CD003807.
28. Gotzsche PC, Johansen HK. Routine versus selective antifungal administration for control of fungal infections in patients with cancer. Cochrane Database Syst Rev 2002;(2):CD000026.
29. Martino P, Venditti M, Petti MC, et al. Cotrimoxazole prophylaxis in patients with leukemia and prolonged granuloytopenia. Am J Med Sci 1984;287(3):7–9.
30. Worthington HV, Clarkson JE, Eden OB. Interventions for treating oral candidiasis for patients with cancer receiving treatment. Cochrane Database Syst Rev 2007;(2):CD001972.
31. Bergmann OJ, Ellermann-Eriksen S, Mogensen SC, et al. Bergmann OJ, Mogensen SC, Br Med J, 1995. Br Med J 1995;310(6988):1169–72.
32. Bergmann OJ, Mogensen SC, Ellermann-Eriksen S, et al. Acyclovir prophylaxis and fever during remission-induction therapy of patients with acute myeloid leukemia: a randomized, double-blind, placebo-controlled trial. J Clin Oncol 1997;15(6):2269–74.
33. Theriault A, Cohen PR. Herpetic geometric glossitis in a pediatric patient with acute myelogenous leukemia. Am J Clin Oncol 1997;20(6):567–8.
34. Barrett AP. A long-term prospective clinical study of orofacial herpes simplex virus infection in acute leukemia. Oral Surg Oral Med Oral Pathol Oral Radiol Endod 1986;61(2):149–52.
35. Carrega G, Castagnola E, Canessa A, et al. Herpes simplex virus and oral mucositis in children with cancer. Support Care Cancer 1994;2(4):266–9.
36. Engelhard D, Morag A, Or R, et al. Prevention of herpes simplex virus (HSV) infection in recipients of HLA-matched T-lymphocyte-depleted bone marrow allografts. Isr J Med Sci 1988;24(3):145–50.
37. Gluckman E, Lotsberg J, Devergie A, et al. Oral acyclovir prophylactic treatment of herpes simplex infection after bone marrow transplantation. J Antimicrob Chemother 1983;12(Suppl B):161–7.
38. James E, Robinson L, Griffiths PD, et al. Acute myeloblastic leukaemia presenting with herpes simplex type-1 viraemia and pneumonia. Br J Haematol 1996;93(2):401–2.
39. O'Meara A, Deasy PF, Hillary IB, et al. Acyclovir for treatment of mucocutaneous herpes infection in a child with leukaemia. Lancet 1979;2(8153):1196.
40. O'Meara A, Hillary IB. Acyclovir in the management of herpes virus infections in immunosuppressed children. Isr J Med Sci 1981;150(3):73–7.
41. Redding SW. Role of herpes simplex virus reactivation in chemotherapy-induced oral mucositis. NCI Monogr 1990;(9):103–5.
42. Vogler WR, Winton EF, Reynolds RC, et al. Factors affecting survival in allogeneic bone marrow transplantation. Am J Med Sci 1989;297(5):300–8.
43. Gomez RS, Carneiro MA, Souza LN, et al. Oral recurrent human herpes virus infection and bone marrow transplantation survival. Oral Surg Oral Med Oral Pathol Oral Radiol Endod 2001;91(5):552–6.
44. Gray JJ, Wreghitt TG, Baglin TP. Susceptibility to acyclovir of herpes simplex virus: emergence of resistance in patients with lymphoid and myeloid neoplasia. J Infect 1989;19(1):31–40.
45. LoPresti AE, Levine JF, Munk GB, et al. Successful treatment of an acyclovir—and foscarnet—resistant herpes simplex virus type 1 lesion with intravenous cidofovir. Clin Infect Dis 1998;26(2):512–3.
46. Snoeck R, Andrei G, Gerard M, et al. Successful treatment of progressive mucocutaneous infection

due to acyclovir—and foscarnet—resistant herpes simplex virus with (S)-1-(3-hydroxy-2-phosphonyl-methoxypropyl)cytosine (HPMPC). Clin Infect Dis 1994;18(4):570–8.
47. Bryant P, Sasadeusz J, Carapetis J, et al. Successful treatment of foscarnet-resistant herpes simplex stomatitis with intravenous cidofovir in a child. Pediatr Infect Dis J 2001;20(11):1083–6.
48. Reusser P. Opportunistic viral infections. In: Cohen J, Powderly WG, Berkley SF, et al, editors. Infectious diseases. 2nd edition. Elsevier; 2004. Available at: http://www.mdconsult.com.libproxy.uthscsa.edu/das/book/body/93451089-4/0/1209/0.html; 2004. Accessed April 29, 2008.
49. Abdelsayed RA, Sumner T, Allen CM, et al. Oral precancerous and malignant lesions associated with graft-versus-host disease: report of 2 cases. Oral Surg Oral Med Oral Pathol Oral Radiol Endod 2002;93(1):75–80.
50. Eggleston TI, Ziccardi VB, Lumerman H. Graft-versus-host disease: case report and discussion. Oral Surg Oral Med Oral Pathol Oral Radiol Endod 1998;86(6):692–6.
51. Bacigalupo A. Antithymocyte globulin for prevention of graft-versus-host disease. Curr Opin Hematol 2005;12(6):457–62.
52. Sharathkumar A, Thornley I, Saunders EF, et al. Allogeneic bone marrow transplantation in children with chronic myelogenous leukemia. J Pediatr Hematol Oncol 2002;24(3):215–9.
53. Goldberg JD, Jacobsohn DA, Margolis J, et al. Pentostatin for the treatment of chronic graft-versus-host disease in children. J Pediatr Hematol Oncol 2003;25(7):584–8.
54. Barrett AP. A long-term prospective clinical study of oral complications during conventional chemotherapy for acute leukemia. Oral Surg Oral Med Oral Pathol Oral Radiol Endod 1987;63(3):313–6.
55. Vidal AM, Sarria JC, Kimbrough RC, et al. Anaerobic bacteremia in a neutropenic patient with oral mucositis. Am J Med Sci 2000;319(3):189–90.
56. Mantadakis E, Danilatou V, Christidou A, et al. Capnocytophaga gingivalis bacteremia detected only on quantitative blood cultures in a child with leukemia. Pediatr Infect Dis J 2003;22(2):202–4.
57. de Oliveira Lula EC, de Oliveira Lula CE, Alves CM, et al. Chemotherapy induced oral complications in leukemic patients. Int J Pediatr Otorhinolaryngol 2007;71(11):1681–5.
58. Elad S, Thierer T, Bitan M, et al. A decision analysis: the dental management of patients prior to hematology cytotoxic therapy or hematopoietic stem cell transplantation. Oral Oncol 2008;44(1):37–42.
59. Worthington HV, Clarkson JE, Eden OB. Interventions for preventing oral mucositis for patients with cancer receiving treatment. Cochrane Database Syst Rev 2007;(4):CD000978.
60. Harris NL, Jaffe ES, Diebold J, et al. World Health Organization classification of neoplastic diseases of the hematopoietic and lymphoid tissues: report of the clinical advisory committee meeting-Airlie House, Virginia, November 1997. J Clin Oncol 1999;17(12):3835–49.

Head and Neck Manifestations of Distant Carcinomas

Luis G. Vega, DDS[a],*, Juliana Dipasquale, DMD[a], Rajesh Gutta, BDS, MS[b]

KEYWORDS

- Metastasis • Head & neck cancer • Distant carcinomas
- Infraclavicular carcinomas

"When you hear hoof beats, think horses, not zebras."

Cancer is a very complex and devastating disease in which basic cell processes are deregulated. Experts have proposed that a malignant tumor is the manifestation of six essential alterations in cell physiology: self-sufficiency in growth signals, insensitivity to growth–inhibitory signals, evasion of programmed cell death (apoptosis), limitless replicative potential, sustained angiogenesis, and tissue invasion and metastasis.[1] The American Cancer Society[2] estimates that 1.4 million new cancer cases and 565 000 deaths from cancer will occur in the United States in 2008 (**Table 1**). Lung cancer followed by breast cancer in women, and prostate cancer in men are the leading causes of cancer-related death (**Table 2**).[3] Despite improvements in early diagnosis, surgical techniques, patient care, and adjuvant therapies, the establishment of distant metastasis is still the most significant turning point in cancer. Patients who have distant metastasis can no longer be cured with local therapy alone and will likely succumb to injury caused by dissemination of the disease (**Table 3**).

Metastatic lesions to the head and neck are rare entities. These lesions are often the first sign of systemic disease, but are generally a sign of widespread systemic disease and poor outcome. This article discusses the general process of metastasis and describes the signs and symptoms of distant carcinomas (infraclavicular) to the oral and maxillofacial region.

METASTATIC PROCESS

The metastatic cascade is an intricate sequence of events necessary to produce a clinically relevant lesion (**Fig. 1**). To effectively spread to a distant site, a cancer cell must complete all steps of the cascade; failure to complete any step results in failure to colonize and proliferate.[4,5] Conventional wisdom assumed that invasion and metastasis are late events. However, current knowledge shows that both events can be early and clinically dormant.[6]

The first step within the metastatic cascade is the development of invasive behavior by the primary tumor cells. Cancer cells will progressively show alterations in cell-to-cell and cell-to-extracellular matrix interactions, leading to initiation of motility. This process drives the tumor cells to trespass the basal lamina and invade the adjacent tissues.[7] Experimental evidence shows that pathophysiologic conditions in the tumor microenvironment, such as low oxygen tension (hypoxia), low glucose concentrations, high lactate concentrations, low extracellular pH (acidity), and high interstitial fluid pressure, play an important role in tumor progression.[8]

Another prerequisite for tumor outgrowth is angiogenesis. Studies have also established that tumor growth beyond 1 to -2 mm depends on angiogenesis.[9] These new blood vessels not only provide the nutrients necessary for tumor growth but also establish an escape route for tumor cells to abandon the primary site and penetrate

---

[a] Division of Oral & Maxillofacial Surgery, Department of Surgery, University of Florida, Health Science Center, 653-1 West 8th Street, Jacksonville, FL 32209, USA
[b] Department of Oral and Maxillofacial Surgery, MSC 7908, University of Texas Health Science Center, 7703 Floyd Curl Drive, San Antonio, TX 78229, USA
* Corresponding author.
E-mail address: luis.vega@jax.ufl.edu (L.G. Vega).

Oral Maxillofacial Surg Clin N Am 20 (2008) 609–623
doi:10.1016/j.coms.2008.06.003
1042-3699/08/$ – see front matter © 2008 Elsevier Inc. All rights reserved.

Table 1
Incidence between primary site and gender of estimated new cancer cases in the United States in 2008

Male		Female	
Prostate	25%	Breast	26%
Lungs	15%	Lungs	14%
Colorectal	10%	Colorectal	10%
Bladder	7%	Uterine corpus	6%
Non-Hodgkin lymphoma	5%	Non-Hodgkin lymphoma	4%
Melanoma	5%	Thyroid	4%
Kidney	4%	Melanoma	4%
Oral cavity and pharynx	3%	Ovary	3%
Leukemia	3%	Kidney	3%
Pancreas	3%	Leukemia	3%

Data from Jemal A, Siegel R, Ward E, et al. Cancer statistics, 2008. CA Cancer J Clin 2008;58(2):71–96.

the circulatory system, a process known as *intravasation*.

Tumor cells might also enter the circulation indirectly through the lymphatic system.[10] Once in the circulatory system, the ability to resist hemodynamic forces or destruction by the immune system dictates the initial fate of the metastatic cells. Blood flow patterns from the primary tumor determine which organ the cells travel to first.[10,11] Tumor cells will travel until they reach a capillary bed and either adhere to the vessel walls or arrest because of size constraints.

Metastatic cells exit the circulatory vessels in a process called *extravasation*. Colonization occurs soon after. Tumor cells must overpower a hostile environment at the distant site to form micrometastases. Hence, only a small proportion of these micrometastases will reach a detectable clinical size after neovascularization of the lesion occurs. Studies have shown that even after successful formation of micrometastasis, macroscopic tumors may not develop because of dormancy.[12] The nature of dormancy is still under investigation. However, genetic or environmental influences might shunt cells out of dormancy into a state of proliferation in which metastatic colonization arises.

Fortunately, the development of metastasis is an extremely inefficient process. Studies have shown that only 0.01% to 0.1% of cancer cells in circulation actually will generate macrometastasis.[11,13] Studies have also shown that apoptosis is the primary contributor to metastatic inefficiency.[14,15] Apoptotic resistance is critical at several

Table 2
Incidence between primary site and gender in estimated cancer deaths in the United States in 2008

Male		Female	
Lungs	31%	Lungs	26%
Prostate	10%	Breast	15%
Colorectal	8%	Colorectal	9%
Pancreas	6%	Ovary	6%
Liver	4%	Pancreas	6%
Leukemia	4%	Non-Hodgkin lymphoma	3%
Esophagus	4%	Leukemia	3%
Bladder	3%	Uterine corpus	3%
Non-Hodgkin lymphoma	3%	Liver	2%
Kidney	3%	Brain	2%

Data from Jemal A, Siegel R, Ward E, et al. Cancer statistics, 2008. CA Cancer J Clin 2008;58(2):71–96.

Table 3
Survival rate from metastatic cancer

Cancer Type	5-Year Survival Rate
Testis	70.0%
Prostate	31.9%
Ovary	29.8%
Breast	26.7%
Uterine corpus	23.1%
Uterine cervix	16.5%
Melanoma	15.3%
Colon and rectum	10.3%
Kidney	9.5%
Urinary bladder	6.4%
Stomach	3.4%
Lung and bronchus	3.0%
Esophagus	2.9%
Liver	2.8%
Pancreas	1.7%

Data from Ries L, Melbert D, Krapcho M, et al. SEER Cancer Statistics Review, 1975–2004, National Cancer Institute. Bethesda, MD. Available at: http://seer.cancer.gov/csr/1975–2004. Accessed July 11, 2008.

metastatic steps, but perhaps the most important stage is resistance to cell death induced by loss of cell-to-cell and cell-to-extracellular matrix contact.

METASTASES TO THE BONE

Metastasis is not a random event. Organ microenvironment is extremely influential in cancer cell metastasis to a specific location.[10,16–18] Bone is the most common location affected by metastatic cancer.[19] Bone is attractive as a primary site for metastasis because of the ability of cancer cells to enter and exit well-vascularized areas of metabolically active bone. Within these areas, normal bone remodeling provides chemotactic and growth factors that attract and support cancer cells. This "vicious cycle" persists when tumor cells control the activity of osteoblasts and osteoclasts to their advantage. Because the bone matrix releases cytokines, the chemoattraction and survival of metastatic cancer cells continue.[20–22] Simply stated, bone metastasis can be characterized either as an osteolytic (breast cancer, myeloma) or osteoblastic lesion (prostate cancer). The consequences of bone metastasis are usually detrimental. Patients present with severe bone pain, hypercalcemia, pathologic fractures, and spinal cord compression.

Sabino and colleagues[23] suggested that bone pain from cancer may be caused by prohyperalgesic factors, such as prostaglandins and endothelins released by the cancer cell that activate nociceptors in the bone marrow. As the tumor grows, sensory neurons involved in the innervation of the marrow are compressed and destroyed, causing neuropathic pain.

Bone metastases occurs in up to 70% of patients who have advanced breast or prostate cancer and 15% to 30% of those who have carcinoma of the lung, colon, stomach, bladder, uterus, rectum, thyroid, or kidney.[21]

Of great clinical importance to oral and maxillofacial surgeons is the fact that bisphosphonates are essential in the treatment regimen of patients who have bone metastases. The reduced incidence and delayed onset of skeletal-related events with the administration of bisphosphonates are well documented.[24,25] In addition to the inhibitory effects on osteoclast-mediated osteolysis,

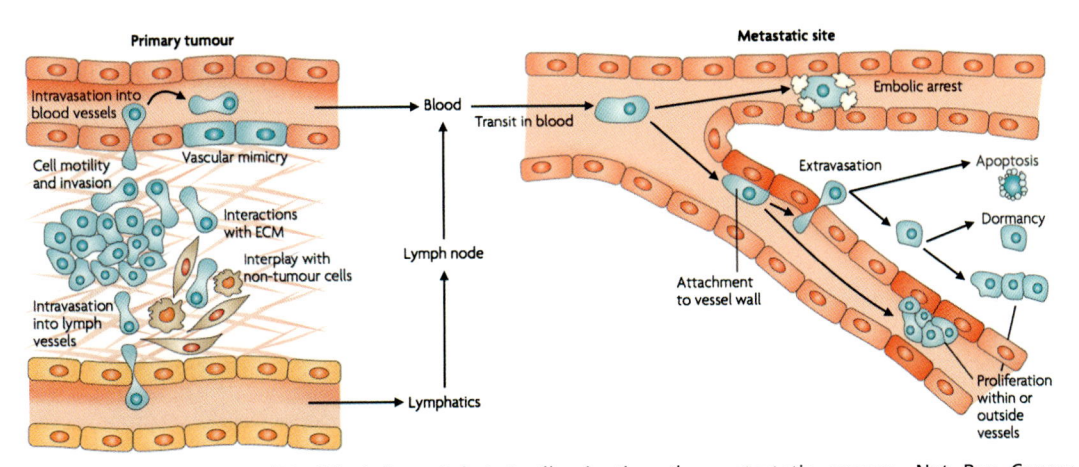

Fig. 1. Metastatic process. (*Modified from* Sahai E. Illuminating the metastatic process. Nat Rev Cancer 2007;7(10):737–49; with permission.)

preliminary studies showed other therapeutic benefits of bisphosphonates, such as inhibition of new blood vessel formation, inhibition of cell invasion by decreasing cell motility and migration, stimulation of specific subset of immune cells, and direct antitumor effect by inhibition of tumor growth.[26]

HEAD AND NECK MANIFESTATIONS OF DISTANT CARCINOMAS

Metastatic lesions to the head and neck are very rare; most oral and maxillofacial surgeons would not see one in their lifetime. When describing metastatic disease to the head and neck, it is better to separate these lesions by location because they have distinct findings. Symptoms vary depending on the location of the metastasis and site of primary cancer.

Metastases to the Oral Region

Metastatic lesions from distant carcinomas to the oral region account for 1% of all oral malignancies.[27,28] Most lesions are found in patients between the fifth and seventh decades of life.[29] Although most metastatic lesions to the head and neck are carcinomas, sarcomas have been reported in the literature.[30]

Diagnosing metastatic lesions from distant carcinomas is challenging for clinicians and pathologists. Several primary intraoral malignancies have similar histologic features to tumors occurring in distant organs. For instance, primary squamous cell carcinoma is difficult to distinguish from metastatic squamous cell carcinoma from the lung, as is distinguishing intraosseous clear cell carcinoma from metastatic renal cell carcinoma.[29]

The criteria for considering a lesion as a metastatic tumor from a distant carcinoma has been established in the literature:[31,32]

- A histologically verified primary tumor must be present
- The secondary lesion must be histologically identical to the primary tumor
- The neoplasm does not occupy a site where primary tumors of oral origin typically arise
- The histopathologic appearance is distinct from that of a typical malignancy of oral origin

Diagnostic algorithms for evaluating patients who have metastasis to the oral region have been described[28,33] and include

- Reviewing clinical history
- Obtaining slides and reports if history of a previous malignant tumor exists
- Reviewing all radiographic material
- Performing a biopsy
- Evaluating the light microscopic feature of the neoplasm and, based on the histologic features, determining the need for special studies, such as immunohistochemistry, histochemical stains, and electron microscopy
- Planning the treatment protocol based on the clinical, pathologic, and radiographic information

In approximately one third of the cases, metastatic lesions were reported as the first sign of systemic disease, initiating pursuit of the primary site.[28,34]

Metastases to the Jaws

It is well established in the literature that metastatic lesions from distant carcinomas affect the jaws more often than the oral soft tissues in a ratio of 2:1. Because the jaws do not contain a lymphatic system, experts believe that metastasis occurs by way of the blood stream. The Batson's vertebral venous plexus has been mentioned as a possible route of metastasis to the head and neck region, explaining why the lungs are not involved in some cases.[27]

The mandible has been identified as the site of predilection, accounting for approximately 80% of cases, with the molar region most frequently involved. In the largest literature review of metastatic lesions to the jaws, Hirshberg and colleagues[29] identified 455 cases of jaw metastasis. Overall, the most common primary metastatic tumor was breast, accounting for 20% of cases, followed by lung (13%), kidney (8%), adrenal (8%), bone (7%), colorectal (6%), prostate (5%), and liver (5%) (**Fig. 2**). The distribution between gender and primary site can be seen in **Table 4**.

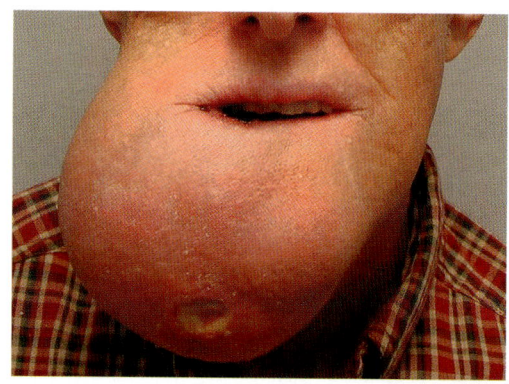

Fig. 2. Metastatic esophageal neuroendocrine tumor to the mandible. (*Courtesy of* Jon Holmes, DMD, MD, FACS, Birmingham, Alabama.)

Table 4
Incidence between primary site and gender for metastatic lesions to the jaw

Male (n = 227)		Female (n = 220)	
Lungs	22.0%	Breast	41.0%
Prostate	11.0%	Adrenal	7.7%
Kidney	9.3%	Genital organs	7.7%
Liver	9.3%	Colorectal	7.3%
Bone	8.8%	Kidney	6.8%
Adrenal	8.3%	Thyroid	6.8%
Colorectal	4.4%	Bone	5.9%
Testes	4.4%	Eye	4.0%
Bladder	3.1%	Lung	3.2%
Esophagus	3.1%	Skin	3.2%
Skin	3.1%	Brain	3.2%
Eye	3.1%	Stomach	0.9%
Thyroid	1.8%	Bladder	0.9%
Stomach	1.8%	Liver	0.5%
Others	6.5%	Others	0.9%

Data from Hirshberg A, Shnaiderman-Shapiro A, Kaplan I, et al. Metastatic tumors to the oral cavity—pathogenesis and analysis of 673 cases. Oral Oncol 2008;44(8):743–52.

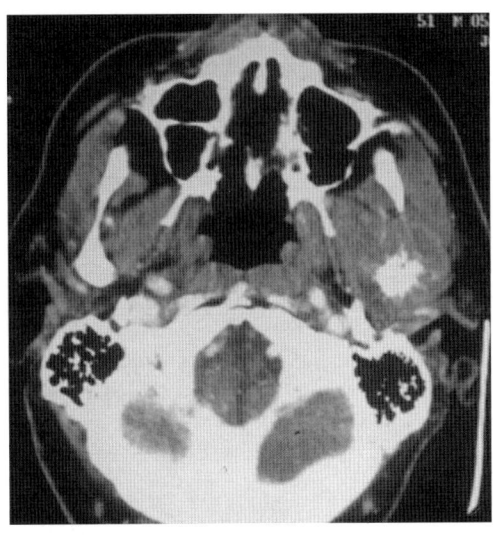

Fig. 3. Metastatic prostate cancer to the mandibular condyle. (*Courtesy of* Jon Holmes, DMD, MD, FACS, Birmingham, Alabama.)

In a review of the Korean literature by Lim and colleagues,[35] lung followed by liver were the most common primary cancers metastasizing to the mandible. The high incidence of hepatocellular carcinoma in Korean population may account for this discrepancy.

Even when the gender distribution is almost the same, D'Silva and colleagues[36] reported that young women exhibited greater incidence of metastases than men in the same age group. However, older men exhibited a significantly greater incidence of metastases than women of the same age group. This shift is mostly likely a reflection of the incidence of breast cancer in younger women, whereas lung carcinomas occur later in life in men.

Interesting cases of bilateral temporomandibular joint involvement from breast cancer and male breast cancer metastasis to the mandible have been reported in the literature.[37,38] In 2005, Kaufmann and colleagues[39] reviewed 23 cases of metastatic lesions to the mandibular condyle. Breast cancer (8 cases) was the most common, followed by lung (6), prostate (2), liver (2), rectum (2), and others (3) (**Fig. 3**).

Pain is the most common symptom in metastatic bone disease.[20] Rapidly progressing swelling, paresthesia, and increasing tooth mobility are other common complaints in patients who have metastatic lesions to the jaws.[40,41] Patients will often present with delayed healing of an extraction socket, pathologic fracture, trismus, masticatory difficulties, and symptoms mimicking temporomandibular joint dysfunction.[35] Of clinical importance is the presence of sensory deficit in areas innervated by the mental nerve, a condition called *mental neuropathy* or *numb chin syndrome*.[42] Mental neuropathy, in the absence of benign origin, represents progression of malignant disease with very poor prognosis.[43]

In most cases, radiographic findings of bony metastatic lesions show a lytic radiolucent lesion with ill-defined margins ("moth-eaten" appearance). Occasionally, lesions present as a pure or mixed radiopacity. Root resorption and widening of the periodontal ligament that might resemble periodontal disease have also been described. In approximately 5% of the cases, radiographs showed no pathologic changes. Although not specific, bone scintigraphy is the most sensitive imaging study for detecting early-stage metabolic alterations caused by cancer in bone.[40]

Survival depends on the nature of the primary lesion. Treatment should focus on improving quality of life. Radiotherapy usually decreases pain and prevents loss of function; radiation has been reported to be the preferred treatment in metastases to the mandible in children.[44] Local resection and chemotherapy have also been used for local control and palliation, but the overall prognosis is poor, with patients surviving less than a year.[27,29,34]

Metastases to Soft Tissues of the Oral Cavity

Metastases to soft tissues of the oral cavity are less common than their counterparts in the jaws. Men are more affected than women in a ratio of 2:1. A review of cases reported that 54% of the 218 metastatic oral soft tissue lesions occurred on the attached gingiva, followed by 22% on the tongue.[29] The role of inflammation in the attraction of metastatic cells toward the attached gingival has been suggested.[28] Lung cancer (25%) was the primary site most commonly involved, followed by kidney (13%), skin (11%), and breast (9%). The distribution between gender and primary site can be seen in **Table 5**.

Clinically, gingival metastases present as a polypoid or exophytic lesion that is highly vascularized and resembles a benign lesion. They are hyperplastic or reactive in nature, much like pyogenic granuloma, peripheral giant cell granuloma, and peripheral ossifying fibroma.[28] Curien and colleagues[45] suggested that malignancy must be suspected when a lesion of the gingiva has a fast evolution, a hemorrhagic tendency, and an ulcerated or necrotic aspect, and based on the general clinical context of the patient. In other parts of the mouth, the most common clinical presentation is a submucosal mass.[46] Several cases of severe hemorrhage have been reported, especially with metastatic lesions of renal cell and hepatocellular carcinoma.[47,48]

As with metastatic lesions to the jaws, prognosis is poor for patients who have metastatic lesions to the oral soft tissue. Treatment efforts are based on disease stage. Local excision, radiation, and chemotherapy are available modalities for local control and palliation.

Metastases to the Eye, Orbit, and Ocular Adnexa

When discussing metastatic tumors to the orbital region, ocular and orbital lesions must be distinguished because of their different incidence and symptomatology.

Ocular metastases

Metastatic ocular tumors are not uncommon; in fact, metastatic tumors to the eye are considered the most common intraocular tumors.[49,50] Reports estimate that metastatic tumors to the globe are more frequent than metastasis to the bony orbit in a ratio of 8:1.[51] Several studies[50,52,53] have tried to identify the incidence of ocular metastasis, but the true incidence has been difficult to estimate, because subclinical disease is frequently unnoticed.[54,55]

It is well established that the uveal tract is the area where most metastatic cancer to the ocular region occurs, with the choroid the most commonly involved site.[49,52,56,57] Choroidal metastases represent the smallest in vivo detectable metastatic lesion. Lesions as small as 1 to 2 mm may produce noticeable functional deficits that can be detected directly with funduscopic examination.[56] Metastasis to the iris, optical disc, and ciliary body are rare, accounting for only 9%, 5%, and 2%, respectively.[49,58]

Practically any cancer that can metastasize through the hematogenous route could gain access to the eye and orbital region. The literature speculates that lymphatic spread is not a route for metastases to the orbit because of its lack of lymphatic channels.[59] However, other reviews described the existence of lymphatics in the lacrimal gland and optic nerve sheath, shedding new light on possible metastatic mechanisms.[60]

In a review of 520 eyes with uveal metastasis in 420 consecutive patients, Shields and colleagues[49] reported that the primary site of malignancy was breast in 47%, lung in 21%, gastrointestinal tract in 4%, kidney in 2%, skin in 2%, and prostate in 2%, and unknown primaries in 17%.

Clinically, patients who have ocular metastasis have clinical complaints of blurring vision, scotomata, metamorphopsia, photopsia, floaters, and pain. Approximately 7% to 14% of patients are

Table 5
Incidence between primary site and gender of metastatic lesions to oral soft tissues

Male (n = 134)		Female (n = 74)	
Lungs	31.3%	Breast	24.3%
Kidney	14.0%	Genital organs	14.9%
Skin	12.0%	Kidney	12.2%
Liver	7.4%	Lung	9.5%
Bone	5.2%	Bone	9.5%
Colorectal	5.2%	Colorectal	6.8%
Esophagus	4.5%	Skin	6.8%
Testes	4.5%	Stomach	4.1%
Stomach	3.7%	Bladder	1.3%
Prostate	1.6%	Liver	1.3%
Bladder	1.6%	Esophagus	1.3%
Breast	1.6%	Brain	1.3%
Thyroid	0.7%	Thyroid	1.3%
Eye	0.7%	Eye	1.3%
Others	6.0%	Others	4.1%

Data from Hirshberg A, Shnaiderman-Shapiro A, Kaplan I, et al. Metastatic tumors to the oral cavity—pathogenesis and analysis of 673 cases. Oral Oncol 2008;44(8):743–52.

asymptomatic at diagnosis.[49,54–57] When no signs of systemic disease are encountered, radiation therapy is effective in reducing or stabilizing the ophthalmic symptoms and size of the lesions. In cases involving systemic disease, chemotherapy or hormone therapy help control ocular metastasis. Metastasis to the vitreous and retina has been reported but are rare.[61,62]

Cancer- and melanoma-associated retinopathy are paraneoplastic syndromes. They are described as manifestations of distant carcinomas in which antibodies directed against tumor antigen cross-react with retinal cells, resulting in visual disturbances. Ocular toxicity can also develop from chemotherapeutic agents during cancer treatment. This potential side effect may have similar clinical presentations to metastatic tumors.[63]

Orbital metastases

Orbital metastases are uncommon. The literature speculates that factors such as an increased median survival of cancer patients and improvement in diagnostic techniques account for the increased incidence of metastatic tumors to the orbit.[64,65] The incidence metastatic tumors to the orbit is estimated to range from 2% to 4.7%.[65] In a review of 1264 patients who had orbital tumors, Shields and colleagues[66] showed a 7% incidence of orbital metastatic tumors.

Orbital metastases are predominantly a condition of adulthood. With increasing age, orbital tumors become more common.[66,67] Orbital metastasis is rare in children. Neuroblastoma and, less commonly, Ewing's sarcoma are the most common orbital metastasis in the pediatric population.[68]

Breast cancer has been established as the primary source of orbital metastasis, with an incidence of 28% to 58%, followed by lung carcinoma (8%–12%), prostate cancer (3%–10%), melanoma (5%–15%), and carcinoid tumors (4%–5%).[59,65,66,69] In Japan, gastrointestinal cancer is a common cause of metastasis to the orbit.[70]

The clinical findings of metastatic tumors to the orbit are well established. They typically manifest one of five clinical presentations: mass, infiltrative, inflammatory, functional, or silent.[64,65] Patients usually complain of limited ocular motility; proptosis; blepharoptosis; palpable or visible mass; blurred or decreased vision; diplopia; and pain. The distinguishing feature of orbital metastases is a progressive course with combined ocular motor and sensory deficits. Cases of enophthalmus have been associated with metastasis in patients who have scirrhous breast cancer.[65,71]

As in any other disease process, a thorough history and clinical examinations are the clinician's most important diagnostic tools. CT scan and MRI are essential aids for diagnosing orbital metastasis. Ultimately, definitive diagnosis of an orbital tumor requires tissue analysis, with fine-needle aspirations and open biopsy the preferred techniques. In cases of widespread cancer, an orbital biopsy is not necessary, because diagnosis can be made based on other findings.

Radiation, chemotherapy, surgical resection, and orbital exenteration are available options for treating orbital metastatic lesions. Treatment modality is selected based on disease stage, extent of orbital involvement, and clinical symptoms. External beam radiation is the most commonly used treatment in orbital metastasis because of its ability to stabilize visual loss, and when used palliatively can improve quality of life with relative low morbidity.[51,59,65,67,72] Patients who have orbital metastasis have a poor prognosis, with long-term survival rare. However, survival up to 10 years has been reported.[72]

Metastases to ocular adnexa

Extraocular muscles Metastases to the extraocular muscles are also rare, and most literature consists of case reports. In the largest literature review from 1864 to 1990, Capone and Slamovits[73] were able to identify 29 cases of extraocular muscles metastasis. Diplopia caused by impaired ocular motility, visual loss, proptosis, and pain were the most common symptoms. Breast cancer was the primary site responsible for 55% of the cases, followed by cutaneous melanoma in 21%. Primary carcinomas of the lungs and gastrointestinal tract have also been reported.[73–76] Reports show the medial (39%) and lateral (33%) recti muscles to be most commonly involved compared with the superior (16%) and inferior (12%) recti muscles. Bilateral muscle involvement was seen in 17% of cases. Similar to other metastatic lesions to the region, tissue diagnosis and palliative radiation seem to be preferred treatments.

Conjunctiva Metastatic tumors to the conjunctiva are rare and are usually not mentioned in literature reviews on ocular metastasis. The bulbar portion of the conjunctiva is the most commonly affected area. Breast cancer, lung cancer, and cutaneous melanoma are the most common primary sites of origin. Most cases reported have been treated with excisional biopsy and radiation.[77,78] Chemotherapy has been used when breast carcinoma was involved.[79]

Eyelid Metastatic lesions to the eyelid represent fewer than 1% of malignant lesions to the area. Mansour[80] reported 49 cases from the Armed Forces Institute of Pathology and reviewed an additional 88 cases from the literature. The most commonly involved primary site was breast (47%), followed by carcinomas of the gastrointestinal tract (12%), lung cancer (7%), melanoma (9%), and urogenital (6%). Approximately 10% were lesions from an unknown primary.

Metastatic lesions to the eyelid from hepatocellular and renal cell carcinoma are extremely rare but have been reported,[81,82] and typically affect patients in the fifth to eighth decades of life. Women are affected more often than men in a ratio of 3:1. This finding could be attributed to the high incidence of breast cancer in women.[80,83] The three most common presentations of eyelid metastasis are a painless nodule, diffuse swelling, or an ulcerated lid.[80,84] Lesions can affect any eyelid, and cases of involvement of all four eyelids have been reported.[85] Surgical excision is the preferred treatment.

Lacrimal gland Only isolated case reports of metastatic lesions to the lacrimal gland have been reported, involving only two instances of carcinoid and two of renal carcinoma.[86] The clinical presentation of these lesions is a mass underneath the upper eyelid that produces a slight proptosis, with downward and nasal displacement of the globe.

Nasolacrimal system A literature review on nasolacrimal system metastatic tumors found three case reports involving cutaneous melanoma, renal cell carcinoma, and hepatocellular carcinoma.[87–89] The clinical presentation of these tumors is a mass in the area, inducing epiphora and mimicking dacryocystitis.

Metastases to Nasal Cavity and Paranasal Sinuses

Metastases to the nasal cavity and paranasal sinuses are uncommon. The highest incidence has been observed in the fifth to sixth decades in men and sixth to seventh decades in women.[90] They are more frequent in men than women in a ratio of 2:1.[91]

The clinical presentation of the metastatic paranasal sinus tumor is similar to that of primary tumors in the same location. Headaches, facial pain, refractory symptoms of sinusitis, and neurologic symptoms secondary to cranial nerve involvement are the most common findings.[92] In the nasal cavity, recurrent epistaxis without history of trauma and nasal obstruction are the most common presenting symptoms. Long-standing nasal and paranasal sinus tumors can extend into the orbital region, resulting in ophthalmic symptoms.[93]

In a review of the literature on metastatic tumors to the paranasal sinuses, Prescher and Brors[94] identified 169 cases, with the maxillary sinus the most commonly affected (33%), followed by sphenoid sinus (22%), ethmoidal sinus (14%), and frontal sinus (9%). In the remaining 22% of cases, two or more sinuses were involved. They also found that renal cell carcinoma (40%) was the most common tumor affecting the paranasal sinuses, which several other studies have confirmed.[93,95,96] The next common primary was lung carcinoma (9%), followed by breast cancer (8%), thyroid cancer (7%), prostate cancer (7%), testicular cancer (5%), and liver cancer (4%). Other lesions originating from the gastrointestinal or genitourinary system have also been described.[91,97,98]

Patients who have single resectable lesions can be treated aggressively.[96] Palliative surgery could be considered for debulking residual disease. Local symptomatic control with radiotherapy is excellent.[92,93]

Metastases to the Ear and Temporal Bone

Metastases to the ear and temporal bone are rare. The literature has suggested that metastasis from distant carcinomas to the temporal bone occurs through hematogenous spread that seeds in the marrow spaces of the petrous bone, or by way of cancer cells in the cerebrospinal fluid that disseminate through the meninges and seed in the internal auditory canal.[99,100]

Gloria-Cruz and colleagues[100] found 47 cases of metastases to temporal bones from autopsy reports of 212 patients who had primary nondisseminated malignant neoplasms. Gender distribution showed a slight male predominance. The average age corresponded to the age at which most primary cancers have their onset, which is the fifth to seventh decades of life.

In a literature review from 1902 to 1994, Streitman and colleagues[99] identified 141 cases of temporal bone metastasis. The most common primary malignancies to metastasize to the temporal bone were breast (24.8%), lung (11.3%), kidney (9.2%), stomach (6.4%), and prostate (5.7%). Approximately 11.3% of lesions were from unidentified primary carcinomas. The petrous portion of the temporal bone was the part most commonly involved (36.5%), followed by the internal auditory canal (17.5%), mastoid area (9.5%), external auditory canal (8.7%), middle ear (4%), and squamous portion (0.8%). Multiple sites of invasion occurred in 23.9% of the cases.

The optic capsule and membranous labyrinth are relatively resistant to metastatic involvement because of their poor vascularity. Thus, vestibular signs and symptoms are less frequent than otologic symptoms.[100] Facial nerve paralysis is the most common clinical manifestation. Other usual presentations include sudden or progressive hearing loss, tinnitus, vertigo, otalgia, otorrhea, and mass in the external canal. Between approximately 30% and 36% of patients had no otologic or vestibular manifestations.

In addition to a thorough history and clinical examination, temporal bone imaging is of paramount importance in diagnosing metastatic lesion to the temporal bone. CT scan helps visualize bony lesions, and MRI should be obtained when internal auditory canal lesions are suspected.

Tumor-specific palliative treatment with radiation or chemotherapy or both might relieve the otologic symptoms. General prognosis is poor.

Metastases to Salivary Glands

Metastatic lesions to the salivary glands represent 8% of all salivary gland malignancies.[101] The literature distinguishes two general types of metastases to the salivary glands: metastatic tumors originating from head and neck region, and metastatic tumors from distant carcinomas. Reports estimate that 80% of metastatic lesions to salivary glands are from the head and neck region. Squamous cell carcinoma and melanoma are the most common primary tumors.[102–105]

Three major patterns of metastasis to the salivary glands have been identified: (1) direct invasion by tumor adjacent to the salivary glands, (2) hematogenous metastases to the parenchyma of the salivary gland, and (3) lymphatic metastases to salivary gland lymph nodes.

Histopathologic diagnosis of metastatic lesions to salivary glands is sometimes challenging. A thorough medical history is the key factor in distinguishing between metastatic salivary gland neoplasms and primary salivary gland neoplasms when histopathologic features are similar.

Metastases to the Parotid Gland

Approximately 80% of metastatic lesions to salivary glands affect the parotid gland.[102] It is well established that metastatic lesions to the parotid gland can manifest as lesions either within the parenchyma of the gland itself or in intraglandular or extraglandular parotid lymph nodes. Experts believe, that secondary to the intricate and rich web of lymphatics in the area, skin malignancies of the scalp and face, especially carcinomas and melanomas, are the most common malignancies associated with metastatic lesions to the parotid gland. Metastatic parotid gland tumors from distant carcinomas are rare.

In a literature review, Pisani and colleagues[103] identified 866 cases of metastatic lesions to the parotid gland, with distant carcinomas representing only 11% of the lesions. Renal cell carcinoma (37%) represented the most common primary site, followed by lung (27%), breast (16%), and prostate cancer (9%) and gastrointestinal tract carcinomas (9%). The literature also contains rare cases of parotid gland metastasis from hepatocellular carcinomas and cases of renal cell carcinoma 10 years after nephrectomy.[106,107]

The most common presenting complaint is a painless mass within the parotid area. Occasionally, fast development of the lesion, pain, and facial weakness are also found. A pulsatile mass with a bruit has been associated with metastasis from renal cell carcinomas.[108] Bilateral parotid gland metastasis has also been reported.[109]

Masses involving the parotid gland should not undergo open biopsy; instead, fine-needle aspiration cytology should be performed to aid diagnosis. Imaging techniques are also valuable to diagnosis. MRI provides the best delineation of soft tissue planes and extension of the tumor into surrounding tissue. Although CT scan with contrast does not provide the same level of soft tissue detail as MRI, imaging is adequate for formulating a treatment plan.[110] Ultrasonography may also be used, but operator experience greatly influences the usefulness of the technique. Moreover, the findings of ultrasonography are not specific. Horii and colleagues[111] found that the combination of fine-needle aspiration cytology, prior history of malignancy, and enhanced MRI had a sensitivity of 100% in diagnosing metastatic parotid tumors.

Surgery is considered the preferred treatment, followed by radiotherapy. Whether to perform a superficial or total parotidectomy with an additional neck dissection remains controversial.[101,103] Furthermore, studies have shown that radical parotidectomy for treating metastasis of melanoma or squamous cell carcinoma does not increase life expectancy and decreases quality of life because of facial paralysis.[112]

As in other cases of head and neck metastasis from distant carcinomas, when salivary gland metastasis is just one focus of a multifocal metastatic disease, prognosis is extremely poor. The salivary gland metastatic lesion is rarely the only metastatic focus. In these cases, cure may be possible by controlling the primary tumor and the salivary metastatic tumor.

Metastases to the Submandibular Gland

Metastatic lesions to the submandibular gland are less common than metastasis to the parotid gland.

When metastases do occur, the lesions are mostly from distant carcinomas, unlike those to the parotid gland. This difference is believed to be caused by the lack of an intricate lymphatic system associated with the submandibular gland.[113]

In a review of 108 patients who had metastatic lesions to salivary glands, Seifert and colleagues[102] reported 33 cases (31%) of submandibular gland involvement, with 10 cases (30%) from distant carcinomas. Further literature review by these authors identified 8 additional cases of metastatic tumors to the submandibular gland. Lung cancer is the most common primary site, followed by renal carcinoma, gastrointestinal tract cancer, and breast cancer. Like the parotid gland, cases of late metastasis to the submandibular gland from renal cell carcinomas 10 years after radical nephrectomy have also been reported.[114]

The most common clinical presentation of metastatic lesions to the submandibular gland is a submandibular gland mass or swelling that is usually painless. Although rare, cases of bilateral submandibular gland metastases have been reported.[113,115]

As with metastatic lesions of the parotid gland, fine-needle aspiration cytology, and MRI, and CT scan with contrast are valuable for diagnosis.

Gland excision has been identified in the literature as the preferred treatment, but radiation or chemotherapy are also good adjuvant therapies.

Metastases to the Sublingual Gland and Minor Salivary Glands

At the time of this writing, no reports of metastatic lesions from distant carcinomas to the sublingual or minor salivary glands exist in the English literature.

Metastases to the Neck

Because of their anatomic proximity, metastatic lesions to the upper and middle neck are typically attributed to primary tumors from the head and neck region.[116,117]

Traditionally, metastatic lesions to the lower neck were associated with primaries from distant carcinomas.[118] In a review of 168 patients who had lymph node metastases of the lower neck, Giridharan and colleagues[119] identified an equal incidence of infraclavicular and head and neck primary tumors.

Metastatic lesions to the neck from infraclavicular cancers are routinely described as metastatic lesions to the supraclavicular region, with no clear localization of the cervical lymph node metastases.[120]

Hess and colleagues[121] identified 320 patients who had supraclavicular lymph node involvement. Breast was the most common primary site (51%), followed by lung (29%), kidney (6%), prostate (3%), colon (3%), ovary (2%), stomach (2%), esophagus (2%), and pancreas (2%) (**Fig. 4**).

Patients generally complain of a painless isolated neck mass, and less commonly of multiple ipsilateral masses or bilateral neck masses. A hard, enlarged, left supraclavicular node indicates the possibility of a metastatic lesion from an infraclavicular primary. This left supraclavicular node is the classical Virchow's node. Because most of the body's lymphatic drainage enters the venous circulation through the left subclavian vein, many tumors tend to metastasize in this region.[122]

Extensive literature on cervical node metastases is dedicated to cancer from unknown primary tumors. Cervical node metastases from an unknown primary deserve special consideration because of the therapeutic challenge; controversy persists when discussing the biology of the unknown primary tumor, optimal diagnostic algorithm, and best treatment.[123,124]

Approximately 3% to 5% of patients who have head and neck cancer will present with cervical metastases from an unknown primary.[125] Studies have identified the most frequent

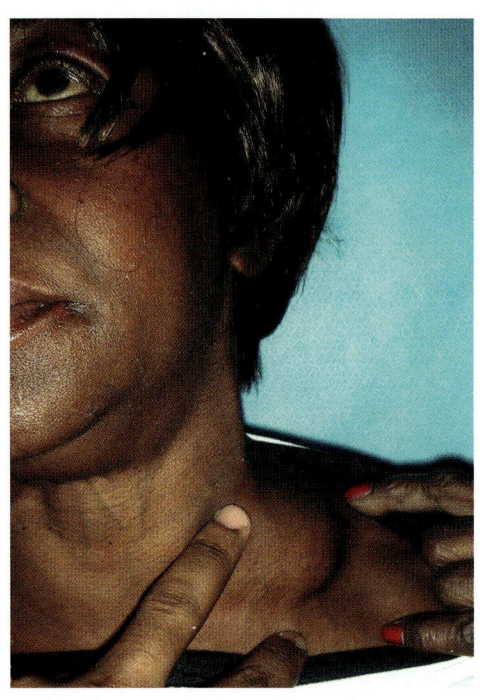

Fig. 4. Metastatic supraclavicular lesion from lung cancer. (*Courtesy of* Rui Fernandes, DMD, MD, FACS, Jacksonville, Florida.)

histopathologic diagnosis to be squamous cell carcinoma (65%–76%), followed by undifferentiated carcinoma (14%–22%) and adenocarcinoma (13%).[123,126,127] The primary tumor is eventually found in 10% to 40% of patients who have cervical node metastases of an unknown primary.

Head and neck primary tumors, especially from the larynx and pharynx, account for approximately 70% of all primary tumors detected.[126,127] When the tumors detected are infraclavicular, lung cancer is most commonly involved, followed by gastrointestinal and genitourinary.[125]

Diagnosis of cervical lymphadenopathy of an unknown primary is a complex process. Several authors have reviewed the approach to evaluating patients who have cancer of an unknown primary.[124,127,128]

Patients who have cervical metastasis from an unknown primary have a reasonable prognosis, resembling that of those who have a known primary tumor at the same N stage.[123] Histopathology, site of nodal metastasis, and the most likely site of the primary tumor must govern treatment.[129]

Metastases to Head and Neck Skin

Cutaneous metastases from distant carcinomas are uncommon. The estimated incidence rates range from 0.7% to 9%. In a meta-analysis including 20,380 cancer cases, Krathen and colleagues[130] reported a 5.3% overall incidence of metastatic skin lesions. Neck skin lesions accounted for 11% of the lesions, follow by 7% scalp lesions and 5% facial lesions (**Fig. 5**). Breast cancer has been reported as the most common primary tumor to metastasize to skin, followed by renal, ovarian, lung, colorectal, bladder, and prostate.

Cutaneous metastatic lesions from distant carcinomas have no specific clinical appearance. Patient can present with a solitary lesion or multiple skin lesions. Lesions have been described as painless or painful nodules or patches that vary from flesh-colored to pink or violaceous. Nonnodular metastatic lesions also have been reported. Cutaneous horns and pyogenic granuloma-like lesions have been described in connection with renal cell carcinoma.[131] Cicatricial alopecia has been described in metastases from breast cancer and gastric carcinomas.[132] A high index of suspicion is necessary, because cutaneous metastases can be mistaken for other common skin lesions.[131]

Patients who have cutaneous metastasis have a poor prognosis, with half succumbing to the disease within 6 months of diagnosis. Patients who have cutaneous metastasis from lung carcinoma have the poorest prognosis.[133]

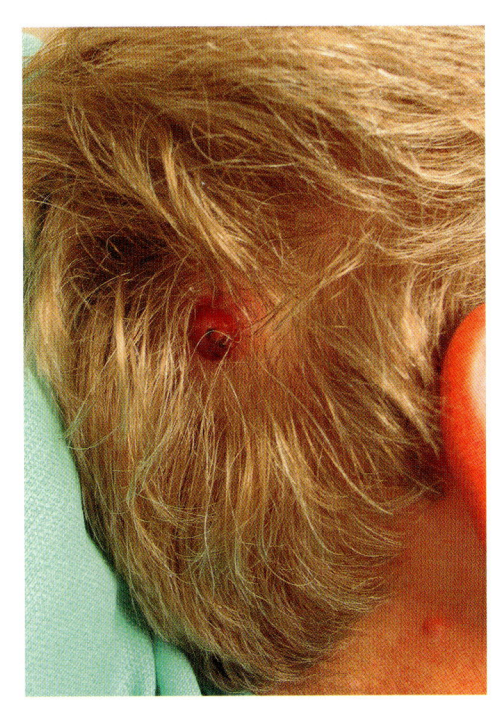

Fig. 5. Metastatic scalp lesion from renal cell carcinoma. (*Courtesy of* Jon Holmes, DMD, MD, FACS, Birmingham, Alabama.)

SUMMARY

Metastatic tumors to the head and neck from distant carcinomas are rare lesions that epitomize the "zebras." They represent a diagnostic and therapeutic challenge for clinicians and health providers. These lesions usually rank low in the differential diagnosis list, but a history of cancer should prompt clinicians about the possibility of a metastatic lesion from a distant carcinoma.

The presence of these lesions usually represents a poor prognosis. The surgeon's role in treating these lesions is to improve or maintain the patient's quality of life, taking into consideration the overall prognosis.

REFERENCES

1. Hanahan D, Weinberg R. The hallmarks of cancer. Cell 2000;100(1):57–70.
2. American Cancer Society. Cancer Facts & Figures 2008. Atlanta: American Cancer Society; 2008;72.
3. Jemal A, Siegel R, Ward E, et al. Cancer statistics, 2008. CA Cancer J Clin 2008;58(2):71–96.
4. Fidler I. Critical factors in the biology of human cancer metastasis: twenty-eighth G.H.A. Clowes memorial award lecture. Cancer Res 1990;50(19):6130–8.

5. Fidler I. Critical determinants of metastasis. Semin Cancer Biol 2002;12(2):89–96.
6. Wittekind C, Neid M. Cancer invasion and metastasis. Oncology 2005;69(Suppl 1):14–6.
7. Liotta L, Stetler-Stevenson W. Tumor invasion and metastasis: an imbalance of positive and negative regulation. Cancer Res 1991;51(Suppl 18): 5054s–9s.
8. Maseide K, Kalliomaki T, Hill R. Microenvironmental effects on tumour progression and metastasis. In: Meadows G, editor. Integration/Interaction of oncologic growth. 1st edition. (Cancer growth and progression, vol. 15). Netherlands: Springer; 2005. p. 1–22.
9. Zetter B. Angiogenesis and tumor metastasis. Annu Rev Med 1998;49:407–24.
10. Chambers A, Groom A, MacDonald I. Dissemination and growth of cancer cells in metastatic sites. Nat Rev Cancer 2002;2(8):563–72.
11. Luzzi K, MacDonald I, Schmidt E, et al. Multistep nature of metastatic inefficiency: dormancy of solitary cells after successful extravasation and limited survival of early micrometastases. Am J Pathol 1998;15(3):865–73.
12. Naumov G, MacDonald I, Chambers A, et al. Solitary cancer cells as a possible source of tumour dormancy? Semin Cancer Biol 2001;11(4):271–6.
13. Sahai E. Illuminating the metastatic process. Nat Rev Cancer 2007;10:737–49.
14. Horak C, Bronder J, Bouadis A, et al. Metastasis. The evasion of apoptosis. In: Srivastava R, editor. Apoptosis, cell signaling, and human diseases. 1st edition. (Molecular mechanisms, vol. 1). Totowa (NJ): Humana Press; 2007. p. 63–96.
15. Mehlen P, Puisieux A. Metastasis: a question of life or death. Nat Rev Cancer 2006;6(6):449–58.
16. Fidler I. The organ microenvironment and cancer metastasis. Differentiation 2002;70(9–10):498–505.
17. Leong S, Cady B, Jablons D, et al. Clinical patterns of metastasis. Cancer Metastasis Rev 2006;25(2): 221–32.
18. Fokas E, Engenhart-Cabillic R, Danillidis K, et al. Metastasis: the seed and soil theory gains identity. Cancer Metastasis Rev 2007;26(3–4):705–15.
19. Coleman R. Metastatic bone disease: clinical features, pathophysiology and treatment strategies. Cancer Treat Rev 2001;27:165–76.
20. Mundy G. Metastasis to bone: causes, consequences and therapeutic opportunities. Nat Rev Cancer 2002;2(8):584–93.
21. Roodman G. Mechanisms of bone metastasis. N Engl J Med 2004;350(16):655–64.
22. Bussard K, Gay C, Mastro A. The bone microenvironment in metastasis; what is special about bone? Cancer Metastasis Rev 2008;27(1):41–55.
23. Sabino M, Mantyh P. Pathophysiology of bone cancer pain. J Support Oncol 2005;3(1):15–24.
24. Costa L. Bisphosphonates: reducing the risk of skeletal complications from bone metastasis. Breast 2007;16(Suppl 3):S16–20.
25. Saad F. New research findings on zoledronic acid: survival, pain, and anti-tumour effects. Cancer Treat Rev 2008;34:183–92.
26. Coleman R. On the horizon: can bisphosphonates prevent bone metastases? Breast 2007;16(Suppl 3): S21–27.
27. Zachariades N. Neoplasms metastatic to the mouth, jaws and surrounding tissues. J Craniomaxillofac Surg 1989;17(6):283–90.
28. Hirshberg A, Buchner A. Metastatic tumours to the oral region. An overview. Eur J Cancer B Oral Oncol 1995;31B(6):355–60.
29. Hirshberg A, Schnaiderman-Shapiro A, Kaplan I, et al. Metastatic tumours to the oral cavity - pathogenesis and analysis of 673 cases. Oral Oncol 2008;44(8):743–52.
30. Chen Y, Chen C, Lin L. Soft-tissue metastasis of osteosarcoma to the submental vestibule. Int J Oral Maxillofac Surg 2006;35(11):1068–71.
31. Fukuda M, Miyata M, Okabe K, et al. A case series of 9 tumors metastatic to the oral and maxillofacial region. J Oral Maxillofac Surg 2002;60(8):942–4.
32. Bodner L, Sion-Vardy N, Geffen D, et al. Metastatic tumors to the jaws: a report of eight new cases. Med Oral Patol Oral Cir Bucal 2006; 11(2):E132–5.
33. Whitaker B, Robinson K, Hewan-Lowe K, et al. Thyroid metastasis to the oral soft tissues: case report of a diagnostic dilemma. J Oral Maxillofac Surg 1993;51(5):588–93.
34. Sánchez Aniceto G, García Peñín A, de la Mata Pages R, et al. Tumors metastatic to the mandible: analysis of nine cases and review of the literature. J Oral Maxillofac Surg 1990;48(3):246–51.
35. Lim S, Kim S, Ahn H, et al. Metastatic tumours to the jaws and oral soft tissues: a retrospective analysis of 41 Korean patients. Int J Oral Maxillofac Sur 2006;35(5):412–5.
36. D'Silva N, Summerlin D, Cordell K, et al. Metastatic tumors in the jaws: a retrospective study of 114 cases. J Am Dent Assoc 2006;137(12):1667–72.
37. Miles B, Schwartz-Dabney C, Sinn D, et al. Bilateral metastatic breast adenocarcinoma within the temporomandibular joint: a case report. J Oral Maxillofac Surg 2006;64(4):712–8.
38. Fontana S, Ghilardi R, Barbaglio A, et al. Male breast cancer with mandibular metastasis. A case report. Minerva Stomatol 2007;56(4):225–30.
39. Kaufmann M, Perren A, Grätz K, et al. Condylar metastasis. Review of the literature and report of a case. Mund Kiefer Gesichtschir 2005;9(5): 336–40.
40. Glaser C, Lang S, Pruckmayer M, et al. Clinical manifestations and diagnostic approach to

40. metastatic cancer of the mandible. Int J Oral Maxillofac Sur 1997;26(5):365–8.
41. Pruckmayer M, Glaser C, Marosi C, et al. Mandibular pain as the leading clinical symptom for metastatic disease: nine cases and review of the literature. Ann Oncol 1998;9(5):559–64.
42. Laurencet F, Anchisi S, Tullen E, et al. Mental neuropathy: report of five cases and review of the literature. Crit Rev Oncol Hematol 2000;34(1):71–9.
43. Sanchis J, Bagán J, Murrilo J, et al. Mental neuropathy as a manifestation associated with malignant processes: its significance in relation to patient survival. J Oral Maxillofac Surg 2008;66(5):995–8.
44. Deutsch M, Wollman M. Radiotherapy for metastases to the mandible in children. J Oral Maxillofac Surg 2002;60(3):269–71.
45. Curien R, Moizan H, Gerard E, et al. Gingival metastasis of a bronchogenic adenocarcinoma: report of a case. Oral Surg Oral Med Oral Pathol 2007; 104(6):e25–8.
46. Tomita T, Inouye T, Shiden S, et al. Palliative radiotherapy for lingual metastasis of renal cell carcinoma. Auris Nasus Larynx 1998;25(2):209–14.
47. Jayasooriya P, Gunarathna I, Attygalla A, et al. Metastatic renal cell carcinoma presenting as a clear cell tumour in the head and neck region. Oral Oncology EXTRA 2004;40:50–3.
48. Pires F, Sagarra R, Pizzigati M, et al. Oral metastasis of a hepatocellular carcinoma. Oral Surg Oral Med Oral Pathol 2004;97(3):359–68.
49. Shields C, Shields J, Gross N, et al. Survey of 520 eyes with uveal metastases. Ophthalmology 1997; 104(8):1265–76.
50. Kreusel K, Bechrakis N, Krause L, et al. Incidence and clinical characteristics of symptomatic choroidal metastasis from breast cancer. Acta Ophthalmol Scand 2007;85(3):298–302.
51. Char D, Miller T, Kroll S. Orbital metastases: diagnosis and course. Br J Ophthalmol 1997;81(5): 386–90.
52. Weiss L. Analysis of the incidence of intraocular metastasis. Br J Ophthalmol 1993;77(3):149–51.
53. Kreusel K, Bechrakis N, Wiegel T, et al. Incidence and clinical characteristics of symptomatic choroidal metastasis from lung cancer. Acta Ophthalmol 2008;86(5):515–9.
54. Wickremasinghe S, Dansingani K, Tranos P, et al. Ocular presentations of breast cancer. Acta Ophthalmol Scand 2007;85(2):133–42.
55. Su H, Chen Y, Perng R. Symptomatic ocular metastases in lung cancer. Respirology 2008;13(2): 303–5.
56. Merrill C, Kaufman D, Dimitrov N. Breast cancer metastatic to the eye is a common entity. Cancer 1991;68(3):623–7.
57. Soysal H. Metastatic tumors of the uvea in 38 eyes. Can J Ophthalmol 2007;42(6):832–5.
58. Shields J, Shields C, Singh A. Metastatic neoplasms in the optic disc: the 1999 Bjerrum lecture: part 2. Arch Ophthalmol 2000;118(2):217–24.
59. Holland D, Maune S, Kovács G, et al. Metastatic tumors of the orbit: a retrospective study. Orbit 2003;22(1):15–24.
60. Dickinson A, Gausas R. Orbital lymphatics: do they exist? Eye 2006;20(10):1145–8.
61. Zaldivar R, Michels M, Grant K, et al. Metastatic breast carcinoma to the vitreous. Retina 2004; 24(2):226–30.
62. Leys A, Van Eyck L, Nuttin B, et al. Metastatic carcinoma to the retina. Clinicopathologic findings in two cases. Arch Ophthalmol 1990;108(10): 1448–52.
63. Solomon S, Hasenyager-Smith J, O'Brien J, et al. Ocular manifestations of systemic malignancies. Curr Opin Ophthalmol 1999;10(6):447–51.
64. Toller K, Gigantelli J, Spalding J. Bilateral orbital metastases from breast carcinoma. A case of false pseudotumor. Ophthalmology 1998;105(10): 1897–901.
65. Ahmad S, Esmaeli B. Metastatic tumors of the orbit and ocular adnexa. Curr Opin Ophthalmol 2007; 18(5):405–13.
66. Shields J, Shields C, Scartozzi R. Survey of 1264 patients with orbital tumors and simulating lesions: the 2002 Montgomery lecture, part 1. Ophthalmology 2004;111(5):997–1008.
67. Demirci H, Shields C, Shields J, et al. Orbital tumors in the older adult population. Ophthalmology 2002;109(2):243–8.
68. Castillo B, Kaufman L. Pediatric tumors of the eye and orbit. Pediatr Clin North Am 2003;50(1): 149–72.
69. Mehta J, Abou-Rayyah Y, Rose G. Orbital carcinoid metastases. Ophthalmology 2006;113(3): 466–72.
70. Amemiya T, Hayashida H, Dake Y. Metastatic orbital tumors in Japan: a review of the literature. Ophthalmic Epidemiol 2002;9(1):35–47.
71. Shields J, Shields C, Brotman H, et al. Cancer metastatic to the orbit: the 2000 Robert M. Curts lecture. Ophthal Plast Reconstr Surg 2001;17(5): 346–54.
72. Mohadjer Y, Holds J. Orbital metastasis as the initial finding of breast carcinoma: a ten-year survival. Ophthal Plast Reconstr Surg 2005;21(1):65–6.
73. Capone A, Slamovits T. Discrete metastasis of solid tumors to extraocular muscles. Arch Ophthalmol 1990;108(2):237–43.
74. Lacey B, Chang W, Rootman J. Nonthyroid causes of extraocular muscle disease. Surv Ophthalmol 1999;44(3):187–213.
75. Couch D, O'Halloran H, Hainsworth K. Carcinoid metastasis to extraocular muscles: case reports and review of the literature. Orbit 2000;19(4):263–9.

76. Lekse J, Zhang J, Mawn L. Metastatic gastroesophageal junction adenocarcinoma to the extraocular muscles. Ophthalmology 2003;110(2):318–21.
77. Kiratli H, Shields C, Shields J, et al. Metastatic tumours to the conjunctiva: report of 10 cases. Br J Ophthalmol 1996;80(1):5–8.
78. Shields C, Demirci H, Karatza E, et al. Clinical survey of 1643 melanocytic and nonmelanocytic conjunctival tumors. Ophthalmology 2004;111(9):1747–54.
79. Skalicky S, Hirst L, Conway R. Metastatic breast carcinoma presenting as a conjunctival lesion. Clin Experiment Ophthalmol 2007;35(8):767–9.
80. Mansour A. Metastatic eyelid disease in 49 cases. Orbit 1988;7(4):245–8.
81. Tailor R, Inkster C, Hanson I, et al. Metastatic renal cell carcinoma presenting as a chalazion. Eye 2007;21(4):564–5.
82. Yeung S, Blicker J, Buffam F, et al. Metastatic eyelid disease associated with hepatocellular carcinoma. Can J Ophthalmol 2007;42(5):752–4.
83. Claessens N, Piérard G. The eyelids and metastatic breast carcinoma. Dermatology 2003;206(2):181–2.
84. Ahamed R, Ram R, Shannon J, et al. Eyelid metastasis from lung carcinoma. Clin Experiment Ophthalmol 2006;34(6):609–10.
85. Douglas R, Goldstein S, Einhorn E, et al. Metastatic breast cancer to 4 eyelids: a clinicopathologic report. Cutis 2002;70(5):291–3.
86. Shields J, Shields C, Eagle R, et al. Metastatic renal cell carcinoma to the palpebral lobe of the lacrimal gland. Ophthal Plast Reconstr Surg 2001;17(3):191–4.
87. Economides N, Page R. Metastatic melanoma of the lacrimal sac. Ann Plast Surg 1985;15(3):244–6.
88. Vozmediano-Serrano M, Toledano-Fernández N, Fernández-Aceñero M, et al. Lacrimal sac metastases from renal cell carcinoma. Orbit 2006;25(3):249–51.
89. Wladis E, Frempong T, Gausas R. Nasolacrimal metastasis from heptocellular carcinoma masquerading as dacryocystitis. Ophthal Plast Reconstr Surg 2007;23(4):333–5.
90. Izquierdo J, Armengot M, Cors R, et al. Hepatocarcinoma: metastasis to the nose and paranasal sinuses. Otolaryngol Head Neck Surg 2000;122(6):932–3.
91. Torrico Román P, Mogollón Cano-Cortés T, López-Ríos Velasco J, et al. Bladder transitional cell carcinoma with metastasis to the maxillary sinus as first symptom. Acta Otorrinolaringol Esp 2001;52(7):622–4.
92. Jiménez Oliver V, Lazarich Valdés A, Dávila Morillo A, et al. Frontal ethmoid metastases of prostatic carcinoma. Report of one case and review of the literature. Acta Otorrinolaringol Esp 2001;52(2):151–4.
93. Simo R, Sykes A, Hargreaves S, et al. Metastatic renal cell carcinoma to the nose and paranasal sinuses. Head Neck 2000;22(7):722–7.
94. Prescher A, Brors D. Metastases to the paranasal sinuses: case report and review of the literature. Laryngorhinootologie 2001;80(10):583–94.
95. Traserra J, Morello G, Traserra-Coderch J. Metastasis of systemic origin in otorhinolaryngology. Rev Neurol 2001;31(12):1265–7.
96. Lee H, Kang H, Lee S. Metastatic renal cell carcinoma presenting as epistaxis. Eur Arch Otorhinolaryngol 2005;262(1):69–71.
97. Molina Ruiz del Portal J, Anaya F, Solis E, et al. Transitional cell carcinoma metastasizing to the sphenoid sinus. Acta Otorrinolaringol Esp 2006;57(2):118–20.
98. Tanaka K. A case of metastases to the paranasal sinus from rectal mucinous adenocarcinoma. Int J Clin Oncol 2006;11(1):64–5.
99. Streitmann M, Sismanis A. Metastatic carcinoma of the temporal bone. Am J Otol 1996;17(5):780–3.
100. Gloria-Cruz T, Schachern P, Paparella M, et al. Metastases to temporal bones from primary nonsystemic malignant neoplasms. Arch Otolaryngol Head Neck Surg 2000;126(2):209–14.
101. Pomar Blanco P, Martín Villares C, San Román Carbajo J, et al. Metastasis to the parotid gland. Acta Otorrinolaringol Esp 2006;57(1):47–50.
102. Seifert G, Hennings K, Caselitz J. Metastatic tumors to the parotid and submandibular glands–analysis and differential diagnosis of 108 cases. Pathol Res Pract 1986;181(6):684–92.
103. Pisani P, Krengli M, Ramponi A, et al. Metastases to parotid gland from cancers of the upper airway and digestive tract. Br J Oral Maxillofac Surg 1998;36(1):54–7.
104. Andreadis D, Poulopoulos A, Nomikos A, et al. Diagnosis of metastatic malignant melanoma in parotid gland. Oral Oncology Extra 2006;42:17–39.
105. Nuyens M, Schüpbach J, Stauffer E, et al. Metastatic disease to the parotid gland. Otolaryngol Head Neck Surg 2006;135(6):844–8.
106. Romanas M, Cherian R, McGregor D, et al. Hepatocellular carcinoma diagnosed by fine-needle aspiration of the parotid gland. Diagn Cytopathol 2004;30(6):401–5.
107. Göğüş C, Kiliç O, Tulunay O, et al. Solitary metastasis of renal cell carcinoma to the parotid gland 10 years after radical nephrectomy. Int J Urol 2004;11(10):894–6.
108. Park Y, Hlivko T. Parotid gland metastasis from renal cell carcinoma. Laryngoscope 2002;112(3):453–6.
109. Garcia Cantera J, Verrier Hernandez A. Bilateral parotid gland metastasis as the initial presentation of a small cell lung carcinoma. J Oral Maxillofac Surg 1989;47(11):1199–201.

110. Malata C, Camilleri I, McLean N, et al. Metastatic tumours of the parotid gland. Br J Oral Maxillofac Surg 1998;36(3):190–5.
111. Horii A, Yoshida J, Honjo Y, et al. Pre-operative assessment of metastatic parotid tumors. Auris Nasus Larynx 1998;25(3):277–83.
112. Jecker P, Hartwein J. Metastasis to the parotid gland: is a radical surgical approach justified? Am J Otolaryngol 1996;17(2):102–5.
113. Cain A, Goodlad J, Denholm S. Metachronous bilateral submandibular gland metastases from carcinoma of the breast. J Laryngol Otol 2001;115(8):683–4.
114. Moudouni S, Tligui M, Doublet J, et al. Late metastasis of renal cell carcinoma to the submaxillary gland 10 years after radical nephrectomy. Int J Urol 2006;13(4):431–2.
115. Böckmann R, Shulz T, Stein H, et al. Bilateral synchronous submandibular lumps in a patient with gastric carcinoma. J Oral Pathol Med 2005;34(2):127–8.
116. Clark S, Sanderson R, McLaren K, et al. Metastatic prostatic carcinoma presenting as cervical lymphadenopathy. J Oral Maxillofac Surg 2001;59(5):571–3.
117. Jereczek-Fossa B, Jassem J, Orecchia R. Cervical lymph node metastases of squamous cell carcinoma from an unknown primary. Cancer Treat Rev 2004;30(2):153–64.
118. Ellison E, Lapuerta P, Martin S. Supraclavicular masses: results of a series of 309 cases biopsied by fine needle aspiration. Head Neck 1999;21(3):239–46.
119. Giridharan W, Hughes J, Fenton J, et al. Lymph node metastases in the lower neck. Clin Otolaryngol 2003;28(3):221–6.
120. Sesterhenn A, Albert U, Barth P, et al. The status of neck node metastases in breast cancer-loco-regional or distant? Breast 2006;15(2):181–6.
121. Hess K, Varadhachary G, Taylor S, et al. Metastatic patterns in adenocarcinoma. Cancer 2006;106(7):1624–33.
122. Hematpour K, Bennett C, Rogers D, et al. Supraclavicular lymph node: incidence of unsuspected metastatic prostate cancer. Eur Arch Otorhinolaryngol 2006;263(9):872–4.
123. Boscolo-Rizzo P, Gava A, Da Mosto M, et al. Carcinoma metastatic to cervical lymph nodes from an occult primary tumor: the outcome after combined-modality therapy. Ann Surg Oncol 2007;14(5):1575–82.
124. Mahoney E, Spegel J. Evaluation and management of malignant cervical lymphadenopathy with an unknown primary tumor. Otolaryngol Clin North Am 2005;38(1):87–97.
125. Donta T, Smoker W. Head and neck cancer: carcinoma of unknown primary. Top Magn Reson Imaging 2007;18(4):281–92.
126. Koivunen P, Laranne J, Viraniem J. Cervical metastasis of unknown origin: a series of 72 patients. Acta Otolaryngol 2002;122(5):569–74.
127. Issing W, Taleban B, Tauber S. Diagnosis and management of carcinoma of unknown primary in the head and neck. Eur Arch Otorhinolaryngol 2003;260(8):436–43.
128. Chorost M, Lee C, Yeoh C, et al. Unknown primary. J Surg Oncol 2004;87(4):191–203.
129. Yalin Y, Pingzhang T, Smith G, et al. Management and outcome of cervical lymph node metastases of unknown primary sites: a retrospective study. Br J Oral Maxillofac Surg 2002;40(6):484–7.
130. Krathen R, Orengo I, Rosen T. Cutaneous metastasis: a meta-analysis of data. South Med J 2003;96(2):164–7.
131. Lim C, Chan R, Regan W. Renal cell carcinoma with cutaneous metastases. Australas J Dermatol 2005;46(3):158–60.
132. Chung J, Namiki T, Johnson W. Cervical cancer metastasis to the scalp presenting as alopecia neoplastica. Int J Dermatol 2007;46(2):188–9.
133. Schoenlaub P, Sarraux A, Grosshans E, et al. Survival after cutaneous metastasis: a study of 200 cases. Ann Dermatol Venereol 2001;128(12):1310–5.

Gastrointestinal Illnesses and Their Effects on the Oral Cavity

Michaell A. Huber, DDS

KEYWORDS
- Reflux disorders
- Gastrointestinal polyposis syndromes
- Inflammatory bowel disease

Anatomically and functionally, the oral cavity represents the beginning of the gastrointestinal (GI) tract. Many disease processes affecting the GI tract may cause observable changes to the oral cavity. In fact, oral cavity changes for which the patient may seek a dental assessment may represent the first clinical manifestation of an underlying GI condition. The astute oral health care provider's recognition and appropriate referral of a possible GI condition contribute to the patient's overall health and wellness. Some of the more important GI conditions that may manifest oral cavity involvement are: reflux disorders, inherited GI polyposis syndromes, and inflammatory bowel disease (IBD). This article briefly reviews the aforementioned topics.

REFLUX DISORDERS

Virtually everyone experiences gastroesophageal reflux (GER) at some time or another, such as after an overindulgent meal.[1,2] This frequently occurring phenomena serves to help relief stomach distention, is short-lived, and not pathologic. Episodes of excessive or extensive GER, however, can damage the tissues of the aerodigestive tract. The etiopathogenesis of reflux disorders is complex and involves interplay of esophageal sphincter function, epithelial tissue sensitivity, and exposure time.[3] Signs and symptoms of reflux localized to the esophagus are termed gastroesophageal reflux disease (GERD), a condition thought to affect 15% to 40% of the population.[4,5] Complications attributed to untreated GERD include reflux esophagitis, esophageal hemorrhage, stricture, Barrett's esophagus, and adenocarcinoma.[2,6]

Manifestations of reflux-induced damage to the laryngopharynx include asthma, cough, hoarseness, globus, dysphagia, throat clearing, sore throat, postnasal drip, earache, and sinusitis.[1–4,7–13] Some authorities consider the laryngopharyngeal involvement of reflux as a distinct entity termed laryngopharyngeal reflux (LPR).[1,2,8] They note the numerous discordant characteristics between GERD and LPR to justify the distinction. Most cases of LPR do not manifest esophageal symptoms or involvement; LPR reflux typically occurs during the day while standing, while GERD reflux typically occurs nocturnally while supine. Traditional therapies for GERD often do not improve LPR. Others, however, dispute these distinctions and consider LPR a protean manifestation of GERD.[3,12] While further study is necessary to define the true relationship of LPR and GERD, the clinical fact is reflux patients experiencing GERD symptoms are likely to seek or be referred for care by a gastroenterologist, while reflux patients experiencing LPR symptoms are likely to seek or be referred for care by an otolaryngologist.[1]

Oral Cavity Features of Reflux Disorders

Potential oral cavity manifestations of reflux include a burning or itching sensation affecting the oral mucosa, mouth ulcers, erosion of tooth structure, halitosis, altered salivary flow, and bad taste.[4,7,10,14–17] Aside from tooth erosion, none of

Division of Oral Medicine, Department of Dental Diagnostic Science, University of Texas Health Science Center, Mail Code 7919, 7703 Floyd Curl Drive, San Antonio, TX 78229-3900, USA
E-mail address: huberm@uthscsa.edu

these findings are specific for reflux. The tooth erosion observed in reflux is characterized as affecting the palatal surfaces of the maxillary teeth first, then the occlusal surfaces of the posterior teeth of both arches, and lastly the lingual surfaces of the mandibular anterior teeth.[18] The teeth typically exhibit a smooth, glazed, dished out appearance of the dentin.[15,16] Affected teeth may become sensitive to thermal insult and prone to fracture. Eventually, the progressive loss in vertical dimension of occlusion may lead to pulp exposure, impaired chewing function, and phonetic disturbances.

Diagnosis of Reflux Disorders

Aside from typical heartburn, most of the presenting signs and symptoms of reflux are nonspecific. In most cases, the diagnosis is established by using a therapeutic trial of a gastric acid inhibitor.[9] Cases responsive to therapy are considered positive for reflux. Various tests, such as endoscopy, laryngoscopy, radiologic studies, and various GI studies may be necessary to diagnose equivocal cases. Conditions to consider in the differential diagnosis for reflux disorders include cardiac disease, biliary tract disease, obstruction, esophageal or gastric cancer, gastroparesis, infectious esophagitis, nonsteroidal anti-inflammatory drug-related gastritis, and peptic ulcer disease.[19]

The presence of the characteristic tooth erosion associated with reflux often is recognized easily by the dental practitioner and warrants referral for medical evaluation. Other conditions to consider as causing tooth erosion include chronic vomiting, eating disorders (bulimia and anorexia), chronic gastritis, and dietary habits.[16] These conditions also warrant a referral for further medical assessment.

Management of Reflux Disorders

Reflux management is usually multifaceted and tailored to address the signs and symptoms of the individual patient. Patients may be advised to:

- Avoid alcohol, caffeine, chocolate, peppermint, fatty foods
- Avoid acidic foods such as citrus, pineapple, and tomatoes
- Avoid spicy foods such as hot sauce, curry, barbecue sauce, hot mustards
- Eat smaller meals throughout the day
- Avoid lying down within 3 hours of eating
- Avoid exercise, bending over, or heavy lifting for several hours after eating
- Take prescribed medications as directed

Products that reduce esophageal sphincter tone or irritate damaged mucosal tissues should be avoided.[9] Although both H2 receptor antagonists (H2RAs) and proton pump inhibitors (PPIs) are superior to placebo, PPIs are more effective than H2RAs.[20] Reflux patients refractory to medical therapy may benefit from surgical interventions to control their disease.[9]

There are no specific limitations on providing dental care for the reflux patient. Both PPIs and H2RAs are associated with numerous drug interactions, and PPIs may cause dry mouth. The reflux patient should be advised to avoid eating a large meal before undergoing dental care and may not tolerate being placed in a fully supine position. The restorative management of reflux-induced tooth erosion should be attempted only after the underlying reflux condition is controlled.[15,16,18]

INHERITED GASTROINTESTINAL POLYPOSIS SYNDROMES

Inherited GI polyposis syndromes represent a diverse group of inherited syndromes often associated with an increased risk for developing colorectal cancer (CRC), in addition to various extraintestinal cancers.[21] Collectively, these syndromes are estimated to account for 1% to 5% of all cases of CRC.[21,22] They traditionally have been classified according to the predominant type of polyp involved (adenomatous or hamartomatous) and their characteristic clinical stigmata, summarized in **Table 1**.[21–24] Adenomatous syndromes occur at 10 times the rate of hamartomatous syndromes.[24] As four of these conditions—Gardner syndrome (GS), tuberous sclerosis (TS), Peutz-Jeghers syndrome (PJS), and Cowden syndrome (CS)—have characteristic orofacial features, they will be discussed in greater detail.

Gardner Syndrome

GS is a well-recognized variant of familial adenomatous polyposis (FAP) and is characterized by the presence of colonic polyposis, osteomas, and numerous soft tissue tumors.[25–28] FAP and its variants predominantly are caused by mutations to the adenomatous polyposis coli (APC) tumor suppressor gene, located on chromosome 5q21. FAP is a highly penetrant autosomal dominant disorder, occurring in an estimated 1 out of 8000 to 1 out of 18,000 live births.[22,29] The occurrence of classical GS is far less frequent and estimated at about 1 in 1,000,000 live births.[25,26]

In addition to the obligatory polyposis, patients who have GS manifest various extraintestinal lesions such as osteomas, epidermoid cysts,

Table 1
Inherited gastrointestinal polyposis syndromes

Syndrome (Susceptibility Gene)	Characteristic Features	Colorectal Cancer (CRC) Risk
Adenomatous type		
Familial adenomatous polyposis (FAP) (APC)	Hundreds to thousands of adenomas throughout the large intestine; congenital pigment of the retinal epithelium; increased incidence of small intestine polyps; increased hepatoblastoma, thyroid cancer, and brain tumor risk	100%
FAP variant phenotypes		
Attenuated FAP	<100 adenomas; more proximal location in colon; delayed CRC risk compared with FAP	69%
Gardner syndrome	FAP plus osteomas, dental abnormalities, multiple skin and soft tissue tumors	100%
Turcot's syndrome	FAP plus central nervous system (CNS) tumors (medulloblastoma, anaplastic astrocytoma, ependymomas)	100%
MYH-associated polyposis (MUTYH)	Similar to attenuated FAP	Unknown
Hamartomatous type		
Familial juvenile polyposis (SMAD4 or BMPR1A)	Multiple hamartomatous polyps of colorectum, occult gastrointestinal (GI) bleeding, chronic bleeding, anemia, hypoproteinemia	20%–60%
Peutz-Jeghers syndrome (*STK11*)	Orofacial melanosis and multiple hamartomatous polyps of small intestine	39%
Cowden syndrome (*PTEN*)	Benign hamartomatous polyps throughout the GI tract, facial tricholemmomas, acral keratosis, oral fibromas, increased breast and thyroid cancer risk	Normal
Bannayan-Riley-Ruvalcaba syndrome (*PTEN*)	Benign hamartomatous polyps throughout the GI tract, microcephaly, lipomas, pigmented penile macules	Normal
Tuberous sclerosis (TSC1, TSC2)	Benign hamartomatous polyps of distal colon and rectum, cutaneous hamartomas, mental retardation, seizure disorders	Normal

Data from Bronner MP. Gastrointestinal polyposis syndromes. Am J Med Genet A 2003;122(4):335–41.
Galiatsatos P, Foulkes WD. Familial adenomatous polyposis. Am J Gastroenterol 2006;101(2):385–98.
Schreibman IR, Baker M, Amos C, et al. The hamartomatous polyposis syndromes: a clinical and molecular review. Am J Gastroenterol 2005;100(2):476–90.
Schulmann K, Pox C, Tannapfel A, et al. The patient with multiple intestinal polyps. Best Pract Res Clin Gastroenterol 2007;21(3):409–26.

desmoid tumors, and numerous dental disorders (odontomas, impacted teeth, supernumerary teeth).[26] Other reported lesions include lipomas, fibromas, and leiomyomas.[22] Most extraintestinal manifestations of GS develop about 10 years before the onset of polyposis.

The osteomas observed in GS may be endosteal or periosteal and most frequently affect the skull and mandible.[30] Most present as bony hard asymptomatic swellings, but tenderness on palpation and interference with function may occur.[28] The presence of three or more osteomas is considered highly suggestive of GS.[26,28,31] The epidermoid cysts often affect the head and neck region and typically present at an early age.[22] Desmoid tumors usually develop after surgical interventions and most commonly occur in the abdominal cavity or retroperitoneum. They are difficult to treat and may become life-threatening through their propensity to extend against or obstruct vital organs and structures.[32] Wijn and colleagues recently published a review of the common dental anomalies observed in FAP/GS (**Table 2**).[28]

The prevalent head and neck manifestations of GS place the dental professional in a unique position to recognize the characteristic findings and initiate a prompt medical referral.[30,31,33] This is especially important for sporadic new cases, in which a family history is absent. The diagnosis of GS is confirmed through endoscopic or genetic testing.[28] First-degree relatives of index patients should undergo annual endoscopic examination beginning at age 10 to 12 years.[21] Contemporary medical strategies to manage GS entail surgical interventions to remove at-risk intestinal tissue. The current gold standard is proctocolectomy with ileal-pouch-anal anastomosis, followed by regular endoscopic assessment of the pouch and remaining upper GI tract.[21] The osteomas associated with GS typically require no treatment, unless they either interfere with normal function or are deemed cosmetically unacceptable.

Tuberous Sclerosis

TS is an autosomal-dominant syndrome characterized by hamartomatous lesions of the brain, heart, lungs, kidneys, and skin.[34] The incidence of TS is approximately 1:10,000, with two thirds of the cases arising sporadically.[35] Most cases are caused by mutations to the tumor suppressor genes TSC1 or TSC2, located at chromosomes 9q34 and 16p13.3, respectively.[35,36] Although the risk of developing cancer in TS appears normal, the patient who has TS is at risk for developing several potentially serious conditions affecting the brain (cortical tubers), kidneys (angiomyolipomas), lungs (lymphangioleiomyomatoses), and heart (rhabdomyomas).[37] Eighty five percent of patients who have TS experience epilepsy at some point, and other commonly observed neurologic concerns include behavioral problems, mental retardation, and learning disabilities.[36]

The most recent diagnostic criteria for TS were published in 1998.[38] The presence of two major criteria, or one major criterion plus two minor criteria is considered diagnostic for TS. Major dermatologic criteria are:

1. Facial angiofibromas or forehead plaques
2. Nontraumatic ungual or periungual fibromas
3. Hypomelanotic macules (more than three)
4. Shagreen patch

Readily visible minor criteria are multiple dental enamel pits, gingival fibromas, and confetti-like macules.[38]

| Table 2 |
| Dental findings in familial adenomatous polyposis and Gardner syndrome |

Finding	Frequency %	Feature
Odontomas	9.4–83.3	Mandible and maxilla equally affected, usually located incisal premolar area; may be multiple
Supernumerary teeth	11–27	Usually small, peg-shaped, and present in alveolar bone between teeth; most prevalent in anterior region of jaw; often associated with impacted teeth
Impacted teeth	4–38	Often associated with coexistent odontoma or supernumerary teeth; canines frequently affected

Data from Wijn MA, Keller JJ, Giardiello FM, et al. Oral and maxillofacial manifestations of familial adenomatous polyposis. Oral Dis 2007;13(4):360–5.

A recent survey of the oral findings in 58 patients who had TS confirmed the high frequency of enamel pitting (97%) and oral fibromas (69%) observed in this patient population.[34] The oral fibromas predominately occur on the gingiva, but other sites such as the buccal mucosa, labial mucosa, tongue, and palate may be affected. The high preponderance of oral findings, combined with the frequently observed facial angiofibromas, affords the dental practitioner a unique opportunity to make the presumptive diagnosis and initiate referral for further medical assessment.

Patients who have TS should undergo routine cranial imaging and renal ultrasonography for the early detection of brain tumors and renal lesions, respectively.[36] In general, necessary dental care can be provided safely to the patient who has TS. The presence of commonly observed comorbidities such as epilepsy, mental handicap, renal disease, and pulmonary disease, however, may necessitate management modifications. Deep sedation or general anesthesia may be relatively contraindicated in the presence of impaired renal or pulmonary function.[39] In this regard, Nott and Halfacre[40] report that using a combination of thiopentone, vecuronium, and nitrous oxide with isoflurane is recommended to obtain adequate general anesthesia in a seizure-prone patient with TS.

Peutz-Jeghers Syndrome

PJS is a rare autosomal dominant hamartomatous polyposis that has an estimated prevalence of 1:50,000 to 1:200,000.[41] PJS cases arise from mutations to the serine/threonine kinase 11 (STK11) tumor suppressor gene located on chromosome 19p13.3.[24,42] This gene is also known as the LKB1 gene, and its inactivation is postulated to contribute to the development of numerous cancers.[41,43] PJS demonstrates a variable penetrance, and approximately 50% of cases represent new mutations. There is no ethnic or racial predisposition.[44] PJS patients are at increased risk for various cancers. The cumulative lifetime risk has been estimated at 54% for breast cancer, 39% for colon cancer, 36% for pancreatic cancer, 29% for stomach cancer, 21% for ovarian cancer, 15% for lung cancer, 13% for small intestine cancer, 10% for cervical cancer, and 9% for uterine and testicular cancers.[41]

The characteristic features of PJS are mucocutaneous melanin pigmentations and a unique type of GI polyp (Peutz-Jeghers polyp).[21,41] The pigmentations present as dark blue to brown macules, 1 to 5 mm in size, predominately on the lip vermilion, buccal mucosa, and hands. Perianal, periorbital, and genital pigmentations also have been reported. PJS pigmentations are usually present at infancy and begin to fade in late adolescence, which is in contrast to the common freckle that develops later in life, never affects the buccal mucosa, and rarely involves the lip vermilion.[24,41] Peutz-Jeghers polyps occur predominately in the small intestine, but the stomach and large intestine also may be affected.[21] They present as 0.1 to 5.0 cm, nondysplastic, coarsely lobulated polyps that exhibit an arborizing pattern of growth.[41,42] They are covered by the appropriate epithelium for the area of the GI tract from which they occur.

Ideally, early recognition of the characteristic mucocutaneous melanosis leads to a thorough medical work-up and the diagnosis of PJS. In reality, most cases of PJS are diagnosed subsequent to the onset of GI complaints such as abdominal pain, obstruction, intussusception, and bloody stools, typically between the ages of 10 and 30 years.[41] Both endoscopic and genetic testing may be used to confirm diagnosis. Treatment of PJS consists of routine endoscopic assessment and surgical removal of rapidly growing, large, or symptomatic polyps. Routine surveillance screening for the associated cancers also is recommended.[41,45] The mucocutaneous pigmentations require no therapy.[46]

Cowden Syndrome

CS, also known as multiple hamartoma syndrome, is a rare autosomal dominant genetic disorder, with an estimated incidence of 1:200,000.[42] Mutations of the tumor suppressor gene phosphate and tensin homolog (PTEN), located on chromosome 10q23.3, underlie the development of CS. The hamartomatous GI polyps observed in CS generally are not associated with an increased cancer risk. Patients who have CS, however, are at an increased risk for developing other cancers, especially cancer of the breast, endometrium, and thyroid.[42,47] Mutations to PTEN also are related to numerous other overlapping syndromes such as Bannayan-Riley-Ruvalcaba syndrome, Lhermitte-Duclos disorder, Proteus syndrome, Proteus-like syndrome, and VATER syndrome.[48,49] As a consequence, many authorities now consider all of the aforementioned syndromes as phenotypic variants of an umbrella syndrome termed PTEN hamartoma-tumor syndrome (PHTS).[49]

Specific diagnostic criteria for CS have been published recently and consist of specific pathognomonic, major, and minor clinical criteria.[50] The most commonly observed findings of CS are facial trichilemmomas, acral keratoses, papillomatous papules, and mucosal lesions (lipomas, neuromas, hemangiomas). The papillomatous papules typically affect the gingival mucosa and buccal mucosa, and frequently impart a cobblestone appearance to the affected tissues.[51] Other findings reported in association with CS include fissured tongue, macrocephaly, high-arched palate, mental retardation, epilepsy, vitiligo, xanthomas, and café au lait spots.[49,51] Aside from potential cosmetic purposes, most of the mucocutaneous lesions of CS require no therapy.[52] The CS patient, however, should undergo routine surveillance screening for breast, endometrial, and thyroid cancer as appropriate.[53]

INFLAMMATORY BOWEL DISEASE

IBD generally encompasses two fairly distinct diseases, ulcerative colitis (UC) and Crohn's disease (CD).[54] An estimated 1.4 million persons in the United States suffer from IBD.[55] The etiopathogenesis of IBD is complex and only partially understood, but it generally is accepted that IBD represents an inappropriate and sustained activation of the mucosal immune system in the milieu of normal luminal GI flora.[56,57] Genetic factors appear to only partially contribute to the development of IBD. First-degree relatives of affected patients have an absolute risk of 7% for developing IBD, while monozygotic twins manifest a 45% concordance for CD and a 6% concordance for UC.[54,56] The lack of a simple mendelian inheritance pattern in twins indicates other unidentified environmental or genetic gene factors likely contribute to disease development. Smoking appears to protect against UC but increases CD risk.[57]

Ulcerative Colitis

By definition, UC affects only the colonic mucosa, and the inflammation is extensive but superficial.[54,58,59] The rectal mucosa invariably is involved, and the inflammation extends proximally in a continuous and confluent manner to the proximal margin. Proximal extension of UC to encompass the entire large bowel (pancolitis) occurs in up to 20% of cases.[58] Common signs and symptoms of UC include bloody diarrhea, abdominal pain, weight loss, anemia, and rectal urgency and frequency.[54] The severity of the signs and symptoms parallels the underlying disease activity. Plain radiographic images typically reveal a colonic diameter exceeding 5 cm.[54] Histologic features include the presence of significant neutrophils within the lamina propria and crypts, microabscesses, and goblet cell depletion.[59]

Crohn's Disease

CD can affect the entire GI tract and typically is characterized by regional transmural granulomatous ulcerations.[60] The most commonly affected sites are the ileocecal area (40%), small intestine (30%), and colon (25%).[54] Signs and symptoms characteristic for ileocecal CD include diarrhea, right lower quadrant pain, low-grade fever, and possible nausea, vomiting, and postprandial pain. Small intestine disease typically manifests abdominal pain, diarrhea, fever, weight loss, obstructive symptoms, and possible malabsorptive disorders (fat-soluble vitamins, Vitamin B12, folate, calcium, magnesium, iron). Characteristic findings of colonic CD are diarrhea, weight loss, fever, and hematochezia. Histologic features of CD include inflammatory infiltration, macrophage aggregation, and noncaseating granulomas.[59]

Extraintestinal Features of Inflammatory Bowel Disease

Various extraintestinal features have been observed in association with IBD and may be the actual concern prompting the patient to seek out care.[61] Potential findings include joint problems (rheumatoid-like arthritis, ankylosing spondylitis, peripheral large joint arthritis), iritis, erythema nodosum, pyoderma gangrenosum, nutritional problems, gallstones, kidney stones, liver disease, and thromboembolic disease. Many of these conditions improve in concert with successful IBD management.

Oral Features of Inflammatory Bowel Disease

A spectrum of putative oral findings has been reported to occur in association with IBD, and it is postulated that these lesions may serve as markers of IBD presence and activity (**Box 1**).[62–65] Overall, oral lesions appear to be observed more frequently in CD than in UC. Commonly referred to conditions such as angular cheilitis, aphthous ulcers, dry mouth, gingivitis, glossitis, and halitosis, however, are commonly observed phenomena, rendering their significance in assessing IBD uncertain. Two recently published studies assessing the association of oral findings and IBD illustrate the lack of clarity on this topic.

Lisciandrano and colleagues[64] examined 198 patients who had IBD (UC = 121, CD = 77) and 89 controls for the presence of oral lesions. At assessment, 44% of UC patients and 38% of CD patients were in clinical remission. Angular cheilitis was noted in 12 who had IBD patients (six UC and six CD) and in no controls. Oral candidiasis was noted in patients who had IBD (one UC and four

> **Box 1**
> **Possible oral findings associated with inflammatory bowel disease**
>
> Pyostomatitis vegetans
> Gingivitis
> Cobblestoning
> Aphthous ulcers
> Tissue tags
> Fissures
> Angular cheilitis
> Oral candidiasis
> Dry mouth
> Nausea
> Halitosis
> Burning mouth
> Dysphagia
> Vomiting
> Regurgitation
> Acidic taste
> Taste changes
> Increased caries
>
> *Data from* Beitman RG, Frost SS, Roth JL. Oral manifestation of gastrointestinal disease. Dig Dis Sci 1981;26(8):741–7.
> Katz J, Shenkman A, Stavropoulos F, et al. Oral signs and symptoms in relation to disease activity and site of involvement in patients with inflammatory bowel disease. Oral Dis 2003;9(1):34–40.
> Lisciandrano D, Ranzi T, Carrassi A, et al. Prevalence of oral lesions in inflammatory bowel disease. Am J Gastroenterol 1996;91(1):7–10.
> Rooney TP. Dental caries prevalence in patients with Crohn's disease. Oral Surg Oral Med Oral Pathol. 1984;57(6):623–4.

CD) and in no controls. Aphthous ulcers were noted in 11 patients who had IBD (seven UC and four CD) and in five controls. No reference to the presence of gingivitis, lip swellings, fissures, mucosal tags, cobblestoning, or pyostomatitis vegetans was noted. The authors concluded that only angular cheilitis and oral candidiasis were significantly associated with IBD, and the presence of aphthous ulcers has limited significance.[64] More recently, Katz and colleagues[63] examined 54 patients who had IBD (UC = 20, CD = 34) and 42 controls for the presence of oral lesions and symptoms associated with IBD. Nausea was noted more frequently in patients who had CD compared with controls, and halitosis was noted more frequently in patients who had UC compared with controls. There were no significant differences regarding the presence of oral ulcerations, geographic tongue, fissured tongue, tongue coating, dry mouth, dysphagia, burning mouth, vomiting, regurgitation, acidic taste, and taste changes among the IBD and control cohorts.[63]

The one oral condition that does appear to strongly correlate with IBD is pyostomatitis vegetans. Pyostomatitis vegetans is the oral variant of pyodermatitis vegetans, and its presence is highly suggestive of IBD, particularly UC.[66–70] It is a unique and rare oral finding characterized by miliary pustular abscesses and erosions affecting the oral mucosa.[70] The pustules may become confluent to form characteristic snail track ulcerations.[68] Frequently affected sites include the labial and buccal mucosa, soft and hard palate, and gingival mucosa, while the floor of the mouth and tongue typically are spared.[68]

Diagnosis of Inflammatory Bowel Disorder

UC and CD have been defined empirically based upon their characteristic clinical, pathologic, endoscopic, and radiological features.[57,59] Up to 15% of patients who have IBD cannot be classified as having either UC or CD, and are classified as having indeterminate colitis.[54] Other conditions to consider in the differential diagnosis for UC include infectious colitis, diversion colitis, pseudomembranous colitis, radiation colitis, and ischemia.[54] For CD, the differential diagnosis should include infectious colitis, appendicitis, carcinoma, lymphoma, and celiac disease.[54]

The presence of pyostomatitis vegetans is highly suggestive of IBD and warrants a prompt referral for medical assessment.[66–70] The histopathologic findings of pyostomatitis vegetans consist of epithelial hyperplasia with focal acantholysis; a dense inflammatory cell infiltrate containing lymphocytes, neutrophils, and eosinophils in the connective tissue; and intraepithelial and subepithelial microabcesses.[68] Immunofluorescent studies are recommended to rule out such autoimmune conditions such as pemphigus and pemphigoid.

The presence of other oral findings putatively associated with IBD should be assessed in the context of the patient's overall health. Patients who have concurrent GI symptoms should be referred for further medical assessment. The need to refer patients without GI symptoms, however, appears to be more dubious, and such patients may be served better by routine monitoring.

Management of Inflammatory Bowel Disease

The management of IBD is predicated on the correct diagnosis and further tailored to address the severity and specific site involved.[57,71] Most physicians use a stepped approach to target therapy in an attempt to obtain adequate disease control with the least amount of intervention. In addition, efforts to ensure adequate nutrition also are undertaken.

5-aminosalicylate compounds remain the mainstay of treatment for mild-to-moderate IBD.[57] These agents appear to act on several aspects of the inflammatory process and various formulations are available that target specific disease locations. In terms of providing sustained maintenance relief, these compounds appear to be of more value in managing UC than CD.[57] Corticosteroids usually are used when patients who have IBD fail to respond to 5-aminosalicylates. Topical and systemic formulations are available and in most cases therapy is limited to treat acute disease flares. Long-term maintenance therapy with corticosteroids has not been proven beneficial and is associated with serious adverse effects such as hypertension, diabetes, and osteoporosis.[54,57] Immunomodulating drugs such as azathioprine, methotrexate, cyclosporine, tacrolimus, and mycophenolate mofetil may be prescribed for patients in whom corticosteroid therapy needs to be reduced.[57,60] The newest drugs under investigation for managing IBD are the biologics. Drugs such as infliximab, certolizumab pegol, and thalidomide all demonstrate tumor necrosis factor α (TNF-α) activity and are being investigated for managing moderate-to-severe IBD, especially CD.[72,73]

Up to 30% of patients who have UC and up to 75% of patients who have CD eventually require surgical intervention to manage their disease.[54] Indications for surgery in UC include cancer, severe hemorrhage, and perforation. For UC, a proctocolectomy is generally curative but results in the lifelong use of an external appliance. For CD, surgery is not curative, and the need for further surgical interventions is common. Indications for surgery in CD include intestinal obstruction, perforation, complicated fistulas, and abscess.[54]

The provision of dental care for the patient who has IBD is predicated on a thorough assessment of the patient's disease status, medication profile, and comorbidities. In general, IBD patients under good medical control can tolerate the delivery of routine outpatient dental care. For more extensive procedures, a consultation with the patient's physician may be warranted. Topical and systemic corticosteroids represent the treatment of choice to manage IBD patients with pyostomatitis vegetans.[68] In addition, the attainment of good medical control of IBD should contribute to regression of pyostomatitis vegetans.

REFERENCES

1. Koufman JA. Laryngopharyngeal reflux is different from classic gastroesophageal reflux disease. Ear Nose Throat J 2002;81(9 Suppl 2):7–9.
2. Lipan MJ, Reidenberg JS, Laitman JT. Anatomy of reflux: a growing health problem affecting structures of the head and neck. Anat Rec B New Anat 2006; 289(6):261–70.
3. Groome M, Cotton JP, Borland M, et al. Prevalence of laryngopharyngeal reflux in a population with gastroesophageal reflux. Laryngoscope 2007;117(8):1424–8.
4. Farrokhi F, Vaezi MF. Extraesophageal manifestations of gastroesophageal reflux. Oral Dis 2007; 13(4):349–59.
5. Voutilainen M, Sipponen P, Mecklin JP, et al. Gastroesophageal reflux disease: prevalence, clinical, endoscopic, and histopathological findings in 1128 consecutive patients referred for endoscopy due to dyspeptic and reflux symptoms. Digestion 2000; 61(1):6–13.
6. Vakil N, van Zanten SV, Kahrilas P, et al. Global Consensus Group. The Montreal definition and classification of gastroesophageal reflux disease: a global evidence-based consensus. Am J Gastroenterol 2006;101(8):1900–20.
7. Chandra A, Moazzez R, Bartlett D, et al. A review of the atypical manifestations of gastroesophageal reflux disease. Int J Clin Pract 2004;58(1):41–8.
8. Franco RA, Andrus JG. Common diagnoses and treatments in professional voice users. Otolaryngol Clin North Am 2007;40(5):1025–61.
9. Hogan WJ, Shaker R. Medical treatment of supraesophageal complications of gastroesophageal reflux disease. Am J Med 2001;111(Suppl 8A):197S–201S.
10. Hogan WJ, Shaker R. Supraesophageal complications of gastroesophageal reflux. Dis Mon 2000; 46(3):193–232.
11. Karkos PD, Benton J, Leong Sc, et al. Trends in laryngopharyngeal reflux: a British ENT survey. Eur Arch Otorhinolaryngol 2007;264(5):513–7.
12. Morice AH. Is reflux cough due to gastroesophageal reflux disease or laryngopharyngeal reflux? Lung 2007 Oct 2; [Epub ahead of print].
13. Qadeer MA, Swoger J, Milstein C, et al. Correlation between symptoms and laryngeal signs in laryngopharyngeal reflux. Laryngoscope 2005;115(11): 1947–52.
14. Groen JN, Smout AJ. Supraoesophageal manifestations of gastro-oesophageal reflux disease. Eur J Gastroenterol Hepatol 2003;15(12):1339–50.
15. Lazarchik DA, Filler SJ. Dental erosion: predominant oral lesion in gastroesophageal reflux disease. Am J Gastroenterol 2000;95(8 Suppl):S33–8.
16. Lazarchik DA, Filler SJ. Effects of gastroesophageal reflux on the oral cavity. Am J Med 1997;103(5A): 107S–13S.

17. Moshkowitz M, Horowitz N, Leshno M, et al. Halitosis and gastroesophageal reflux disease: a possible association. Oral Dis 2007;13(6):581–5.
18. Van Roekel NB. Gastroesophageal reflux disease, tooth erosion, and prosthodontic rehabilitation: a clinical report. J Prosthodont 2003;12(4):255–9.
19. Ray SW, Secrest J, Ch'ien AP, et al. Managing gastroesophageal reflux disease. Nurse Pract 2002;27(5):36–53.
20. Khan M, Santana J, Donnellan C, et al. Medical treatments in the short-term management of reflux oesophagitis. Cochrane Database Syst Rev 2007;(2):CD003244.
21. Schulmann K, Pox C, Tannapfel A, et al. The patient with multiple intestinal polyps. Best Pract Res Clin Gastroenterol 2007;21(3):409–26.
22. Galiatsatos P, Foulkes WD. Familial adenomatous polyposis. Am J Gastroenterol 2006;101(2):385–98.
23. Bronner MP. Gastrointestinal polyposis syndromes. Am J Med Genet A 2003;122(4):335–41.
24. Schreibman IR, Baker M, Amos C, et al. The hamartomatous polyposis syndromes: a clinical and molecular review. Am J Gastroenterol 2005;100(2):476–90.
25. Bilkay U, Erdem O, Ozek C, et al. Benign osteoma with Gardner syndrome: review of the literature and report of a case. J Craniofac Surg 2004;15(3):506–9.
26. Fotiadis C, Tsekouras DK, Antonakis P, et al. Gardner's syndrome: a case report and review of the literature. World J Gastroenterol 2005;11(34):5408–11.
27. Payne M, Anderson JA, Cook J. Gardner's syndrome: a case report. Br Dent J 2002;193(7):383–4.
28. Wijn MA, Keller JJ, Giardiello FM, et al. Oral and maxillofacial manifestations of familial adenomatous polyposis. Oral Dis 2007;13(4):360–5.
29. Rowley PT. Inherited susceptibility to colorectal cancer. Annu Rev Med 2005;56:539–54.
30. Baykul T, Heybeli N, Oyar O, et al. Multiple huge osteomas of the mandible causing disfigurement related with Gardner's syndrome: case report. Auris Nasus Larynx 2003;30(4):447–51.
31. Fonseca LC, Kodama NK, Nunes FC, et al. Radiographic assessment of Gardner's syndrome. Dentomaxillofac Radiol 2007;36(2):121–4.
32. Lynch HT, Shaw TG, Lynch J. Inherited predisposition to cancer: a historical overview. Am J Med Genet C Semin Med Genet 2004;129(1):5–22.
33. Öner AY, Pocan S. Gardner's syndrome: a case report. Br Dent J 2006;200(12):666–7.
34. Sparling JD, Hong CH, Brahim JS, et al. Oral findings in 58 adults with tuberous sclerosis complex. J Am Acad Dermatol 2007;56(5):786–90.
35. Narayanan V. Tuberous sclerosis complex: genetics to pathogenesis. Pediatr Neurol 2003;29(5):404–9.
36. Sparagana SP, Roach ES. Tuberous sclerosis complex. Curr Opin Neurol 2000;13(2):115–9.
37. Hyman MH, Whittemore VH. National Institutes of Health consensus conference: tuberous sclerosis complex. Arch Neurol 2000;57(5):662–5.
38. Roach ES, Gomez MR, Northrup H. Tuberous sclerosis complex consensus conference: revised clinical diagnostic criteria. J Child Neurol 1998;13(12):624–8.
39. Cutando A, Gil JA, Lopez J. Oral health management implications in patients with tuberous sclerosis. Oral Surg Oral Med Oral Pathol Oral Radiol Endod 2000;89(4):430–5.
40. Nott MR, Halfacre J. Anaesthesia for dental conservation in a patient with tuberous sclerosis. Eur J Anaesthesiol 1996;13(4):413–5.
41. Giardiello FM, Trimbath JD. Peutz-Jeghers syndrome and management recommendations. Clin Gastroenterol Hepatol 2006;4(4):408–15.
42. Doxey BW, Kuwada SK, Burt RW. Inherited polyposis syndromes: molecular mechanisms, clinicopathology, and genetic testing. Clin Gastroenterol Hepatol 2005;3(7):633–41.
43. Sanchez-Cespedes M. A role for LKB1 gene in human cancer beyond the Peutz-Jeghers syndrome. Oncogene 2007 Jun 18; [Epub ahead of print].
44. Pereira CM, Coletta RD, Jorge J, et al. Peutz-Jeghers syndrome in a 14-year-old boy: case report and review of the literature. Int J Paediatr Dent 2005;15(3):224–8.
45. Hearle N, Schumacher V, Menko FH, et al. Frequency and spectrum of cancers in the Peutz-Jeghers syndrome. Clin Cancer Res 2006;12(10):3209–15.
46. Kauzman A, Pavone M, Blanas N, et al. Pigmented lesions of the oral cavity: review, differential diagnosis, and case presentations. J Can Dent Assoc 2004;70(10):682–3.
47. Schaffer JV, Kamino H, Witkiewicz A, et al. Mucocutaneous neuromas: an under-recognized manifestation of PTEN hamartoma–tumor syndrome. Arch Dermatol 2006;142(5):625–32.
48. Gustafson S, Zbuk KM, Scacheri C, et al. Cowden syndrome. Semin Oncol 2007;34(5):428–34.
49. Scheper MA, Nikitakis NG, Sarlani E, et al. Cowden syndrome: report of a case with immunohistochemical analysis and review of the literature. Oral Surg Oral Med Oral Pathol Oral Radiol Endod 2006;101(5):625–31.
50. Eng C. Will the real Cowden syndrome please stand up: revised diagnostic criteria. J Med Genet 2000;37(11):828–30.
51. Hand JL, Rogers RS 3rd. Oral manifestations of genodermatoses. Dermatol Clin 2003;21(1):183–94.
52. Leão JC, Batista V, Guimarães PB, et al. Cowden's syndrome affecting the mouth, gastrointestinal, and central nervous system: a case report and review

53. Zbuk KM, Eng C. Hamartomatous polyposis syndromes. Nat Clin Pract Gastroenterol Hepatol 2007;4(9):492–502.
54. Chutkan RK. Inflammatory bowel disease. Prim Care 2001;28(3):539–56.
55. Loftus EV. Clinical epidemiology of inflammatory bowel disease: incidence, prevalence, and environmental influences. Gastroenterology 2004;126(6):1504–17.
56. Gaya DR, Russell RK, Nimmo ER, et al. New genes in inflammatory bowel disease: lessons for complex diseases? Lancet 2006;367(9518):1271–84.
57. Podolsky DK. Inflammatory bowel disease. N Engl J Med 2002;347(6):417–29.
58. Moses PL, Moore BR, Ferrentino N, et al. Inflammatory bowel disease. 1. Origins, presentation, and course. Postgrad Med 1998;103(5):77–84.
59. Xavier RJ, Podolsky DK. Unravelling the pathogenesis of inflammatory bowel disease. Nature 2007;448(7152):427–34.
60. Ponsky T, Hindle A, Sandler A. Inflammatory bowel disease in the pediatric patient. Surg Clin North Am 2007;87(3):643–58.
61. Gitnick G. Inflammatory bowel diseases: Part II. Extraintestinal involvement and management. Am Fam Physician 1989;39(2):225–33.
62. Beitman RG, Frost SS, Roth JL. Oral manifestation of gastrointestinal disease. Dig Dis Sci 1981;26(8):741–7.
63. Katz J, Shenkman A, Stavropoulos F, et al. Oral signs and symptoms in relation to disease activity and site of involvement in patients with inflammatory bowel disease. Oral Dis 2003;9(1):34–40.
64. Lisciandrano D, Ranzi T, Carrassi A, et al. Prevalence of oral lesions in inflammatory bowel disease. Am J Gastroenterol 1996;91(1):7–10.
65. Rooney TP. Dental caries prevalence in patients with Crohn's disease. Oral Surg Oral Med Oral Pathol 1984;57(6):623–4.
66. Calobrisi SD, Mutasim DF, McDonald JS. Pyostomatitis vegetans associated with ulcerative colitis. Temporary clearance with fluocinonide gel and complete remission after colectomy. Oral Surg Oral Med Oral Pathol Oral Radiol Endod 1995;79(4):452–4.
67. Philpot HC, Elewski BE, Banwell JG, et al. Pyostomatitis vegetans and primary sclerosing cholangitis: markers of inflammatory bowel disease. Gastroenterology 1992;103(2):668–74.
68. Soriano ML, Martinez N, Grilli R, et al. Pyodermtitis–pyostomatitis vegetans: report of a case and review of the literature. Oral Surg Oral Med Oral Pathol Oral Radiol Endod 1999;87(3):322–6.
69. Storwick GS, Prihoda MB, Fulton RJ, et al. Pyodermatitis–pyostomatitis vegetans: a specific marker for inflammatory bowel disease. J Am Acad Dermatol 1994;31(2 Pt 2):336–41.
70. Thornhill MH, Zakrzewska JM, Gilkes JJ. Pyostomatis vegetans: report of three cases and review of the literature. J Oral Pathol Med 1992;21(3):128–33.
71. Veloso FT, Ferreira JT, Barros L, et al. Clinical outcome of Crohn's disease: analysis according to the Vienna classification and clinical activity. Inflamm Bowel Dis 2001;7(4):306–13.
72. Sandborn WJ, Feagan BG, Stoinov S, et al. PRECISE 1 Study Investigators. Certolizumab pegol for the treatment of Crohn's disease. N Engl J Med 2007;357(3):228–38.
73. Schreiber S, Khaliq-Kareemi M, Lawrance IC, et al. PRECISE 2 Study Investigators. Maintenance therapy with certolizumab pegol for Crohn's disease. N Engl J Med 2007;357(3):239–50.

Head and Neck Manifestations of Tuberculosis

LTC Robert G. Hale, DDS*, CPT David I. Tucker, DDS

KEYWORDS

- Tuberculosis • Scrofula • Head and neck • Treatement

Tuberculosis (TB) is a communicable disease caused by *Mycobacterium tuberculosis*, which is transmitted by aerosolized saliva droplets among individuals in close contact with the expelled sputum of a diseased patient. The bacteria enter the body through the respiratory tract, causing a primary pulmonary infection, manifested by bacteremia with potential to infect nearly all organs within the first weeks of infection. Symptoms are usually a mild respiratory illness with initial inoculation. In most cases, cell-mediated defenses contain the bacteria in a dormant lung focus of macrophages, and the patient becomes asymptomatic with a positive tuberculin skin test. Secondary TB is reactivation of dormant bacteria. Secondary TB accounts for 90% of TB cases in HIV-negative patients in the United States. Up to 40% of HIV-positive patients will progress to primary progressive tuberculosis once infected.[1] Infected patients can develop progressive TB with erosion of tuberculin granulomatous lesions beyond the lung parenchyma into nearby lymphatics or blood vessels. Head and neck manifestations of TB are caused by the hematogenous or lymphatic spread of the bacteria to affect the larynx, oropharynx, maxillofacial structures, ear, mastoid, and cervical spine.[2] Other cases of TB of the head and neck are from self-inoculation of open lesions of the aero–digestive tract with infected sputum.[3] This article describes the history, epidemiology, bacteriology, pathophysiology, diagnosis, and treatment of TB with emphasis on head and neck manifestations of this systemic disease.

HISTORY OF TUBERCULOSIS

Evidence of TB is present in ancient mummies with spinal deformities and calcified lung lesions characteristic of the disease. Hippocrates identified TB as phthisis, and he advised followers to avoid treating late-stage disease to avoid damage to their reputations, because it was almost always fatal.[4] The earliest recorded symptoms of pulmonary TB—cough, expectoration, hemoptysis, and wasting—were found in the library of Assurbanipal (668 to 626 BC), king of Assyria.[4] Later descriptions of TB labeled the disease as lupus vulgaris (TB of the skin), Pott disease (TB of the bones) or, simply consumption.

Urbanization of Europe in the 16th and 17th centuries led to conditions favorable for an epidemic of TB until it became the leading cause of death (white plague) in Western Europe during the late 18th and early 19th centuries.[5] TB is estimated to have caused 30% of deaths in 19th century Paris.[4] The disease was so common that it was fashionable to glamorize the disease as a tragic event in operas as seen reiterated in the popular 2001 film Moulin Rouge.[6] Undoubtedly, the singer/dancer exposed everyone to danger with each cough, which is interesting in light of a recently published outbreak of TB among dancers and patrons in a Kansas bar.[7]

TB was romanticized as the "Gentle Death" in the 19th century, because the victim often appeared to slowly and gracefully fade away.[4] Rene Dubos, MD, a renowned scholar of that era, wrote "to be consumptive was almost

---

The views expressed in this article are those of the authors and do not necessarily represent the official policy or position of the United States Army, the Department of Defense, or the United States government.
OMS Residency, Brooke Army Medical Center, Fort Sam Houston, TX 78234, USA
* Corresponding author.
E-mail address: robert.g.hale@us.army.mil (R.G. Hale).

a mark of distinction, and the pallor caused by the disease was part of the standard beauty." He went on to say, "languid pallor was then such a desirable feminine attribute that the use of rouge was abandoned and replaced by lightening powders; during the 19th and 20th centuries, tuberculosis was truly the white plague".[8]

John Henry Holliday,[9,10] who lost his mother to TB in 1866, went to Pennsylvania College of Dental Surgery. Shortly after his graduation in 1872, "Doc Holliday" discovered he was ill with consumption and moved west to drier climates. He started a practice in Dallas, Texas, but a hacking cough interrupted patient treatment and prevented a successful practice of dentistry. The soon-to-be-famous gunslinger found a gambling and whisky habit as he moved further west, eventually to Tombstone, Arizona, to participate in the celebrated shootout at the OK Corral. At the age of 36, the pale and thin "Doc" met his end more peacefully than his foes as he passed away from consumption.

Although not as aggressive as the bubonic plague of medieval times, TB has killed more people in history than the black plague, leprosy, or HIV. In 1882, Dr. Robert Koch proved a bacterial infection caused TB, and later investigations demonstrated secretions from consumptive lungs contained live bacteria. Effective treatment for TB had to wait until streptomycin in 1944,[4] but the combination of vaccination of children, improved sanitation, and, perhaps, the sequestration of infected individuals led to the decline of tuberculosis in the 20th century.

EPIDEMIOLOGY

The Centers for Disease Control and Prevention (CDC) reported 84,304 new TB cases in the United States in 1953 (**Fig. 1**).[5] This rate steadily declined to 20,000 per year until the emergence of HIV in the mid-1980s.[10] Over the following 20 years, despite an overall and continual fall in TB cases, there was a surge of TB among HIV-positive patients. In 2005, for persons reported with TB aged 25 to 44 years, 13% had an HIV coinfection.[11] Although there has been the appearance of multidrug-resistant TB (MDR-TB) and extensively drug-resistant TB (XDR-TB), the numbers have been small, and there is no apparent trend in the number of cases over time.[12]

The 2006 CDC statistics reported the annual number of new TB cases in the United States was 13,779. California, New York, Texas, and Florida account for 48% of the national TB caseload. African Americans accounted for 44% of United States-born cases; Hispanics and Asians accounted for 80% of foreign-born cases. The top five countries of origin for TB-positive foreign-born cases were Mexico, Philippines, Vietnam, India, and China (**Fig. 2**). There were 646 TB deaths in the United States in 2005.[12]

Worldwide, the situation is more ominous, with the World Health Organization (WHO) reporting 9 million new cases in 2004. TB is believed to be present in one third of the world's population and accounts for 2 million deaths a year. Sub-Saharan Africa and Asia account for 80% of worldwide TB cases. According to WHO, the number of reported TB cases is stable in the world except in Africa, where a TB epidemic is being driven by the spread of HIV. The number of MDR-TB and XDR-TB cases is increasing, but the scale of the problem globally is unknown.[13]

BACTERIOLOGY

TB's causative organism, *M tuberculosis*, is a nonmobile, nonspore- forming rod-shaped bacillus, 1 to 4 μm long and 0.3 to 0.5 μm wide, which stains

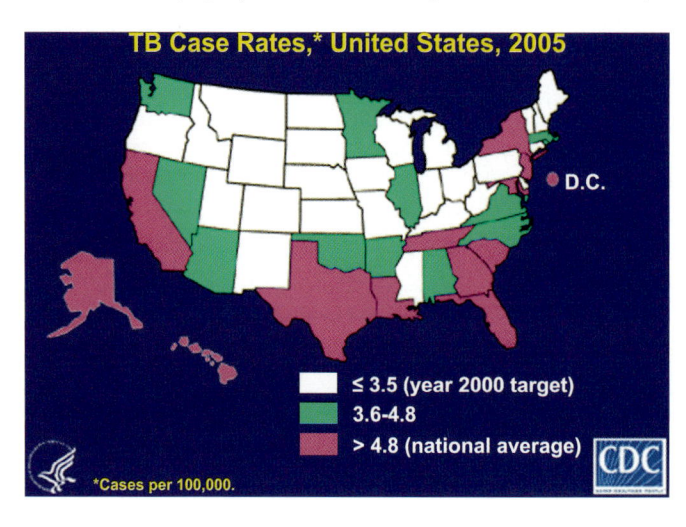

Fig. 1. Tuberculosis case rates 2005. (*Courtesy of* Centers for Disease Control and Prevention, Atlanta).

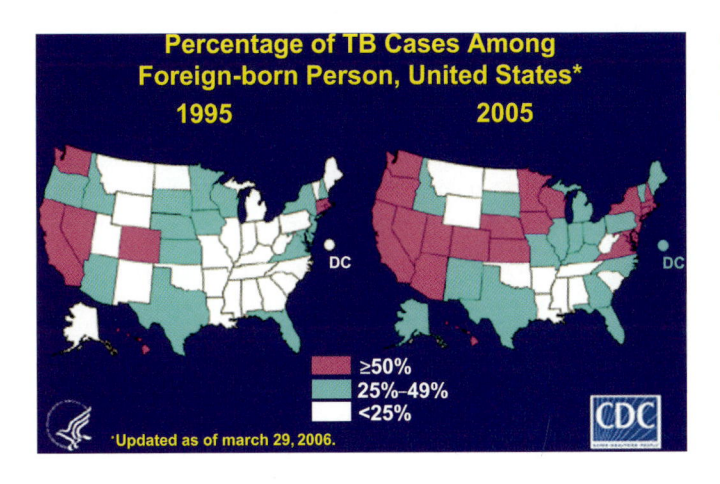

Fig. 2. Percentage of tuberculosis case rates among foreign persons. (*Courtesy of* Centers for Disease Control and Prevention, Atlanta.)

weakly gram positive. The cell wall is rich in lipids and retains carbolfuchsin red dye after acid washing; therefore, the *Mycobacterium* bacilli is said to be acid fast.[14] These bacteria are slow-growing, obligate aerobes, usually causing chronic disease and surviving as intracellular parasites once engulfed by macrophages. The thick protein–phospholipid wall is responsible for the bacilli resistance to phagocytosis.[14] Other important Mycobacterium are *M leprae*, which causes leprosy, *M avium*, which is a serious disseminated disease in patients who have HIV, and *M bovi*, which is a form of cattle TB infecting people in places where pasteurization is not practiced.[15] The bacteria should be cultured in Löwenstein-Jensen or Middlebrook media, which take at least 8 weeks to detect growth. These cultures are required for accurate diagnosis and antibiotic susceptibilities.[16] The bacteria also may be grown in liquid media, which is more rapid and can detect *Mycobacterium* growth in as few as 7 days. Further speciation is confirmed with DNA/RNA probe or high-pressure liquid chromatography (HPLC). Concentration and decontamination of sputum specimens followed by auramine–rhodamine or auramine-O-fluorescence staining, permit rapid scanning of the slides and are more sensitive than the older Ziehl-Nielsen method.[17] The average number of organisms is reported by the laboratory, and this should be available to the clinician within 24 hours of specimen submission.

The virulence of *M tuberculosis* is related to a number of structural and physiologic properties unique to this bacterium. It has the ability to bind directly to macrophages; once ingested *M tuberculosis* grows intracellularly and essentially evades the immune system. The high lipid concentration in the cell wall resists antibiotic penetration and lysis through complement deposition and dissolution by lysozyme. The infected macrophage then becomes surrounded by giant cells and forms an area of caseous necrosis.[14] The immunocompromised population may not be capable of producing this inflammatory response, particularly patients who have advanced AIDS.[16]

PATHOPHYSIOLOGY

M tuberculosis is acquired by susceptible persons by inhalation of aerosolized droplets containing the bacteria. Primary infection is in the lung parenchyma and adjacent lymph nodes. The disease usually resolves after symptoms of a mild respiratory illness, but the organisms remain alive, contained in a lung focus by host cell-mediated defenses. Reactivation can occur through subsequent illnesses or immune suppression, leading to disease. In some cases, the primary TB infection becomes progressive, and subsequent bacteremia results in TB meningitis or a debilitating generalized acute infection called miliary TB. Miliary TB is so named because the radiographic lesions look like disseminated millet seeds.[17] Organs with high oxygen tension are most susceptible to TB infection, including lung, kidney, and bone (**Fig. 3**).[18]

Only 5% to 15% of patients who have TB infection progress to disease because of underlying host-specific factors.[15] Disease is more prevalent in infants, children, adolescents, elderly, and in individuals who have immunosuppressive diseases.[19] Common symptoms include fever, fatigue, malaise, and anorexia. Fever is common in the afternoon and evening, falling at night with drenching night sweats. A chronic hacking cough produces hemoptysis 20% of the time.[20]

Pulmonary TB may involve the pleura, bronchi, trachea, and larynx. Clinical examination of the patient who has pulmonary tuberculosis should focus on a complete history and physical

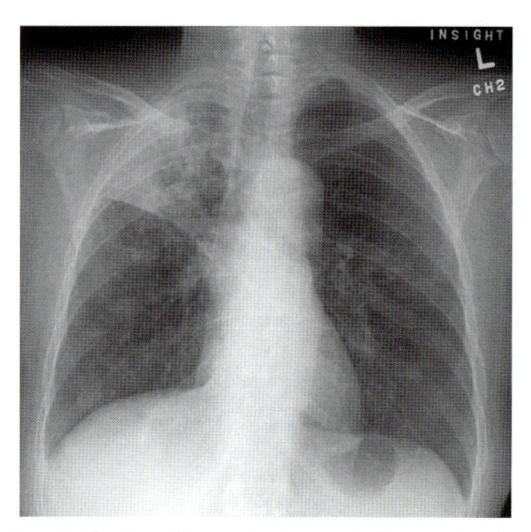

Fig. 3. Chest radiograph demonstrating extensive right upper lobe consolidation and hilar adenopathy often seen with tuberculosis.

examination. Physical findings may include fever, muscle weakness, focal rales or findings of a pleural effusion, or a focal mass or lymphadenopathy. Thorough evaluation of the suspected TB patient is paramount, as it may be present in almost any organ system. In extrapulmonary TB, symptoms may include an obvious mass or lesion with local pain, swelling, and occasionally fistula formation. Extrapulmonary lesions may be ulcerative, but granulomatous disease is more common.[21] Specific symptoms should be evaluated thoroughly with radiographs and CT to evaluate the major organ systems and skeleton for the presence of disease.

Lymphatic spread of TB may involve the cervical and hilar lymph nodes. The infected cervical lymph nodes are usually unilateral, matted, painless, and soft; if left untreated, the neck masses fistulate and exude caseous material.[22] Scrofula or TB lymphadenitis is a term used to describe cervical lymph node involvement. Scrofula in children in the United States usually is caused by *M scrofulaceum*.[23] Suspicious lymph nodes should be biopsied and cultured. Excision of nonhealing, fistulous, or nonresponsive lesions should be considered.[24]

TB of bones and joints is caused by hematogenous spread of the organisms. Joint involvement is manifested as chronic and progressive swelling of the wrists and hands.[25] TB of the TMJ also has been reported.[26] Biopsies of intra-articular soft tissue lesions increase the likelihood of diagnosing TB as a cause of the arthritis.[25] Vertebral involvement commonly causes back pain; TB osteomyelitis destroys the disc space and causes TB spondylitis, also called Pott disease.[27] Cervical spine involvement has been reported from direct extension of infected lymph nodes.[28] TB also can infect the mandible secondarily by means of bacterial entry into the bone through an exposed dental pulp or a fresh extraction site. Pain and subperiosteal swelling are accompanied by diffuse radiographic lesions of the mandible.[29]

TB of the head and neck has been documented extensively. A 10-year retrospective study in India documented 165 cases of TB of the head, neck, and oral cavity. Of these patients, 121 (73.3%) had isolated tubercular lymphadenitis; 24 (14.5%) had laryngeal TB, and four (2.4%) had tubercular otitis media. Three (1.8%) had cervical spine involvement; three (1.8%) had parotid gland involvement, and eight (5%) had oral cavity involvement. One patient had temporomandibular joint involvement, and one had TB of the nose.[30]

Only about 0.05% to 5% of patients who have active TB will present with oral lesions.[16] Primary oral TB occurs by direct inoculation of the oral mucosa from an infected individual, and it is exceptionally rare. Primary oral TB is more common in younger patients, and only a few case reports have been reported.[29] The secondary oral TB is far more prevalent and arises from mycobacterium-contaminated sputum self-inoculating the oral structures, or by means of hematogenous spread in miliary TB.[16] Oral TB may have a range of presentations. Typically ulcerative or granulomatous in form, these lesions are most common on the dorsum of the tongue or palate and may cause destruction of underlying bone in the maxilla or mandible, which may mimic squamous cell carcinoma (**Fig. 4**).[31]

Localized pain is the most common symptom, with odynophagia present in 61.1% of patients who have oral TB.[16] Squamous cell carcinoma,

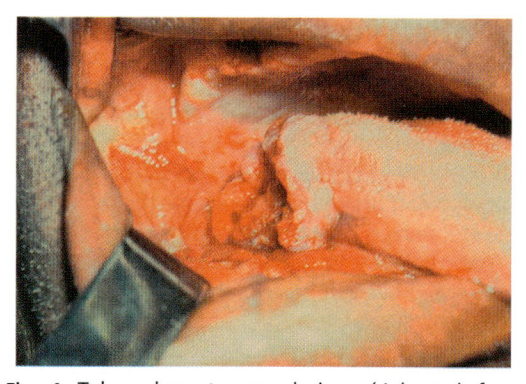

Fig. 4. Tuberculous tongue lesion. (*Adapted from* Marx RE, Stern D. Oral and maxillofacial pathology: a rationale for diagnosis and treatment. Carol Stream (IL): Quintessence Publishing Company; 2003; with permission.)

traumatic ulceration, primary syphilis, and pulmonary fungal diseases may show a similar clinical presentation and should be included in the differential diagnosis.[32]

DIAGNOSIS

Risk factors for TB include immunodeficiency disorders, immunosuppressive medications, hematologic or reticuloendothelial malignancies, end-stage renal disease, hemodialysis, alcoholism, and malnutrition. Solid organ transplant recipients are also at increased risk. Populations at high risk for contracting TB are medically underserved, low-income populations, homeless, intravenous drug abusers, and residents of long-term care facilities, correctional institutions, and mental institutions.[33]

Koch laid the foundation for TB testing in 1890. By boiling a filtrate of tubercle bacilli and inoculating patients with this serum, he observed a significant skin reaction in those infected with TB.[34] The standard screening test for TB performed today is essentially the same tuberculin skin test (TST).

There are two methods of tuberculin skin testing. The intradermal Mantoux method is used in the United States, and the multiple-puncture test is preferred in some countries because of the ease of administration. The Mantoux method involves injection of purified protein derivative (PPD) intradermally into the skin. The multiple-puncture test uses old tuberculin and is used commonly in underdeveloped countries because of ease of administration; however, it is less sensitive and specific.[34]

Routine tuberculin testing programs are discouraged in the asymptomatic United States general population because of the high rate of false-positive results and the low prevalence of disease. Indications for annual screening tuberculin skin testing in asymptomatic individuals, however, include: HIV infection, close contact with cases of active TB, health care workers, prison guards, bacteriology laboratory personnel, and head and neck cancer patients. A group of patients at Sloan-Kettering Cancer Center had a rate of TB over 20 times that of the general population.[35]

A TST cannot be used to confirm active TB infection and should not be performed in suspected TB patients, because it may cause a necrotizing skin reaction in those who have active disease. A positive skin test will occur in individuals who have active TB, who have received the BCG (Bacille Calmette Guerin vaccine), who were previously exposed but not infected, and those who have received successful treatment of TB. A negative reaction may occur in patients who have HIV, miliary TB, metabolic derangements, malnutrition, lymphoma, corticosteroid use, and autoimmune diseases.[36]

A whole blood interferon (IFN)-gamma assay has been developed to overcome the limitations of the TST. T-cells of individuals previously sensitized with TB antigens will produce IFN-gamma when they reencounter mycobacterium antigens. A result with high levels of IFN-gamma production is presumed to be indicative of TB infection. Early assays used PPD as the stimulating antigen; however, newer assays use antigens specific to M tuberculosis (RD1 antigens, antigens not shared with BCG, or most nontuberculous Mycobacterium species). There are two methods for detecting the IFN-gamma released by the T-cell, an ELISA and an enzyme-linked immunospot assay (ELISPOT).[37]

The chest radiograph is no longer a good screening tool for TB disease among the general population. In high-risk environments, however, the radiograph may be a useful tool for screening contacts and symptomatic persons.[38] Classically, pulmonary TB presents as a focal infiltration of the upper lobe(s), usually of the apical or posterior segments, or of the superior apical segment(s) of the lower lobe(s). Disease may be unilateral or bilateral. Cavitation may be present, and inflammation and tissue destruction may result in fibrosis with traction or enlargement of hilar and mediastinal lymph nodes. One-third of adult cases of pulmonary TB do not present with classic findings on chest radiograph. These atypical presentations may show scattered lobar or segmental infiltration, with or without hilar adenopathy, lung mass lesions (tuberculoma), or pleural effusions.[39] This is especially true for patients who have advanced HIV disease, where an atypical radiographic presentation is common.[40] Active versus inactive TB usually cannot be determined by radiography; indeed, reports of scarring consistent with old granulomatous disease may be associated with active TB. A frontal view chest radiograph is usually sufficient to evaluate a patient for latent TB infection, because lateral views add little to diagnosis.[41,42]

Histologic evidence of granuloma formation or caseation will be evident on hematoxylin and eosin (H&E) processed specimens; however, the diagnosis of TB cannot be made based on routine (H&E) processed tissue specimens and gram staining.

Despite advances in testing, the diagnosis of TB often is made based on clinical presentation. For 15% to 20% of patients given a diagnosis of TB, no specific bacteriologic confirmation ever is established.[43] Miziara[16] demonstrated that the diagnosis of TB in patients who have HIV can be difficult. In some patients who have oral TB, sputum analysis, tuberculin skin testing, and histologic examination were negative, and the diagnosis only could be confirmed with biopsy specimen cultures. These cultures often take several weeks, but treatment should be started with strong clinical suspicion.

TREATMENT

Although TB has been endemic in the human population for thousands of years, no real effort was undertaken to cure the disease until 1854, when Hermann Brehmer postulated that TB was curable with good nutrition, isolation, and exposure to fresh air. These approaches led to widespread use of sanitariums, where patients were isolated in remote areas and provided rest, clean air, and other treatments as technology and science advanced.[44] These sanitariums served a dual purpose; they isolated the infected from the general population and enforced rest, a proper diet, and hospital life, which assisted the healing processes.

Early surgical attempts at treating TB focused on decreasing the volume of the lung. In 1888, Forlanini used a needle to create a pneumothorax in patients who had TB to allow the lung to recover.[45] Advances in surgical techniques led to techniques such as phrenicostomy (crushing of the phrenic nerve) and thoracoplasty (removal of ribs). These procedures often were performed in the sanatorium in combination with traditional therapy.

Development of the BCG vaccine was very useful in preventing TB meningitis in children, but had poor results for pulmonary TB. Although first administered to people in 1921, it was not widely available until World War II. Even today, BCG seems to have its greatest effect in preventing miliary TB or TB meningitis, which is the reason it remains extensively used in countries where efficacy against pulmonary TB is negligible.[46]

The discovery of streptomycin in 1943 was a significant breakthrough in the treatment of TB. Ototoxicity and resistant TB, however, limited its use. These problems were solved in the 1950s with multidrug regimens involving combinations of isoniazid (INH), pyrazinamide (PZA), ethambutol (EMB), and rifampin (RIF), which still are used today.

INH is nearly ideal for treating TB. It is bactericidal, easily tolerated orally in a single daily dose, and inexpensive. The major toxicity is hepatitis, which is rare in persons younger than 20 years of age. It should not be taken with alcohol, as this increases hepatotoxicity.

RIF is another effective drug in treating TB. It is also bactericidal and is tolerated well. Although not hepatotoxic, it affects the clearance of other drugs by the liver. Patients also may be concerned about the orange colored urine, sweat, and stool, as it is excreted as a reddish-orange compound.

PZA is also bactericidal and effective orally, but gastrointestinal intolerance complaints are common. Like INH, liver toxicity is a concern, and liver function tests should be monitored initially to avoid hepatitis. EMB generally is tolerated well with minimal adverse effects.

The biggest challenge in treating TB lies in patient compliance (**Fig. 5**).[47] A typical course of treatment for TB involves 6 months of multiple medications. Directly observed therapy (DOT) was developed in the 1980s to ensure patient compliance with a standard protocol of antibiotic therapy. DOT has resulted in significantly lower rates of drug resistance and relapses and should be considered for all patients infected with TB.[48]

The American Thoracic Society currently recommends the use of a combination of EMB, PZA, INH, and RIF in patients who do not have HIV for the first 2 months of treatment. Patients who have HIV and those who have resistant disease are treated with a separate protocol with different dosing and combinations of the same drugs.[49] At 2 months, sensitivities of the microorganisms

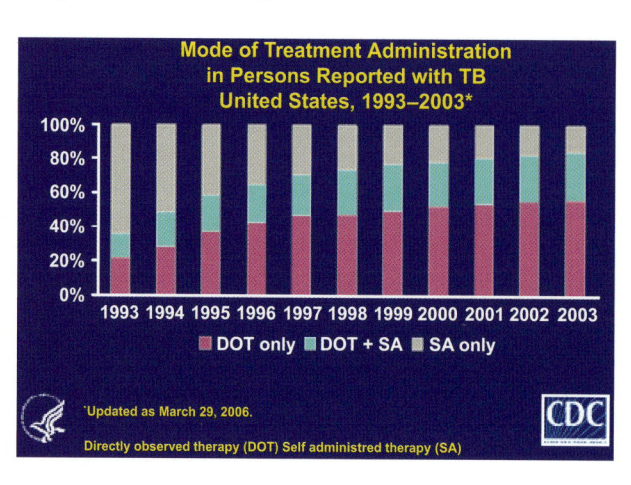

Fig. 5. Treatment methodology in the United States. (*Courtesy of* Centers for Disease Control and Prevention, Atlanta.)

and repeat clinical examination will determine if the patient will receive an additional 4 or 7 months of therapy. Drugs used to treat TB have various adverse effects, and are tolerated poorly by some. When this occurs, a drug with comparable spectrum should be substituted to ensure appropriate coverage.

Because of the relative rarity of head and neck TB, an established protocol has not been developed regarding the treatment of this disease. Studies performed comparing 6- and 9-month therapy for treating the more common TB lymphadenitis showed no difference in remission rates between the shorter versus longer therapy.[50] Another trial demonstrated two 6-month regimens that were equal in efficacy for treating TB lymphadenitis.[51] The treatment for other head and neck manifestations is generally the same, but should be individualized based on cultures and in patients not tolerating INH or RIF.

In immunocompromised patients or those who have drug resistant forms or adverse drug reactions, therapy will have to be individually tailored. Persistent oral lesions should be rebiopsied and cultured if they do not respond to the initial phase of treatment and should be monitored throughout drug therapy.

SUMMARY

TB is a serious communicable disease that causes 2 million deaths a year worldwide. It is estimated one third of the world's population is infected with TB. TB has proved difficult to eradicate. Laboratory testing also has been challenging, with as many as 19% of TB cases failing to show positive bacteriology tests. Head and neck masses and oral lesions always should be included in the differential diagnosis of TB, especially in high-risk patient populations. A combination of clinical suspicion, extensive laboratory analysis, and radiographic examination is invaluable in treating and preventing the spread of this insidious but deadly disease that has plagued mankind for ages.

REFERENCES

1. Cantwell MF, Snider DE, Cauthen GM, et al. Epidemiology of tuberculosis in the United States, 1985 through 1992. JAMA 1994;272(7):535–9.
2. Bailey BJ, Calhoun KH, Healy GB, et al. Otologic manifestations of systemic diseases. In: Schleuning AJ, Andersen PE, Fong KJ, editors. Head and neck surgery—otolaryngology. 3rd edition. Philadelphia: Lippincott Williams, and Wilkins; 2001. p. 1861.
3. Sezer B, Zeytingolu M, Tuncay U, et al. Oral mucosal ulceration. J Am Dent Assoc 2004;135(3):336–40.
4. Koehler CW. Consumption, the great killer. Modern Drug Discovery 2002;5(2):47–9. Available at: http://pubs.acs.org/subscribe/journals/mdd/v05/i02/html/02timeline.html. Accessed February 10, 2008.
5. Geiter LJ. TB epidemiology. Available at: http://www.aeras.org/tb/epidemiology/index.html. Accessed February 10, 2008.
6. Luhrman B, Pearce C. Moulin Rouge. Bazmark Films, Twentieth Century Fox Film Corp; 2001.
7. Magruder C, Woodruff R, et al. Cluster of tuberculosis cases among exotic dancers and their close contacts—Kansas, 1994–2000. MMWR Weekly 2001; 50(15):291–3.
8. The romantic death; in the 19th century, tuberculosis was so prevalent that poets, artists, and musicians glorified the spirituality of the disease—special issue: tuberculosis. Nutrition Health Review; Summer 1991. Available at: http://findarticles.com/p/articles/mi_m0876/is_n59/ai_11243007. Accessed January 31, 2008.
9. John Henry Holliday family history. Available at: http://www.kansasheritage.org/families/holliday.html. Accessed February 10, 2008.
10. Final resting place of Doc Holliday. Available at: http://www.hollywoodusa.co.uk/GravesOutofLA/docholliday.htm. Accessed February 10, 2008.
11. Marks S, Magee E, Robison V, et al. Reported HIV status of tuberculosis patients—United States, 1993–2005. MMWR Weekly 2007;56(42):1103–6.
12. Robison V, Althoomsons S, Pratt R, et al. 2006 surveillance slides. Reported tuberculosis in the United States 2007. Available at: http://www.cdc.gov/tb/surv/surv2006/pdf/FullReport.pdf. Accessed February 10, 2008.
13. Coninx R. Tuberculosis in complex emergencies. Bull World Health Organ 2007;85(8):569–648.
14. Todar K. Tuberculosis. University of Wisconsin—Madison, Department of Bacteriology 2005. Available at: http://www.textbookofbacteriology.net/tuberculosis.html. Accessed February 10, 2008.
15. Andreoli TE, Carpenter C, Griggs R, et al. Infections of the lower respiratory tract. In: Lederman MM, editor. Cecil. essentials of medicine. 6th edition. Philadelphia: W.B. Saunders; 2004. p. 867.
16. Miziara ID. Tuberculosis affecting the oral cavity in Brazilian HIV-infected patients. Oral Surg Oral Med Oral Pathol Oral Radiol Endod 2005;100(2): 179–82.
17. Miliary tuberculosis. Available at: http://pathhsw5m54.ucsf.edu/case32/image328.html. Accessed February 10, 2008.
18. Mistr SK. Tuberculosis. Available at: http://www.emedicine.com/oph/topic458.htm. Accessed March 9, 2008.
19. Jerant AF, Bannon M, Rittenhouse S. Identification and management of tuberculosis. Am Fam Physician 2000;61(9):2667–78, 2681–82.

20. Martin G, Lazarus A. Epidemiology and diagnosis of tuberculosis. Postgrad Med 2000;108(2):42–4, 47–50, 53–4.
21. Fanning A. Tuberculosis: 6. Extrapulmonary disease. CMAJ 1999;160(11):1597–603.
22. Bailey BJ, Calhoun KH, Healy GB, et al. Granulomatous diseases of the head and neck. In: Littlejohn MC, Bailey BJ, Yoo KJ, editors. Head and neck surgery—otolaryngology. 3rd edition. Philadelphia: Lippincott Wiliams, and Wilkins; 2001. p. 167.
23. Swanson DS, Pan X, Musser JM. Identification and subspecific differentiation of mycobacterium scrofulaceum by automated sequencing of a region of the gene (hsp65) encoding a 65-kilodalton heat shock protein. J Clin Microbiol 1996;34(12):3151–9.
24. McClay JE. Scrofula. Available at: http://www.emedicine.com/ent/topic524.htm. Accessed February 10, 2008.
25. Watts HG, Lifeso RM. Current concepts review—tuberculosis of bones and joints. J Bone Joint Surg Am 1996;78(2):288–98.
26. Soman D, Davies SJ. A suspected case of tuberculosis of the temporomandibular joint. Br Dent J 2003;194(1):23–4.
27. Hidalgo JA, Alangaden G. Pott disease (tuberculous spondylitis). Available at: http://www.emedicine.com/MED/topic1902.htm. Accessed February 10, 2008.
28. Fang D, Leong JC, Fang HS. Tuberculosis of the upper cervical spine. Br Ed Soc Bone Joint Surg 1983;65(1):47–50.
29. Ito FA, de Andrade CR, Vargas PA, et al. Primary tuberculosis of the oral cavity. Oral Dis 2005;11(1):50–3.
30. Prasad KC, Sreedharan S, Chakravarthy Y, et al. Tuberculosis in the head and neck: experience in India. J Laryngol Otol 2007;121(10):979–85.
31. Eng HL, Lu SY, Yang CH, et al. Oral tuberculosis. Oral Surg Oral Med Oral Pathol Oral Radiol Endod 1996;81(4):415–20.
32. Mignogna MD, Muzio L, Favia G, et al. Oral tuberculosis: a clinical evaluation of 42 cases. Oral Dis 2000;6(1):25–30.
33. Screening for tuberculosis and tuberculosis infection in high-risk populations. Recommendations of the Advisory Council for the Elimination of Tuberculosis. MMWR 1995;44(RR-11):19–34.
34. Shashidhara AN, Chaudhuri K. The tuberculin skin test—emerging 100 years since its first use. NTI Newsletter 1990;26(1&2):1–18.
35. Kamboj M, Sepkowitz KA. The risk of tuberculosis in patients with cancer. Clin Infect Dis. 2006;42(11):1592–5.
36. Basgoz N. Clinical manifestations, diagnosis, and treatment of military tuberculosis. Available at: http://www.utdol.com/utd/content/topic.do?topicKey=tubercul/8624&view=print. Accessed February 10, 2008.
37. Pai M, Riley LW, Colford JM. Interferon-gamma assays in the immunodiagnosis of tuberculosis: a systematic review. Lancet Infect Dis 2004;4(12):761–76.
38. Reported tuberculosis in the United States, 2004. Atlanta (GA): U.S. Department of Health and Human Services, CDC; 2005.
39. Daley CL, Gotway MB, Jasmer RM. Radiographic manifestations of tuberculosis: a primer for clinicians. 2nd edition. University of California, San Francisco: Francis J Curry National TB Center; 2006.
40. Perlman DC, el-Sadr WM, Nelson ET, et al. Variation in chest radiographic patterns in pulmonary tuberculosis by degree of human immunodeficiency virus-related immunosuppression. Clin Infect Dis 1997;25(2):242–6.
41. Meyer M, Clarke P, O'Regan AW. Utility of the lateral chest radiograph in the evaluation of patients with a positive tuberculin skin test result. Chest 2003;124(5):1824–7.
42. Steingart KR, Henry M, Ng V, et al. Fluorescence versus conventional sputum smear microscopy for tuberculosis: a systematic review. Lancet Infect Dis 2006;6(9):570–81.
43. Stumpe KD, Dazzi H, Schaffner A, et al. Infection imaging using whole-body FDG-PET. Eur J Nucl Med 2000;27(7):822–32.
44. Brief history of tuberculosis. Available at: http://www.umdnj.edu/~ntbcweb/history.htm. Accessed February 10, 2008.
45. Sakula A. Carlo Forlanini, inventor of artificial pneumothorax for treatment of pulmonary tuberculosis. Thorax 1983;38(5):326–32.
46. Rodrigues LC, Diwan VK, Wheeler JG. Protective effect of BCG against tuberculous meningitis and miliary tuberculosis: a meta-analysis. Int J Epidemiol 1993;22(6):1154–8.
47. Addington WW. Patient compliance: the most serious remaining problem in the control of tuberculosis in the United States. Chest 1979;76(6 Suppl):741–3.
48. Weis SE. The effect of directly observed therapy on rates of drug resistance and relapse in tuberculosis. N Engl J Med 1994;330(17):1179–84.
49. Blumberg HM, Burman WJ, Chaisson RE, et al. American Thoracic Society/Centers for Disease Control and Prevention/Infectious Diseases Society of America. Treatment of tuberculosis. Am J Respir Crit Care Med 2003;167(4):603–62.
50. Yuen AP, Wong SH, Tam CM, et al. Prospective randomized study of thrice weekly six-month and nine-month chemotherapy for cervical tuberculous lymphadenopathy. Otolaryngol Head Neck Surg 1997;116(2):189–92.
51. Jawahar MS, Rajaram K, Sivasubramanian S, et al. Treatment of lymph node tuberculosis—a randomized clinical trial of two 6-month regimens. Trop Med Int Health 2005;10(11):1090–8.

Wegener's Granulomatosis

Lawrence W. Weeda, Jr, DDS*, Stephen A. Coffey, DDS

KEYWORDS
- Wegener's granulomatosis • Vasculitides
- Strawberry gingivitis

Wegener's granulomatosis (WG) is an uncommon systemic disease characterized by necrotizing granulomatous lesions of the upper and lower respiratory tracts, skin, and eyes, and focal necrotizing glomerulonephritis. It is an immune-based process in which antibodies develop to cytoplasmic components in the neutrophil, causing lysis and release of enzymes and proteases, which induce further inflammation and local tissue necrosis.[1] First described by Klinger in 1931 and subsequently by Wegener in 1936 and 1939, WG is one of a number of small vessel vasculitides that are characterized by circulation of the abnormal antibody ANCA (antineutrophil cytoplasmic antibody) and antibodies against proteinase 3 (PR-3), a serine proteinase found in neutrophils. WG is a distinct entity with clinical and histopathologic criteria including:

Necrotizing granulomas of the upper and lower respiratory tracts
Generalized necrotizing vasculitis of small arteries and veins
Renal involvement with rapidly progressing necrotizing glomerulonephritis leading to renal failure and death within an average of 6 months.[2]

Since the original description of the disease, it has been recognized that there are limited forms of the process that may remain localized for prolonged periods before multiorgan involvement occurs. One of the identified limited forms has respiratory, but not renal involvement. There is also a superficial form in which lesions are limited to the skin and mucosa.[3] It is important to recognize that oral lesions may be the initial presenting feature in any of the forms of WG.[4]

ETIOLOGY

The cause of WG is unknown. No isolated genetic marker, environmental agent, microorganism, or other entity has been identified as causing this disease process. Familial reports of first-degree relatives exist, but these are rare. Because of the widespread occurrence of upper and lower airway involvement in these patients, granuloma formation caused by inhaled antigen and altered immune reactivity, genetic predisposition, and host factors are thought to play significant roles in causing the disease. Inhalation of a stimulant causes activation of neutrophils leading to transfer of PR-3 to cell membranes and increased levels of c-ANCA, gammaglobulins, and circulating immune complexes.[5] Vasculitis results from increased cellular and humoral immune factors that also contribute to granuloma formation, tissue destruction, and the other clinical factors of the disease process.

INCIDENCE/PREVALENCE

A prevalence of 3 cases per 100,000 people has been reported.[6] WG affects men and women equally, and has a wide age range of 9 to 78 years (mean 41 years).[7] Patients who have WG are predominantly Caucasian, with Caucasians representing approximately 90% of those affected.

INITIAL CLINICAL PRESENTATION

The clinical manifestations of WG are broad and often involve multiple organ systems. Nonspecific symptoms including fatigue, lethargy, weight loss, loss of appetite, fever, and night sweats may be

Department of Oral and Maxillofacial Surgery, University of Tennessee, College of Dentistry, 875 Union Avenue, Memphis, TN 38163, USA
* Corresponding author.
E-mail address: lweeda@utmem.edu (L.W. Weeda).

seen. Limited or mild presentations of WG involve arthralgias and upper and lower airway involvement without renal lesions. Presentation of the classic form of the disease includes sinusitis, serous otitis media, rhinitis with nasal ulcerations, cough, and hemoptysis. Patients who have the fulminant type of WG present with the preceding signs and symptoms and experience rapidly progressive respiratory failure and renal failure. Approximately 75% of patients diagnosed with WG initially seek care because of upper and lower respiratory complaints such as severe or persistent rhinorrhea, seasonal or allergic rhinitis, recurrent epistaxis, oral or nasal ulcerations, ear pain, hearing difficulty, cough, or fever. Sinusitis is the most common symptom and is seen in the initial presentation 73% of the time, and eventually develops in 85% of those who have WG.[8] Otitis media with eustachian tube blockage and altered hearing is seen as a presenting complaint in 25% of cases. Renal impairment is an uncommon initial complaint, and nonrenal manifestations almost always precede functional renal disease. Constitutional symptoms such as fevers, weight loss, anorexia, arthralgias, myalgias, and fatigue are nonspecific but common in patients who have WG (**Tables 1** and **2**).[9]

LUNG DISEASE

Virtually all WG patients will have upper airway and lung involvement, and often both in the course of their disease. Patients may complain of cough, dyspnea, pleuritic chest pain, or hemoptysis; alternatively, they may be completely asymptomatic. Common radiographic findings include pulmonary infiltrates of the upper lobes (often confused with pneumonia) and solitary or multiple pulmonary nodules, with more than half of these patients being asymptomatic. The most common lung findings are multiple, bilateral nodal infiltrates that tend to cavitate. Lung biopsy usually demonstrates granulomata and vasculitis.[10]

RENAL DISEASE

Kidney involvement is noted 18% of the time on presentation, and 85% of the time during the course of the disease.[8] The degree of kidney involvement ranges from mild focal and segmental glomerulonephritis with minimal urinary findings and little functional impairment, to fulminant diffuse necrotizing glomerulonephritis. Extrarenal findings invariably precede renal disease. Once present, however, renal disease can progress quickly to severe glomerulonephritis in a matter of weeks or even days.[10]

Table 1
Presenting signs and symptoms in Wegener's granulomatosis

Sign or Symptom	Patients n	%
Pulmonary infiltrates	60	71
Sinusitis	57	67
Joint (arthralgia or arthritis)	37	44
Otitis	21	25
Cough	29	34
Rhinitis or nasal symptoms	19	22
Hemoptysis	15	18
Ocular inflammation	14	16
Weight loss	14	16
Skin rash	11	13
Epistaxis	9	11
Renal failure	9	11
Chest discomfort	7	8
Anorexia or malaise	7	8
Proptosis	6	7
Dyspnea	6	7
Oral ulcers, hearing loss, pleuritis or effusion, headache	5	6

Adapted from Fauci A, Haynes B, Katz P, et al. Wegener's granulomatosis: prospective clinical and therapeutic experience with 85 patients for 21 years. Ann Intern Med 1983;98:77; with permission.

Table 2
Organ system involvement in Wegener's granulomatosis

Organ System	Patients n	%
Lung	80	94
Paranasal sinuses	77	91
Kidney	72	85
Joints	57	67
Nose or nasopharynx	54	64
Ear	52	61
Eye	49	58
Skin	38	45
Nervous system	19	22
Heart	10	12

Adapted from Fauci A, Haynes B, Katz P, et al. Wegener's granulomatosis: prospective clinical and therapeutic experience with 85 patients for 21 years. Ann Intern Med 1983;98:78; with permission.

UPPER AIRWAY DISEASE

Sinusitis is the most common complaint. Biopsy specimens of the upper airway frequently show nonspecific changes of acute and chronic inflammation with necrosis rather than the hallmark granulomatous vasculitis of WG. Development of a saddle nose deformity caused by collapse of nasal support is fairly common, but bony erosion through the walls of the maxillary sinus or palatal perforation is uncommon in WG.[10]

Either of these findings strongly indicates another midline destructive disease (ie, midline granuloma or a midline neoplasm). Secondary infections related to the sinusitis are common, with *Staphylococcus aureus* being the predominant cultured organism. Sinus disease may be responsive to antibiotic therapy initially, but recurrent episodes may require surgical intervention.

JOINT DISEASE

Most patients suffer from musculoskeletal manifestations such as diffuse polyarthralgias, arthritis of one or more joints, or a rheumatoid-like arthritis involving the wrists, metacarpophalangeal joints, interphalangeal joints, knees, ankles, and other small joints.[10] Arthralgias are typically polyarticular, involving small and large joints symmetrically. Arthritis most commonly is associated with large joints, especially the knees and ankles, and is seldom deforming. The extent of joint involvement usually parallels the disease process in other organ systems.

EYE DISEASE

Ocular involvement is present in 50% to 66% of patients who have symptoms, including conjunctivitis, episcleritis, uveitis, optic nerve vasculitis, retinal artery occlusion, nasolacrimal duct obstruction, and proptosis.[11] Most ocular symptoms are caused by vasculitis. Proptosis results from tracking of the granulomatous lesions laterally through the lamina papyracea of the ethmoid bone into the medial orbit, and is frequently refractory to treatment even with complete remission in other organ systems.

SKIN DISEASE

Skin disease occurs in 30% to 50% of patients who have WG. The incidence falls to 27% when uremic skin disease is excluded. Skin involvement may include various nonspecific cutaneous lesions, including palpable purpura, subcutaneous nodules, pustules, vesicles, macules, petechiae, and splinter hemorrhages of the fingernails.[12]

The extremities are the most common sites of skin lesions, especially the legs and feet. Raynaud's phenomenon, digital ischemia, and necrosis not caused by vasospasm can been found in patients who have the fulminant type of WG. Skin disease is usually nonspecific, but four histopathologic subgroups have been identified: (1) necrotizing vasculitis, (2) necrotizing palisading granuloma, (3) granulomatous vasculitis, and (4) lymphomatoid granulomatosis. Hu and colleagues[13] noted a clinicopathologic link to progress. Vesicles and ulcers correlated with severe onset and extensive disease, and necrotizing vasculitis or lymphomatoid granulomatosis had the worst prognosis.

NERVOUS SYSTEM DISEASE

Nervous system disease is seen in about 20% of patients who have WG. Involvement is divided equally between peripheral nervous system involvement and cranial nerve abnormalities. In a study by Drachman,[14] the facial nerve was the most frequently involved cranial nerve.

MISCELLANEOUS ORGAN SYSTEM INVOLVEMENT

Other organ system involvement that has been reported includes acute pericarditis, granulomata of major salivary glands, acute thyroiditis, and necrotizing granulomata of the cervical vertebrae.

ORAL PRESENTATION

Oral lesions occur in 6% to 13% of WG cases, and are the initial presenting feature in only 2% of cases.[15–17] The prevalence of oral lesions tends to increase in patients who have more advanced disease. Oral symptoms may include a painful cobblestone or ulcerative appearance of the palatal mucosa or gingival. Palatal bony erosion is overstated and rarely occurs.[1] Oroantral fistulae and labial mucosa nodules are also uncommon oral findings. Oral signs and symptoms are commonly suggestive of fungal disease. There have been reports of the initial presenting feature of pain and swelling involving the major salivary glands.[18,19] The most common oral lesion in WG is a hyperplastic gingivitis, which is red to purple with many petechiae, and usually limited to the attached mucosa. It has been given the name strawberry gingivitis, because it resembles the appearance of over-ripe strawberries (**Fig. 1**). It is rarely an early manifestation, but its microscopic features of pseudoepitheliomatous hyperplasia (PEH), multinucleated giant cells, and microabscesses in a patient who had severe systemic upset are virtually diagnostic of WG.[20] The lesion

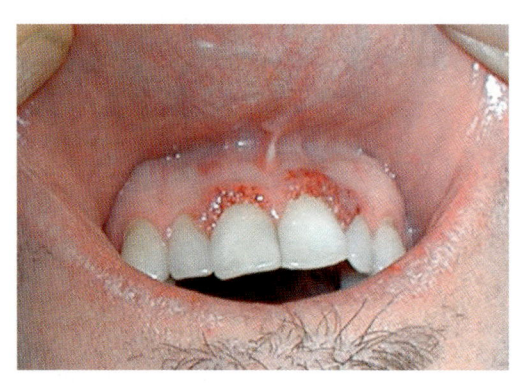

Fig. 1. Hyperplastic gingivitis.

begins at the interdental papilla as an exophytic hyperplasia with petechial flecks and a red friable granular appearance. Pain and bleeding are common symptoms. It spreads quickly, accompanied by alveolar bone loss and tooth mobility.[21] Extraction sites associated with the lesion fail to heal. Often involvement of the lower respiratory tract and/or kidney can be detected at the time of oral presentation, yielding a worse prognosis than isolated oral involvement.[3]

DIFFERENTIAL DIAGNOSIS

Although oral findings are an uncommon initial finding in WG, oral involvement becomes more frequent as the systemic disease process progresses. Because the oral manifestations of WG are frequently clinically nonspecific, patients who have only oral findings may provide a clinical picture resembling several different processes.

There have been reported cases in which the initial findings were limited to pain and swelling of one or more major salivary glands. In these cases, the differential diagnosis would include infectious diseases, both viral (mumps) and bacterial (tuberculosis, actinomycosis, syphilis), and noninfective processes (Sjögren's, sarcoidosis).[18]

In cases presenting as oral ulcers or hyperplastic gingivitis, entities to consider include fungal disease, squamous cell carcinoma, lymphoma, infectious granulomatous processes (tuberculosis, actinomycosis, syphilis), Langerhans cell histocytosis, peripheral giant cell lesion, necrotizing ulcerative gingivitis, necrotizing sialometaplasia, and pyogenic granuloma.[3,20]

In most instances, special stains of biopsy material, cultures, or antibody titer can rule out fungal disease or bacterial infection.[4] The histopathological characteristics of the oral lesions of WG (ie, PEH, necrosis with microabscess formation, and multinucleated giant cells [which are different than the giant cells encountered in the peripheral giant cell lesion) usually will rule out other processes that may share some of the histopathological characteristics of WG.[20]

PATHOLOGY

The classic necrotizing granulomatous pattern of WG can be found in the small arteries and veins, and in biopsies of involved lung and renal tissues. Biopsies of the upper respiratory tract including nasal, sinus, and tracheal mucosa typically demonstrate nonspecific acute and chronic inflammation without true vasculitis and with or without giant cells.[8] Bronchoalveolar lavage shows phagocytosis of neutrophils by monocytes, neutrophilic alveolitis, and high levels of c-ANCA compared with serum levels. Renal biopsies display crescentic focal segmental glomerulonephritis with necrosis in severe forms.[9]

ORAL HISTOPATHOLOGY

The histopathology noted in the classic description of WG includes vasculitis, ill-defined granulomata, multinucleated giant cells, and necrosis. These criteria, however, usually are seen only on thorascopic lung biopsy and are notably absent from oral lesions.[15] Vasculitis is the most common missing component in oral lesion histopathology. The most common histopathologic features encountered in oral lesions are:

Intense acute or chronic inflammation with microabscesses
Multinucleated giant cells
PEH

These findings are considered nonspecific, and make diagnosing WG from only microscopic criteria difficult. This reinforces the importance of seeking other evidence of systemic disease to aid in the diagnosis. Even with these histopathologic variables, the previously noted oral microscopic criteria associated with the strawberry gingivitis lesion is highly suggestive of WG when no other organ system involvement is apparent.[20]

DIAGNOSIS

The diagnosis of WG requires analyzing the combination of supportive clinical and histopathologic features, and laboratory confirmation. WG should be suspected with a patient who presents with multisystem illness involving upper and/or lower respiratory tract disease, glomerulonephritis, and vasculitis of any organ system. Historically, the gold standard for diagnosis of WG was necrotizing granulomatous inflammation on lung biopsy, but this method is not always effective because of the fact that active lung involvement is not always present initially.[9] Presence of the classic triad of necrotizing granulomas of the upper and lower respiratory tract including the ears, nose and throat; necrotizing or granulomatous vasculitis of small arteries and veins; and necrotizing glomerulonephritis along with a positive c-ANCA easily confirms the diagnosis.[12] In early or limited disease, however, the diagnosis of WG may become more difficult. Destructive upper airway disease has to be distinguished from fungal or bacterial infection, substance abuse, malignancy, and trauma.[8] The American College of Rheumatology suggests that the diagnosis of WG requires at least two of the following: (1) oral ulcers or nasal discharge; (2) nodules, fixed infiltrate, or cavities on chest films; (3) nephritic urinary sediment (red cell cast or greater than 5 red blood cells [RBC] per high power field); and (4) granulomatous inflammation on biopsy.[15]

LABORATORY STUDIES

Davies first described testing for ANCA in 1982. Van der Woude and colleagues[22] confirmed the connection between WG and ANCA in 1985. ANCA is a laboratory marker that is sensitive and specific for WG. Indirect immunofluoresecnce reactions exist for the antineutrophil cytoplasmic antibodies in either a perinuclear pattern (p-ANCA) or a cytoplasmic pattern (c-ANCA). Cytoplasmic localization confirmed with c-ANCA is present in approximately 90% to 95% of cases of acute generalized WG.[5] Positive c-ANCA may be present in 60% of early or localized forms of WG. In the presence of clinical findings, a positive c-ANCA confirms the diagnosis, while a negative result does not rule out WG necessarily. A positive c-ANCA should be confirmed by a more specific ELISA test for PR-3 and antimyeloperoxidase (MPO). PR3 is a serine proteinase found in the granules of neutrophils and is the major antigen for c-ANCA. MPO is a lysosomal enzyme also found in neutrophils, and it is the major antigen for p-ANCA.[15]

Hematologic laboratory abnormalities found in patients who have WG include normochromic anemia, normocytic anemia, leukocytosis, eosinophilia, and an elevated erythrocyte sedimentation rate.[8] Urinalysis reveals microhematuria, proteinuria, and cellular casts.[9] Blood chemistries reveal hypoalbuminemia and mild to severe renal insufficiency. As previously mentioned, serologic studies may include positive c-ANCA and positive rheumatoid factor and antinuclear antibodies, hypergammaglobulinemia, and an elevated C-reactive protein.[9]

GENERAL MANAGEMENT

For 35 years, the gold standard for treatment for WG has been the combination of prednisone and cyclophosphamide (cyc).[23] This therapy brings an immediate response to most patients within the first week. The typical treatment protocol is oral administration of prednisone, 1 mg/kg/d, and cyc 2 to 3 mg/kg/d. Once remission is achieved, the prednisone is tapered gradually over 3 months to 60 mg on alternate days, and then tapered until discontinued. The cyc is continued for at least 1 year following complete remission. Complete remission is indicated by resolution of oral lesions, clearing of pulmonary infiltrates with evidence of stable scarring, and no further evidence of active renal sediment.[15] Following the year of remission, the cyc dose is lowered in 25 mg increments every 2 to 3 months until discontinuance, or disease activity is noted.[8] Using this protocol yields an initial remission rate of over 90%. There is a 30% rate of relapse following complete remission, which usually occurs during tapering of immunosuppressant therapy, requiring readjustment of dosages. c-ANCA levels may be used to follow disease activity. Patients are less prone to relapse if their antineutrophilic antibodies disappear during treatment. If c-ANA levels persist, there is a greater risk of relapse.

As in all immunosuppressive protocols, there is significant risk for therapy-related morbidity. The most common complication is cystitis (34%), but this usually does not have long-term impact.[11] Other therapy-related morbidities include bladder cancer, myelodysplastic syndrome, severe infections, squamous cell carcinoma, Kaposi sarcoma, and basal cell carcinoma.[15] These morbidities are dose-related to the immunosuppressive agents. Commonly noted adverse effects include marrow suppression, particularly leukopenia, hair loss, gonadal dysfunction, and herpes zoster.[11]

The myelosuppressive adverse effects of cyc and the infectious morbidities can be decreased by monitoring the white blood cell count and keeping the leukocyte count above 3000/mm^3 and the total neutrophil count in the 1000 to 1500/mm^3 range. Increasing the prednisone dose in patients who can tolerate only a subtherapeutic dose of cyc allows the cyc dose to be increased and limits the degree of leukopenia.[11]

The typically seen adverse effects associated with long-term glucocorticoid therapy may occur during prednisone therapy. Short-term adverse effects of prednisone therapy include hyperglycemia and fluid retention. Osteoporosis, infections, and severe joint or abdominal pain are some of the potential long-term adverse effects.[24]

Most alternatives to the standard prednisone/cyc regimen are aimed at treatment of resistant cases of WG, or substitutions for cyc that may decrease the therapy-related morbidity while still offering the benefits of remission. Intermittent pulse intravenous cyc administration has proven as effective as oral administration while decreasing treatment-related morbidity, but relapse is more common. Trimethoprim sulfamethoxazole (Bactrim) has been added to the standard regimen to reduce relapse rate and infection incidence.[15] Substituting 25 mg of oral methotrexate weekly for the cyc once the disease process has been controlled has maintained remission.[1]

Recent studies have looked at new agents to replace cyc in the treatment equation. Rituximab, a monoclonal antibody that selectively depletes B lymphocytes; Infliximab, a monoclonal antitumor necrosis factor α drug; and the immunosuppressive drug, Leflunomid may play a therapeutic role in the future.[25–28]

ORAL MANAGEMENT

Once a diagnosis of WG is established, it is important to perform a thorough oral evaluation to identify any potential infectious sources that should be addressed before instituting immunosuppressive therapy. Intralesional steroid injections (triamcinolone acetonide 10 mg/mL) may assist in the prompt resolution of gingival disease.[8] During induction therapy, only emergency dental treatment should be performed. Daily antimicrobial mouth rinses may be helpful during induction and maintenance therapy. During remission, frequent recall and prophylaxis should be performed. Before any invasive procedure, the managing physician should be consulted. Antibacterial prophylaxis and corticosteroid supplementation should be employed as required. If oral lesions suggestive of relapse appear, immediate specialist referral is indicated.

SUMMARY

WG is an uncommon disease process with considerable risk of mortality if diagnosis and treatment are delayed. Skin, sinus, or oral mucosal lesions may be part of the initial presentation. This article provided the clinician with information concerning recognition, diagnosis, and treatment of WG. Early recognition and treatment are essential in limiting the potentially life-threatening aspects of the disease.

REFERENCES

1. Marx RE, Stern D. Wegener's granulomatosis. In: Bywaters LC, editor. Oral and maxillofacial pathology: rationale for diagnosis and treatment. Chicago: Quintessence; 2003. p. 199–201.
2. Eufinger H, Machtens E, Akuamoa-Boateng E. Oral manifestations of Wegener's granulomatosis: review of the literature and report of a case. Int J Oral Maxillofac Surg 1992;21:50–3.
3. Handlers J, Waterman J, Abrams A, et al. Oral features of Wegener's granulomatosis. Arch Otolaryngol 1985;111:267–70.
4. Allen C, Camisa C, Salewski C, et al. Wegener's granulomatosis: report of three cases with oral lesions. J Oral Maxillofac Surg 1991;49:294–8.
5. Neville BW, Damm DD, Allen CM, et al. Wegener's granulomatosis. In: Alvis K, editor. Oral and maxillofacial pathology. 2nd edition. Philadelphia: WB Sanders; 2002. p. 297–300.
6. Hoffman GS, Kerr GS, Leavitt RY. Wegener's granulomatosis: an analysis of 158 patients. Ann Intern Med 1992;116:488–98.
7. Cotch MF, Hoffman GS. The epidemiology of Wegener's granulomatosis: how rare is it? [abstract]. Arthritis Rheum 1994;37(Suppl 9):S408.
8. Lilly J, Juhlin T, Lew D, et al. Wegener's granulomatosis presenting as oral lesions: a case report. Oral Surg Oral Med Oral Pathol Oral Radiol Endod 1998;85:153–7.
9. Allen NB. In: Bennett CJ, Plum F, editors. Wegener's granulomatosis. In: Cecil textbook of medicine. 20th edition. Philadelphia: WB Saunders; 1996. p. 1495–8.
10. Fauci A, Haynes B, Katz P, et al. Wegener's granulomatosis: prospective clinical and therapeutic experience with 85 patients for 21 years. Ann Intern Med 1983;98:76–85.
11. Haynes BE, Fishman ML, Fauci AS, et al. The ocular manifestations of Wegener's granulomatosis: fifteen years experience and review of the literature. Am J Med 1977;63:131–41.
12. Patten S, Tomecki K. Wegener's granulomatosis: cutaneous and oral mucosal disease. J Am Acad Dermatol 1993;28:710–8.
13. Hu C, O'Loughlin S, Winkelmann R. Cutaneous manifestations of Wegener's granulomatosis. Arch Dermatol 1977;113:175–82.
14. Drachman DA. Neurological complications of Wegener's granulomatosis. Arch Neurol 1963;8:145–55.
15. Ponniah I, Shaheen A, Shankar K, et al. Wegener's granulomatosis: the current understanding. Oral Surg Oral Med Oral Pathol Oral Radiol Endod 2005;100(3):265–70.
16. Parsons E, Macleod R, Nand N, et al. Wegener's granulomatosis. J Clin Periodontol 1992;19:64–6.

17. Cohen R, Cardoza T, Drinnan A, et al. Gingival manifestations of Wegener's granulomatosis. J Periodontol 1990;61:705–9.
18. Vanhauwaert B, Roskams T, Vanneste S, et al. Salivary gland involvement as initial presentation of Wegener's disease. Postgrad Med J 1993;69:643–5.
19. Ah-See K, McLaren K, Maran A. Wegener's granulomatosis presenting as major salivary gland enlargement. J Laryngol Otol 1996;110:691–3.
20. Napier S, Allen J, Irwin C, et al. Strawberry gums: clinicopathological manifestation diagnostic of Wegener's granulomatosis? J Clin Pathol 1993;46:709–12.
21. Lutcavage GJ, Schaber SJ, Arendt DA, et al. Gingival mass with massive soft-tissue necrosis. J Oral Maxillofac Surg 1991;49:1332–8.
22. Van der Woude FJ, Rasmussen N, Lobatto S, et al. Autoantibodies against neutrophils and monocytes: tool for diagnosis and marker of disease activity in Wegener's granulomatosis. Lancet 1985;425–9.
23. Fauci AS, Wolff SM. Wegener's granulomatosis: studies in eighteen patients with a review of the literature. Medicine 1973;52:535–61.
24. deSilva DJ, Cole C, Luthert P, et al. Masked orbital abscess in Wegener's granulomatosis. Eye 2007;21:246–8.
25. Keogh K, Ytterberg S, Fervenze F, et al. Rituximab for refractory Wegener's granulomatosis. Am J Respir Crit Care Med 2006;173:180–7.
26. Jayne D. Leflunomide versus methotrexate in Wegener's granulomatosis. Rheumatology 2007;46(7):1047–8.
27. Metzler C, Miehle N, Manger K, et al. Elevated relapse rate under oral methotrexate versus leflunomide for maintenance in Wegener's granulomatosis. Rheumatology 2007;46(7):1087–91.
28. Lamprecht P, Voswinkel J, Lilienthal T, et al. Effectiveness of TNF-α blockade with infliximab in refractory Wegener's granulomatosis. Rheumatology 2002;41:1303–7.

Systemic Lupus Erythematosus and Discoid Lupus Erythematosus

David B. Powers, DMD, MD[a,b,*]

KEYWORDS

- Lupus erythematosus • Discoid lupus
- Treatment • Medications • Surgical implications

Systemic lupus erythematosus (SLE) is an autoimmune disorder of unknown etiology that affects numerous organ systems including the renal, cardiovascular, gastrointestinal, and central and peripheral nervous systems. This inflammation leads to damage of the affected organ systems and a myriad of symptoms which can sometimes lead to delay or confusion with the diagnosis of the disorder. The primary cause of tissue injury is due to autoantibodies and immune complexes mediating destruction of host tissue cell nuclei. The practicing oral and maxillofacial surgeon (OMS) needs to understand the potential complications of SLE and the alterations in treatment protocols which would be necessary to safely treat a patient with SLE. This article outlines the disease process, prevalence and presentation, and specific variants, and discusses treatment regimens available for incorporation into current practice.

DESCRIPTION AND PREVALENCE

In SLE, tissues and cells are damaged by host-induced antibodies and immune complexes. Over 90% of cases occur in women, usually of child-bearing age, but the disease can also strike the elderly, men, and children.[1] In the United States the prevalence of SLE ranges from 15 to 50 cases per 100,000 population, with an incidence of 1.5 to 7.6 cases per 100,000 population per year, with African Americans have a higher incidence (1:250) when compared with Caucasians (1:1000).[2] Patel and colleagues[3] recently reported a significant ethnic variance in biopsy-proven cases of lupus nephritis in the United Kingdom as follows: 110.3 cases per 100,000 Chinese patients, 99.2 cases per 100,000 Afro-Caribbean patients, 21.4 cases per 100,000 Indo-Asian patients, and 5.6 cases per 100,000 white/Caucasian patients.

Johnson and colleagues[4] reported the Afro-Caribbean incidence as 206.0 cases per 100,000 population, which is consistent with the US experience. Regardless of the study, a definite variability in the incidence and prevalence of SLE has been established based on ethnic background. Genetics has an important role in the presentation of SLE. Grisolia[5] noted that if a mother had SLE, her daughter's potential for developing the disease was 1:40, whereas her son's potential would be 1:250. Significant progress has been made in isolating genomes to the presentation of SLE, as well as in identifying pathogenic autoantibodies and

---

This is a United States Government work. The views expressed by the author do not represent the official position of the United States Air Force, the Department of Defense, or any other branch of the United States Government.

[a] US Air Force Center for Sustainment of Trauma and Readiness Skills (C-STARS), Baltimore, MD, USA
[b] R. Adams Cowley Shock Trauma Center, University of Maryland Medical Center, Baltimore, MD, USA
* C-STARS Baltimore, 22 S. Greene Street, Room T5R46, R. Adams Cowley Shock Trauma Center, Baltimore, MD 21201-1544.
E-mail address: DPowers@umm.edu

their main clinical effects.[2] Although these findings convey a greater understanding of the disease, an in-depth discussion of this research is beyond the scope of this article and does not significantly alter the treatment regimen provided by the surgeon.

VARIANTS

Several distinct variations and presentations of lupus are seen in a review of the medical literature.[1,2,6]

Systemic Lupus Erythematosus

SLE is generally accepted as the most common form of the disease that patients and physicians refer to when discussing this disorder. Autoantibodies, circulating immune complexes, and T lymphocytes all convey the presence of the disease. The primary focus of this article revolves around this particular presentation (**Fig. 1**).

Cutaneous Lupus Erythematosus

Rheumatologists have broken down cutaneous lupus into specific and nonspecific skin lesions found in patients with lupus erythematosus (LE). These categories are acute cutaneous LE, subacute cutaneous LE, and chronic cutaneous LE.[6]

Acute cutaneous Lupus Erythematosus
Acute cutaneous LE usually presents as a butterfly rash localized to the face but can occur anywhere on the body. Systemic manifestations of the disease are common with this entity (**Fig. 2**).

Subacute cutaneous lupus erythematosus
In subacute cutaneous LE, skin lesions occur on portions of the body that are exposed to the sun. A key characteristic of this condition is the lack

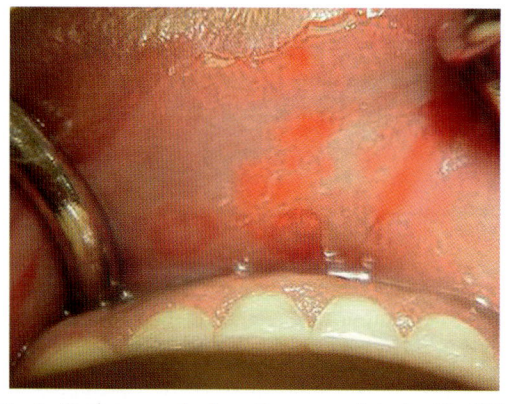

Fig. 1. Oral mucosal ulcerations associated with SLE. These ulcerations are generally painless and can present on other cutaneous tissues.

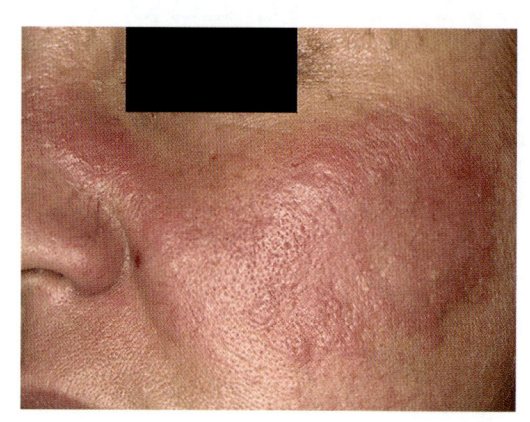

Fig. 2. Classic presentation of malar rash associated with SLE.

of scarring associated with the rash with resolution. Subacute cutaneous LE occurs in three forms: annular, psoriasiform, or a combination of both.

Annular Ringlike lesions commonly appear in the chest region. These lesions are symmetric in shape and are usually associated with systemic findings of LE.

Psoriasiform In the psoriasiform condition, thick and scaly lesions similar in appearance and development to psoriasis can develop anywhere on the body, although they usually appear at the knees.

Chronic cutaneous lupus erythematosus
Discoid lupus erythematosus Discoid LE is the most common of the chronic cutaneous forms of LE, constituting between 50% and 80% of all forms of presentation. A skin disorder occurs in which a red, raised rash appears on the body, primarily in the facial region, which may result in scarring. The length of duration of the rash varies from days to weeks or years, and recurrence is a distinct possibility. In a small percentage of patients with discoid LE, usually less than 5%, SLE may ultimately develop (**Figs. 3** and **4**). One of the more concerning aspects of this disorder is the development of scarring alopecia. Patients with discoid LE (**Fig. 5**) rarely meet the published criteria for the diagnosis of SLE. Discoid LE can occur at any age but is most often seen between the ages of 20 and 40 years with a male-to-female ratio of 1:2. There is a slight racial predilection for the African American population over those of Caucasian heritage.[1,7]

Hypertrophic lupus Hypertrophic lupus is caused by a raised bump similar to a wart and consistently develops at the site of trauma.

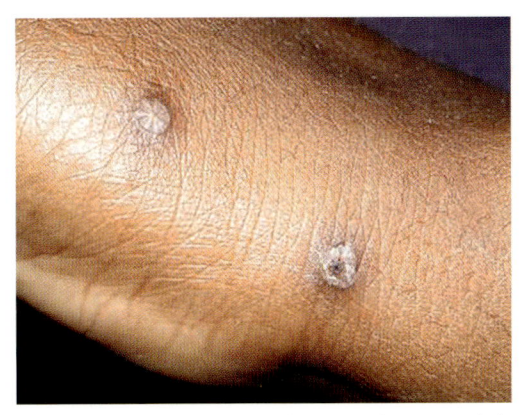

Fig. 3. Discoid LE lesions on the lateral aspect of the hand.

Lupus profundus In lupus profundus, a deep dermal or subcutaneous nodule arises in which the overlying skin may be attached to the developing lesion, but it generally heals without scarring.

Lupus tumidus Lupus tumidus presents with indurated plaques or broad, slow-healing lesions.

Chilblain lupus Chilblain lupus presents with itchy, cold sensations of the extremities, including the fingers and toes, as well as dark red, painful swelling.

Drug-Induced Lupus

Drug-induced lupus is an iatrogenic form of the disease caused by the ingestion of different medications. Numerous medications can cause a drug-induced form of lupus, but the symptoms generally resolve after termination of the drug. Common medications found to induce a lupus reaction are listed in **Table 1**.[1,8–10]

There are significant differences between drug-induced lupus and SLE. The ratio of presentation between the sexes is roughly equivalent, renal

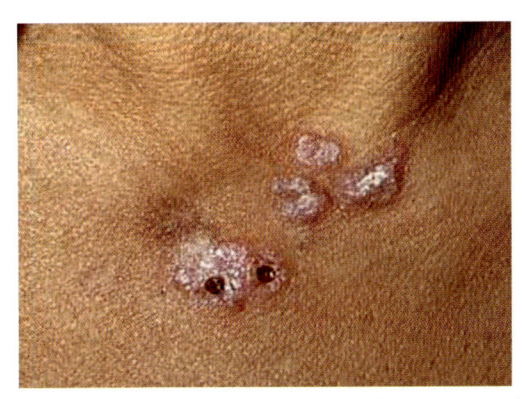

Fig. 4. Raised red rash in the region of the suprasternal notch consistent with the presentation of discoid LE.

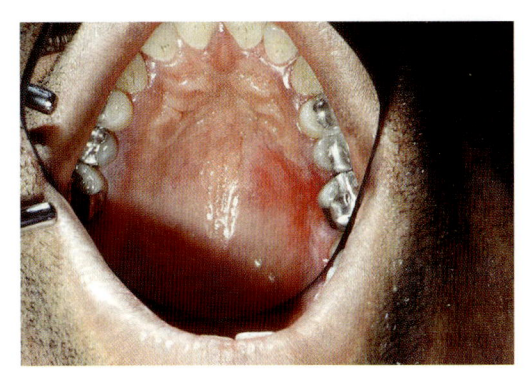

Fig. 5. Discoid LE on the palatal mucosa.

and central nervous system involvement is rare, and there is no development of autoantibodies to native DNA or hypocomplementemia. Repeat laboratory studies should be accomplished after discontinuing the medication causing the condition to verify the return to normal values and justify the diagnosis of drug-induced lupus.

Neonatal Lupus

Neonatal lupus is an unusual disorder that can occur in newborn babies of women with SLE, Sjögren's syndrome, or even in individuals with no history of the presence of autoimmune disorders. It is believed that neonatal lupus is caused by autoantibodies called anti-Ro (SSA) and anti-La (SSB). At birth, the infants have a skin rash, liver disorders, and anemia. These symptoms gradually resolve over several months. In rare instances, infants with neonatal lupus may have a serious heart condition that causes a persistent bradycardia. Neonatal lupus is rare, and most infants of mothers with SLE are born healthy. All women who are pregnant and known to have anti-Ro (SSA) or anti-La (SSB) antibodies should be monitored by echocardiograms during week 16 and 30 of pregnancy for detection of the possible development of fetal bradycardia.[2]

PHYSICAL FINDINGS

At the onset of symptoms, the patient may display a single organ system involvement or multisystem involvement. The most common presenting symptoms are listed in **Table 2**.[1]

The description of fever and malaise is a challenging diagnostic dilemma in the determination of SLE. It can be a manifestation of active SLE or a marker of infection, malignancy, or a drug-induced reaction. An elevation of temperature greater than 102°F should merit a thorough evaluation of the patient to rule out possible active

Table 1
Common medications that induce a lupus reaction

Definite Association	Possible Association	Unlikely Association
Anti-TNF biologics	Beta-blockers	Allopurinol
Chlorpromazine	Captopril	Chlorthalidone
Hydralazine	Carbamazepine	Gold salts
Isoniazid	Cimetidine	Griseofulvin
Methyldopa	Ethosuximide	Methysergide
Minocycline	Hydrazines	Oral contraceptives
Procainamide	Levodopa	Penicillin
Quinidine	Lithium	Phenylbutazone
	Methimazole	Reserpine
	Nitrofurantoin	Streptomycin
	Penicillamine	Tetracyclines
	Phenytoin	
	Propylthiouracil	
	Sulfasalazine	
	Sulfonamides	
	Trimethadione	

infection or malignancy, because the temperature elevation in SLE is generally below that threshold.

The malar rash is a fixed erythematous area which cannot be wiped off, sparing the nasolabial folds (see **Fig. 2**). Classically described as a "butterfly rash" that can be flat or raised over the cheeks and bridge of the nose, it often involves the chin and ears. A discoid rash can occur in up to 20% of patients with SLE and can lead to significant disfigurement secondary to scarring (see **Figs. 3** and **4**).[1] The discoid rash presents as erythematous patches with keratotic scaling over sun-exposed areas of the skin, which may occur in the presence or absence of any other systemic manifestations (**Fig. 6**) (**Table 3**).

The presence of intraoral mucosal ulcerations is a valuable diagnostic tool for the diagnosis of SLE. The practicing OMS may be called upon to evaluate these patients as a referral from general medical and dental practitioners. These ulcers, usually painless, can also appear in the vaginal tissues of female patients, and a thorough medical history and discussion of overall presenting symptoms exclusive of the head and neck region is imperative.

Gastrointestinal findings may include vague abdominal complaints of discomfort, nausea, and diarrhea. Acute abdominal pain, vomiting, and severe diarrhea may signify vasculitis of the intestine. Musculoskeletal manifestations of the disease include tenderness, edema, and effusions.[1] Arthritis is usually symmetric, nonerosive, and usually nondeforming, frequently involving the proximal interphalangeal and metacarpophalangeal joints of

Table 2
Common presenting symptoms of lupus

Symptom	Percentage of Patients Positive During Disease
Fever/malaise	95
Arthralgia/myalgia	95
Anemia	70
Photosensitivity	70
Malar rash	50
Oral ulcers	40

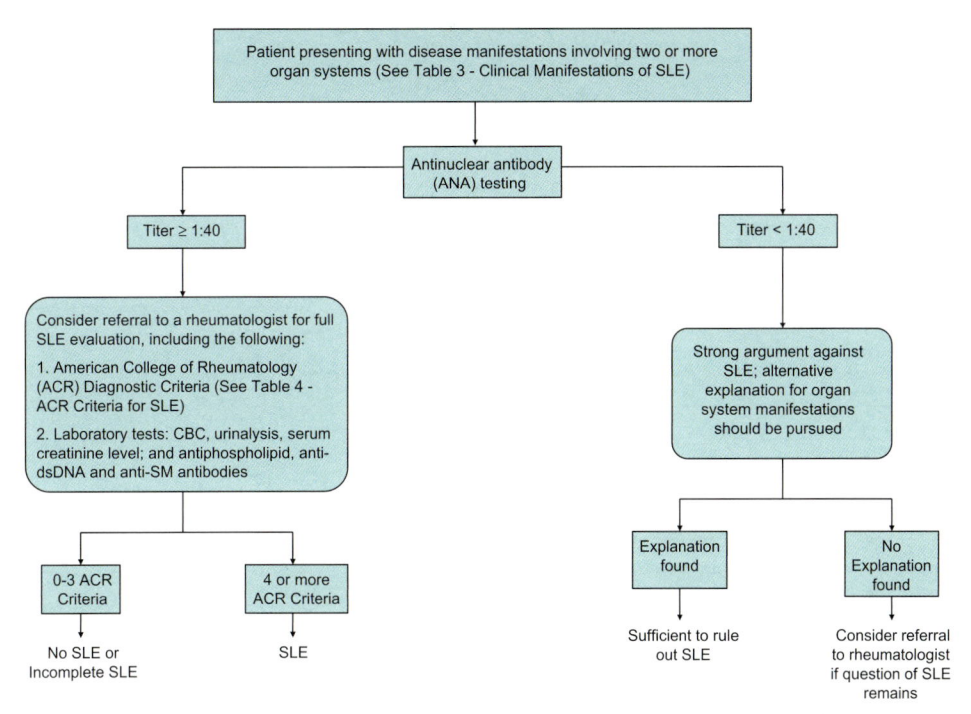

Fig. 6. Algorithm for the diagnosis of SLE. (*From* Gill JM, Quisel AM, Rocca PV, et al. Diagnosis of systemic lupus erythematosus. Am Fam Physician 2003;68:2179–86; with permission. Available at: http://www.aafp.org/afp/20031201/2179.html. Accessed July 19, 2008; with permission.)

the hands, as well as the wrists and knees. Evaluation of the digital extremities may also show evidence of vasculitis and splinter hemorrhages.[1]

Fundoscopic examination is another evaluation that is within the scope of the OMS and is an important component of the SLE work-up in patients with visual complaints. Retinal vasculitis can lead to blindness and is demonstrated by sheathed narrow retinal arterioles with white exudates adjacent to the vessels (**Fig. 8**).[11]

As is common with other renal diseases, signs and symptoms of renal impairment may not be apparent in SLE until advanced nephrotic syndrome or renal failure is present. Obtaining a baseline urinalysis, serum blood urea nitrogen (BUN), and creatinine levels would be a prudent step in the preliminary evaluation of a patient with SLE, or to monitor progression of the disease in a patient known to have the disorder.[1] A comprehensive evaluation must occur to evaluate for possible pulmonary effusions, pericarditis, systolic murmurs, and other sequela of the progression of SLE within the cardiopulmonary system.

DIAGNOSIS OF SYSTEMIC LUPUS ERYTHEMATOSUS

In 1982 the American College of Rheumatology accepted the criteria for the definition of SLE as published by Tan and colleagues (**Table 4**).[12]

Eleven separate findings were presented, and a patient was determined to have SLE if they showed four or more of these components.

DIFFERENTIAL DIAGNOSIS

During the determination of SLE, a comprehensive differential diagnosis (**Box 1**) must be considered by the OMS if a patient acutely needs surgical intervention or management in a clinic setting. Each of these medical conditions should be considered when treating a patient who presents with the signs and symptoms of SLE without a formal diagnosis and are presented in no particular order.[1,9]

The list in **Box 1** is not exclusive, and other medical conditions could be present or should be considered. A comprehensive history and physical examination paying particular attention to the description of symptoms by the patient is paramount to the safe treatment of an individual who presents with symptoms suggestive of SLE but who does not have a definitive diagnosis at the time of evaluation.

MORBIDITY AND MORTALITY

Once the diagnosis of SLE has been confirmed, the survival rate for patients with the disease is 90% to 95% at 2 years, 82% to 90% at 5 years, 71% to 80% at 10 years, and 63% to 75% at 20

Table 3
Clinical manifestations of SLE

Clinical Manifestation	Percentage of Patients Positive During Course of Disease
Systemic	95
Fatigue, malaise, fever, anorexia, nausea, weight loss	
Musculoskeletal	95
Arthralgia/myalgia	95
Nonerosive polyarthritis	60
Myopathy/myositis	40
Hematologic	85
Anemia of chronic disease	70
Leukopenia	65
Lymphopenia	50
Lymphadenopathy	20
Cutaneous	80
Photosensitivity	70
Malar rash	50
Oral ulcers	40
Other rashes (urticarial, bullous, maculopapular)	40
Alopecia	40
Vasculitis	20
Discoid rash	15–20
Neurologic	60
Cognitive dysfunction	50
Organic brain syndromes	35
Seizures	20
Psychosis	10
Headache	25
Cardiopulmonary	60
Pleurisy	50
Pericarditis	30
Pleural effusions	30
Endocarditis (Libman-Sacks)	10
Renal	50
Proteinuria	50
Cellular casts	50
Nephritic syndrome	25
Gastrointestinal	45
Abnormal liver enzymes	40
Nonspecific (anorexia, nausea, mild pain, diarrhea)	30
Fetal loss	30
Thrombosis	15
Venous	10
Arterial	5
Ocular	15
Sicca syndrome	15
Conjunctivitis	10

Data from Hahn BH Systemic lupus erythematosus. In: Harrison's principles of internal medicine. 17th edition. New York: McGraw-Hill; 2008. p. 2075–83.

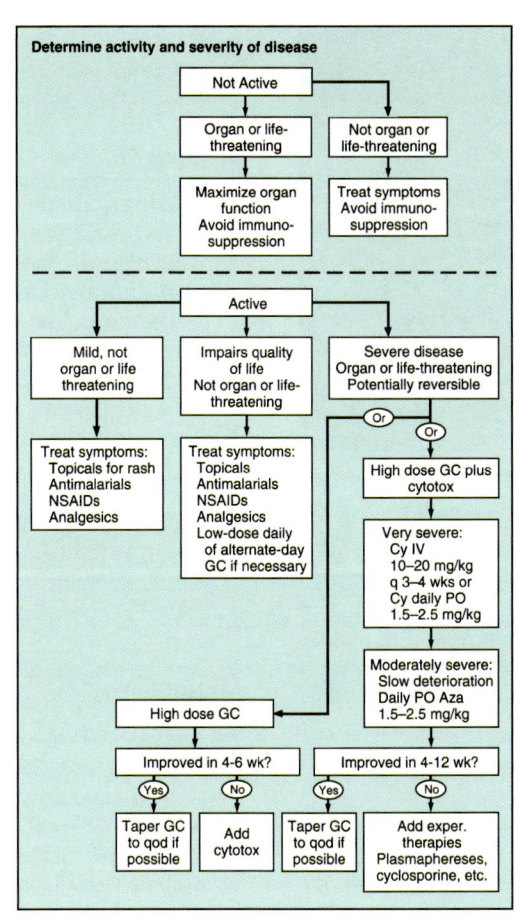

Fig. 7. Algorithm for the treatment of SLE. (*From* Q-Notes for Adult Medicine. SLE-Systemic Lupus Erythematosus. Available at: http://enotes.tripod.com/sle.htm. Accessed July 19, 2008; with permission.)

years.[1] High serum creatinine levels (>1.4 mg/dL), hypertension, nephrotic syndrome (24-hour urine protein excretion >2.6 g), anemia, low socioeconomic class, and hypocomplementemia have been associated with an approximately 50% mortality rate at 10 years.[1] Infections and renal failure are the leading causes of death in the first decade of disease, whereas thromboembolic events are frequently the cause of death in the second and later decades. Providers must consider avascular necrosis, which is common in patients receiving glucocorticoids for SLE, or septic arthritis when one joint is inflamed out of proportion to all other joints as a possible site of infection from an unknown origin.[13] Atherosclerosis occurs prematurely in patients with SLE and is an independent risk factor for cardiovascular disease and potential cardiovascular causes of death.[14]

LABORATORY AND IMAGING STUDIES

The diagnosis of SLE is a difficult process. It may take months or even years for physicians to piece together the various components of the disorder and symptoms to adequately complete the diagnosis. Although the OMS generally will not be involved in the primary diagnosis of SLE, an understanding of relevant laboratory and imaging studies is necessary to initiate necessary medical referrals, to determine the disease severity of an SLE patient referred for surgical intervention, or to identify a potential flare-up of the disease before surgery. Certain laboratory tests, such as the antinuclear antibody test, anti-DNA, anti-Sm, anti-RNP, anti-Ro (SSA), and anti-LA (SSB), are important in the initial diagnosis of the disease and also have roles as markers of specific disease activities. These tests have limited practicality for the OMS in a clinic referral setting and are not within the scope of this article for the purpose of managing an SLE patient as an in-patient referral. As previously mentioned, of paramount importance is a comprehensive history and physical examination paying particular attention to the patient's description of symptoms, precipitating events such as sun exposure, and a determination

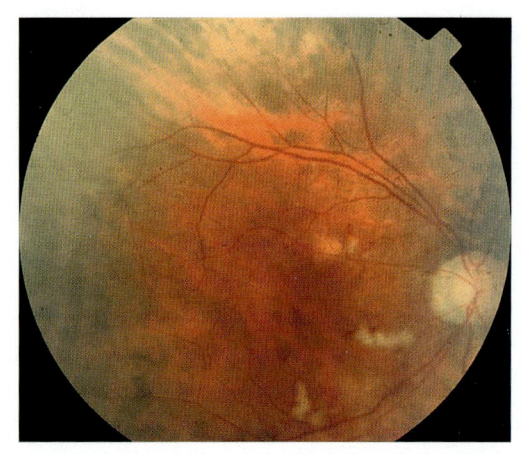

Fig. 8. Uveitis noted in a fundoscopic examination of a patient with SLE.

of current medications the patient is taking. A review of easily obtainable laboratory and imaging tests with a rationale for their use is presented in the following sections.

Laboratory Studies

1. A complete blood count is effective for the evaluation of anemia, hemolytic anemia, leukopenia, lymphopenia, or thrombocytopenia.
2. The partial thromboplastin time (PTT) can be elevated secondary to lupus anticoagulant, which is associated with thrombosis. Mild-to-moderate PTT elevations necessitate an additional work-up due to the potential for serious consequences from a thromboembolic event.
3. The erythrocyte sedimentation rate is a marker for inflammatory processes such as vasculitis or infection and can be elevated during periods of SLE flare-ups.
4. C-reactive protein is a marker for inflammatory processes such as vasculitis or infection and can be elevated during periods of SLE flare-ups.
5. Urinalysis is used to evaluate for proteinuria and cellular casts.
6. Blood chemistries, specifically BUN and creatinine, can be important markers of renal involvement and the progression of disease. Liver function studies are rarely affected by SLE. Elevations of hepatocellular enzymes would most likely indicate a medication-induced disorder, viral hepatitis, or biliary obstruction.
7. Complement levels are generally decreased during periods of SLE flare-ups.
8. The presence of anticardiolipin is a marker for increased risk of miscarriage in pregnant women with SLE.

Imaging Studies

1. Chest radiography is used to evaluate for pulmonary effusions, infiltrates, or cardiomegaly. Conventional chest films are generally sufficient, but abnormal findings may necessitate further evaluation with CT.
2. If chest radiology is concerning for effusions, an echocardiogram can be beneficial to confirm signs of pulmonary hypertension.
3. CT or magnetic resonance is used on patients who present with central nervous system findings. All types of seizures have been reported in patients with SLE. The incidence of stroke is high in the first 5 years of disease. Patients with antiphospholipid antibodies are at higher risk for such events.[15]

MANAGEMENT

Because there is no cure for SLE and complete remissions are rare, the patient and medical treatment team should devise strategies to control acute flares of the disease and develop medication protocols in which symptoms are maintained at an acceptable level, usually resulting in some type of secondary drug side effect. Environmental factors causing exacerbations of SLE are largely unknown with the exception of ultraviolet B and A light, with as many as 70% of patients being photosensitive.[1] For this reason patients are routinely counseled to avoid sunlight and to wear large hats, long sleeves and pants, and sunblock when outdoors, especially in portions of the country where the sun can be intense. Corticosteroids have been the mainstay in the treatment of patients with SLE. Medications such as prednisone and dexamethasone are used to manage the severely disabling presentations of SLE and for life-threatening symptoms. Undesirable side effects of these medications are extensive and include weight gain, hypertension, infection, ischemic necrosis of the bone, a propensity for the development of diabetes mellitus, osteoporosis, and psychosis.[1] Patients without life-threatening symptoms should be managed with non-steroidal anti-inflammatory drugs (NSAID) such as ibuprofen and naproxen. Careful and close monitoring of symptoms should occur because increased incidences of elevated serum transaminases, aseptic meningitis, and renal impairment have been seen with NSAID use.[1]

Patients with dermatopathic manifestations of disease, fatigue, and lupus arthritis appear to

Table 4
American College of Rheumatology criteria for SLE[12]

Criterion	Definition
1. Malar rash	Fixed erythema, flat or raised, over the malar eminences tending to spare the nasolabial folds
2. Discoid rash	Erythematous raised patches with adherent keratotic scaling and follicular plugging; atrophic scarring may occur in older lesions
3. Photosensitivity	Skin rash as a result of unusual reaction to sunlight, by patient history or physician observation
4. Oral ulcers	Oral or nasopharyngeal ulceration, usually painless, observed by physician
5. Arthritis	Nonerosive arthritis involving two or more peripheral joints characterized by tenderness, swelling, or effusion
6. Serositis	a) Pleuritis–convincing history of pleuritic pain or rubbing heard by a physician or evidence of pleural effusion
	OR
	b) Pericarditis–documented by electrocardiogram or rub or evidence of pericardial effusion
7. Renal disorder	a) Persistent proteinuria >0.5 g per day or >3+ if quantitation not performed
	OR
	b) Cellular casts–may be red cell, hemoglobin, granular, tubular, or mixed
8. Neurologic disorder	a) Seizures–in the absence of offending drugs or known metabolic derangements (eg, uremia, ketoacidosis, or electrolyte imbalance)
	OR
	b) Psychosis–in the absence of offending drugs or known metabolic derangements (eg, uremia, ketoacidosis, or electrolyte imbalance)
9. Hematologic disorder	a) Hemolytic anemia–with reticulocytosis
	OR
	b) Leukopenia–<4000/mm total on two or more occasions
	OR
	c) Lymphopenia–<1500/mm on two or more occasions
	OR
	d) Thrombocytopenia–<100,000/mm in the absence of offending drugs
10. Immunologic disorder	a) Positive LE cell preparation
	OR
	b) Anti-DNA–antibody to native DNA in abnormal titer
	OR
	c) Anti-Sm–presence of antibody to Sm nuclear antigen
	OR
	d) False-positive serologic test for syphilis known to be positive for at least 6 months and confirmed by *Treponema pallidum* immobilization or fluorescent treponemal antibody absorption test
11. Antinuclear antibody	An abnormal titer of antinuclear antibody by immunofluorescence or an equivalent assay at any point in time and in the absence of drugs known to be associated with drug-induced lupus syndrome

Box 1
Differential diagnosis list for SLE
Chronic fatigue syndrome
Multiple sclerosis
Fibromyalgia
Lyme disease
Drug-induced lupus
Discoid lupus
Depression
Hypochondria
Rheumatoid arthritis
Rosacea
Vasculitis
Scleroderma
Endocarditis
Metastatic malignancy
Fever of unknown origin
Mixed connective tissue disease
Hemoptysis

respond well to treatment with antimalarial medications such as hydroxychloroquine.[9] These medications if used for a prolonged period of time can lead to retinal degeneration.[1] Immunosuppressive agents such as cyclophosphamide and mycophenolate mofetil have proven effective for patients who develop renal or central nervous system disorders. Risks of these medications include an increased incidence of cancer and infection.[10]

POTENTIAL COMPLICATIONS FOR THE ORAL AND MAXILLOFACIAL SURGEON

Many potential complications exist for the OMS treating a patient with SLE. First, a determination of disease status and the potential for an active flare-up need to be established as discussed in the previous sections on history and physical examination and laboratory and imaging studies. Warning signs of a flare-up include increased fatigue, pain, rash, fever, abdominal discomfort, headache, and dizziness. If an active flare-up of the disorder is occurring, elective surgical intervention should be delayed until the symptoms are under control. Emergency treatment should be performed after adequately discussing the planned procedure with the patient and their physician of record to determine the need for potential medications (**Table 5**) such as supplemental steroids or advanced monitoring equipment available in a hospital setting.

Box 2 lists some of the common complications and treatment decisions an OMS may have to make in the treatment of a patient with SLE.[1]

Table 5		
Medications used in the management of SLE		
Class	Indications	Complications
NSAID Ibuprofen Naproxen	Arthralgias, arthritis, myalgias, fever, mild serositis	Elevated serum transaminases, aseptic meningitis, renal impairment, gastrointestinal distress
Glucocorticoids Prednisone Methylprednisolone Prednisolone Dexamethasone	Life-threatening manifestations of SLE, severe manifestations of disease, management of acute flare-ups	Cushingoid appearance, weight gain, hypertension, immunocompromised state, capillary fragility, acne, diabetes mellitus, ischemic necrosis of bone, osteoporosis, myopathy, psychosis, need for stress-dose supplement
Antimalarials Hydroxychloroquine	Dermatologic manifestations of disease, fatigue, lupus arthritis	Retinal toxicity, rash, myopathy, neuropathy
Cytotoxic agents Azathioprine Chlorambucil Cyclophosphamide Mycophenolate mofetil Methotrexate	Controlling active disease, reducing the rate of flares, reducing steroid requirements	Bone marrow suppression, increased opportunistic infections (eg, herpes zoster), irreversible ovarian failure, bladder toxicity, increased risk of malignancy

Data from Hahn BH. Systemic lupus erythematosus. In: Harrison's principles of internal medicine. 17th edition. New York: McGraw-Hill; 2008. p. 2075–83; and Appenzeller S, Cendes F Costallat LT. Epileptic seizures in systemic lupus erythematosus. Neurology 2004;63(10):1808–12.

> **Box 2**
> **SLE complications and treatment decisions**
>
> Vasculitis
>   Intestinal perforations
> Initiation of SLE exacerbation post surgery
> Pericarditis
>   Cardiac tamponade
> Myocarditis
>   Arrhythmias
>   Sudden cardiac death
> Lupus pneumonitis
>   Anesthesia considerations
> Acute intra-alveolar/pulmonary
> Adult respiratory distress syndrome
> Pulmonary hypertension
>   Anesthesia considerations
> Renal disease
>   Nephrotic syndrome
>   Renal dose medications
>   Fluid/medication restrictions during surgery
> Anemia
>   Anemia of chronic disease
>   Hemolytic anemia
> Thrombocytopenia
>   Bleeding time elevation
> Intravascular thrombosis
>   Stroke
>   Myocardial infarction
>   Potential anticoagulation
> Complications of high-dose glucocorticoid therapy
>   Need for supplemental "stress-dose" steroids
>   Diabetes
>   Immunocompromised state
>   Increased infection rates
> Complications of cytotoxic agents

SUMMARY

The management of a patient with SLE presents the OMS with a challenging array of decisions to make in regards to treatment sequencing. Careful reviews of the patient's medical history, the presentation of the illness, and the medication profile, and an open discourse with medical colleagues are necessary to ensure the safety of patients. By becoming comfortable with the medical treatment the patient is undergoing as well as having a firm understanding of where the patient is along the cascade of disease severity (see **Fig. 7**), appropriate decisions can be made in regards to the patient's outcome and prognosis. Proceeding into surgical treatment without following these guidelines could potentially result in catastrophic consequences for the patient.

REFERENCES

1. Hahn BH. Systemic lupus erythematosus. In: Fauci AS, Braunwald E, Kasper DL, editors. Harrison's principles of internal medicine. 17th edition. New York: McGraw-Hill; 2008. p. 2075–83.
2. Rahman A, Isenberg DA. Systemic lupus erythematosus. N Engl J Med 2008;358:929–39.
3. Patel M, Clarke AM, Bruce IN, et al. The prevalence and incidence of biopsy-proven lupus nephritis in the UK: evidence of an ethnic gradient. Arthritis Rheum 2006;54(9):2963–9.
4. Johnson AE, Gordon C, Palmer RG, et al. The prevalence and incidence of systemic lupus erythematosus in Birmingham, England: relationship to ethnicity and country of birth. Arthritis Rheum 1995;38(4):551–8.
5. Grisolia JS. Systemic lupus erythematosus. Available at: www.emedicine.com/neuro/topic360.htm. Accessed July 19, 2008.
6. Sinha AA. Lupus and the skin: manifestations, causes, treatments and research horizons. Available at: www.hss.edu/print/conditions_14362.htm. Accessed July 19, 2008.
7. Yell JA, Mbuagbaw J, Burge SM. Cutaneous manifestations of systemic lupus erythematosus. Br J Dermatol 1996;135(3):355–62.
8. McPhee SJ, Papadakis MA, Tierney LM. Current medical diagnosis and treatment. Columbus (OH): McGraw-Hill Publishers; 2007. p. 846–64.
9. Lupus: a patient care guide for nurses and other health care professionals. National Institute of Health, National Institute of Arthritis and Musculoskeletal and Skin Diseases handout. 3rd edition. Bethesda (MD): 2008. Available at: www.niams.nih.gov. Accessed July 19, 2008.
10. Physicians desk reference. 62nd edition. Montvale (NJ): Thomson Healthcare; 2008.
11. Kayazawa F, Honda A. Severe retinal vascular lesions in systemic lupus erythematosus. Ann Ophthalmol 1981;13(11):1291–4.

12. Tan EM, Cohen AS, Fries JF, et al. The 1982 revised criteria for the classification of systemic lupus erythematosus. Arthritis Rheum 1982;25: 1271–7.
13. Abu-Shakra M, Buskila D, Shoenfeld Y. Osteonecrosis in patients with SLE. Clin Rev Allergy Immunol 2003;25(1):13–24.
14. Rho YH, Chung CP, Oeser A, et al. Novel cardiovascular risk factors in premature coronary atherosclerosis associated with systemic lupus erythematosus. J Rheumatol 2008 Jul 15; [Epub ahead of print].
15. Appenzeller S, Cendes F, Costallat LT. Epileptic seizures in systemic lupus erythematosus. Neurology 2004;63(10):1808–12.

Index

Note: Page numbers of article titles are in **boldface** type.

A

Acquired immunodeficiency syndrome (AIDS),
   and HIV in adolescents and adults, **535–565**
     antiretroviral therapy, 551–552
     oral manifestations of, 552–560
        bacterial infections, 557–559
        fungal infections, 554–555
        neoplasms, 559–560
        viral infections, 555–557
     pathogenesis, 535–536
     skeletal, 548
     skin, 540–542
     systemic complications in, 539–551
        cardiovascular risk factors in, 545–546
        clinical course of infection, 536–538
        diagnosis, 538–539
        endocrine/metabolic, 547–548
        gastrointestinal, 543–544
        genitourinary, 542–543
        hematologic, 545
        immune reconstitution inflammatory syndrome, 551
        liver, 544
        Mycobacterium avium complex, 551
        neurologic, 548–550
        psychiatric, 550–551
        pulmonary, 546–547
        renal, 544–545
Acute cutaneous lupus erythematosus, 650
Acute lymphocytic leukemia, oral manifestations of, 595–596
Acute myelogenous leukemia, oral manifestations of, 598–600
Adolescents, HIV and AIDS in, **535–565**
AIDS. *See* Acquired immunodeficiency syndrome *and* Human immunodeficiency virus.
Angiocentric lymphoma, 590
Annular cutaneous lupus erythematosus, 650
Antiretroviral therapy, in adolescents and adults with HIV and AIDS, 551–552
Aphthous ulcers, oral, in adolescents and adults with HIV and AIDS, 560

B

Bacillary epithelioid angiomatosis, oral, in adolescents and adults with HIV and AIDS, 558
Bacterial infections, oral, in adolescents and adults with HIV and AIDS, 557–559
   bacillary epithelioid angiomatosis, 558–559
   linear gingival erythema, 557–558
   necrotizing ulcerative gingivitis, 558
   necrotizing ulcerative periodontitis, 558
Biopsy, in Sjögren syndrome diagnosis, 570–571
Bone, metastases of distant carcinomas to, 609–610
Burkitt's lymphoma, 589–590

C

Candidiasis, oral, in adolescents and adults with HIV and AIDS, 554–555
   in patients with leukemia, 602
Carcinoma, head and neck manifestations of distant, **609–623**
   metastases to, 609–617
     bone, 609–610
     ear and temporal bone, 614–615
     eye, orbit, and ocular adnexa, 612–614
     jaws, 610–611
     nasal cavity and paranasal sinuses, 614
     neck, 616–617
     oral region, 610
     parotid gland, 615
     salivary glands, 615
     skin of head and neck, 617
     soft tissues of the oral cavity, 612
     sublingual gland and minor salivary glands, 616
     submandibular gland, 615–616
   metastatic process, 607–609
Cardiovascular disease, in adolescents and adults with HIV and AIDS, 545–546
Chilblain lupus, 651
Chronic cutaneous lupus erythematosus, variants of, 650
Chronic lymphocytic leukemia, oral manifestations of, 596–597
Chronic myelogenous leukemia, oral manifestations of, 600
Colitis, ulcerative, effects on oral cavity, 628
Conjunctiva, metastases of distant carcinomas to, 613
Connective tissue disorders, in Sjögren syndrome, 569
Cowden syndrome, effects on oral cavity, 627–628
Crohn's disease, effects on oral cavity, 628
Cutaneous lesions, in adolescents and adults with HIV and AIDS, 540–542
   infectious, 540–541
   inflammatory, 542
   neoplastic, 541–542

Index

Cutaneous lupus erythematosus, variants of, 650
Cytomegalovirus, oral, in adolescents and adults with HIV and AIDS, 557

D

Dementia, AIDS dementia complex, 548
Discoid lupus erythematosus, 650
 See also Systemic lupus erythematosus.
Drug-induced lupus, 651

E

Ear, metastases of distant carcinomas to, 614–615
Endocrine disease, in adolescents and adults with HIV and AIDS, 547–548
Extranodal marginal zone B-cell lymphoma, 590–591
Extraocular muscles, metastases of distant carcinomas to, 613
Eye, disease, in Wegener's granulomatosis, 643
 metastases of distant carcinomas to, 612–614
Eyelid, metastases of distant carcinomas to, 613–614

F

Fungal infections, oral, in adolescents and adults with HIV and AIDS, 554–555
 deep, 555
 oral candidiasis, 554–555

G

Gardner syndrome, effects on oral cavity, 624–625
Gastrointestinal complications, of HIV and AIDS in adolescents and adults, 543–544
Gastrointestinal illnesses, effects on the oral cavity, **625–634**
 inflammatory bowel disease, Crohn's disease, 628
  ulcerative colitis, 628
 inherited gastrointestinal polyposis syndromes, 624–628
  Cowden syndrome, 627–628
  Gardner syndrome, 624–626
  Peutz-Jeghers syndrome, 626–627
  tuberous sclerosis, 626
 reflux disorders, 623–624
Gastrointestinal manifestations, of Sjögren syndrome, 568–569
Genitourinary complications, of HIV and AIDS in adolescents and adults, 542–543
Gingival erythema, linear, in adolescents and adults with HIV and AIDS, 554–555
Gingivitis, necrotizing ulcerative, in adolescents and adults with HIV and AIDS, 558
Graft-versus-host disease, oral manifestations in patients with leukemia, 603

H

Hairy leukoplakia, oral, in adolescents and adults with HIV and AIDS, 555–556
Head and neck, manifestations of distant carcinoma in, **609–623**
 metastases to, 609–617
  bone, 609–610
  ear and temporal bone, 614–615
  eye, orbit, and ocular adnexa, 612–614
  jaws, 610–611
  nasal cavity and paranasal sinuses, 614
  neck, 616–617
  oral region, 610
  parotid gland, 615
  salivary glands, 615
  skin of head and neck, 617
  soft tissues of the oral cavity, 612
  sublingual gland and minor salivary glands, 616
  submandibular gland, 615–616
 metastatic process, 607–609
Head and neck manifestations, of tuberculosis, **635–642**
 bacteriology, 634–635
 diagnosis, 637–638
 epidemiology, 634
 history of, 633–634
 pathophysiology, 635–637
 treatment, 638–639
Hematologic disease, in adolescents and adults with HIV and AIDS, 545
Hematologic manifestations, of Sjögren syndrome, 569
Herpes simplex virus, oral manifestations in patients with leukemia, 602–603
 oral, in adolescents and adults with HIV and AIDS, 557
HIV. See Human immunodeficiency virus.
Hodgkin's lymphoma, 585–586
Human immunodeficiency virus (HIV), in adolescents and adults, **535–565**
 antiretroviral therapy, 551–552
 oral manifestations of, 552–560
  bacterial infections, 557–559
  fungal infections, 554–555
  neoplasms, 559–560
  viral infections, 555–557
 pathogenesis, 535–536
 skeletal, 548
 skin, 540–542
 systemic complications in, 539–551
  cardiovascular risk factors in, 545–546
  clinical course of infection, 536–538
  diagnosis, 538–539
  endocrine/metabolic, 547–548
  gastrointestinal, 543–544
  genitourinary, 542–543

hematologic, 545
immune reconstitution inflammatory
  syndrome, 551
liver, 544
Mycobacterium avium complex, 551
neurologic, 548–550
psychiatric, 550–551
pulmonary, 546–547
renal, 544–545
Human papillomavirus, oral, in adolescents and adults with HIV and AIDS, 556–557
Hypertrophic lupus, 650

I

Immune reconstitution inflammatory syndrome, in adolescents and adults with HIV and AIDS, 551
Immune-mediated lesions, oral, in adolescents and adults with HIV and AIDS, 560
  aphthous ulcers, 560
  neutropenic ulceration, 560
Infectious complications, of HIV and AIDS in adolescents and adults, 539–540
  oral, 554–559
    bacterial, 557–559
    fungal, 554–555
    viral, 555–557
  skin, 540–541
Inflammatory bowel disease, effects on oral cavity, 628–630
  Crohn's disease, 628
  diagnosis, 629
  extraintestinal features, 628
  management, 629–630
  oral features, 628–629
  ulcerative colitis, 628
Inflammatory complications, of HIV and AIDS in adolescents and adults, 542
Inherited gastrointestinal polyposis syndromes, effects on oral cavity, 624–628
  Cowden syndrome, 627–628
  Gardner syndrome, 624–626
  Peutz-Jeghers syndrome, 626–627
  tuberous sclerosis, 626

J

Jaws, metastases of distant carcinomas to, 610–611
Joint disease, in Wegener's granulomatosis, 643

K

Kaposi's sarcoma, in adolescents and adults with HIV and AIDS, oral lesions of, 559
  skin lesions of, 541–542

L

Lacrimal gland, metastases of distant carcinomas to, 614
Larynx, in Sjögren syndrome, 568
Leukemia, **597–608**
  lymphoid, 595–597
    acute lymphocytic, 595–596
    chronic lymphocytic, 596–597
  myelodysplastic syndromes, 600–601
  myeloid, 597–600
    acute myelogenous, 597–600
    chronic myelogenous, 600
  normal development of white blood cells, 595
  treatment of oral manifestations, 601–604
    candidiasis, 602
    graft-*versus*-host disease, 603
    mucositis, 603–604
    oral herpes, 602–603
    surgical management of leukemic patients, 604
Linear gingival erythema, in adolescents and adults with HIV and AIDS, 554–555
Liver disease, in adolescents and adults with HIV and AIDS, 544
Lung disease, in Wegener's granulomatosis, 642
Lupus profundus, 651
Lupus tumidus, 651
Lupus. *See* Systemic lupus erythematosus.
Lymphoid leukemias, 595–597
  acute lymphocytic, 595–596
  chronic lymphocytic, 596–597
Lymphoproliferative diseases, systemic, **585–596**
  basic pathophysiology, 583–584
  Burkitt's lymphoma, 589–590
  complications of treatment, 591
  extranodal marginal zone B-cell/
    mucosa-associated lymphatic tissue lymphoma, 590–591
  Hodgkin's lymphoma, 585–587
  medical evaluation, 584
  nasal T/NK cell lymphoma, 590
  non-Hodgkin's lymphoma, 587–588

M

Metabolic disease, in adolescents and adults with HIV and AIDS, 547–548
Metastases, of distant carcinoma to head and neck, **609–623**
  bone, 609–610
  ear and temporal bone, 614–615
  eye, orbit, and ocular adnexa, 612–614
  jaws, 610–611
  metastatic process, 607–609
  nasal cavity and paranasal sinuses, 614
  neck, 616–617

Index

Metastases (*continued*)
    oral region, 610
    parotid gland, 615
    salivary glands, 615
    skin of head and neck, 617
    soft tissues of the oral cavity, 612
    sublingual gland and minor salivary glands, 616
    submandibular gland, 615–616
Mucosa-associated lymphatic tissue (MALT) lymphoma, 590–591
Mucositis, oral manifestations in patients with leukemia, 603–604
Mycobacterium avium complex, in adolescents and adults with HIV and AIDS, 551
Myelodysplastic syndromes, oral manifestations of, 600–601
Myeloid leukemias, oral manifestations of, 597–600
    acute myelogenous, 597–600
    chronic myelogenous, 600

N

Nasal cavity, metastases of distant carcinomas to, 614
Nasal T/NK cell lymphoma, 590
Nasolacrimal system, metastases of distant carcinomas to, 614
Neck. *See also* Head and neck.
    metastases of distant carcinomas to, 616–617
Necrotizing ulcerative gingivitis, in adolescents and adults with HIV and AIDS, 558
Neonatal lupus, 651
Neoplastic complications, of HIV and AIDS in adolescents and adults, 539–540
    oral, 559–560
    skin, 541–542
Nervous system disease, in Wegener's granulomatosis, 643
Neurologic disorders, in adolescents and adults with HIV and AIDS, 548–550
Neurologic manifestations, of Sjögren syndrome, 569
Neutropenic ulceration, oral, in adolescents and adults with HIV and AIDS, 560
Non-Hodgkin's lymphoma, 587–589
    in adolescents and adults with HIV and AIDS, 540
    oral lesions of, 560

O

Ocular adnexa, metastases of distant carcinomas to, 613
Ocular metastases, of distant carcinomas, 612–614
Ophthalmologic findings, in Sjögren syndrome, 567–568
Oral cavity, findings in Sjögren syndrome, 566–567
    gastrointestinal illnesses and their effects on, **625–634**

lesions of, in adolescents and adults with HIV and AIDS, 552–560
    bacterial infections, 557–559
        bacillary epithelioid angiomatosis, 558–559
        linear gingival erythema, 557–558
        necrotizing ulcerative gingivitis, 558
        necrotizing ulcerative periodontitis, 558
        syphilis, 559
    fungal infections, 554–555
        deep, 555
        oral candidiasis, 554–555
    immune-mediated, 560
        aphthous ulcers, 560
        neutropenic ulceration, 560
    neoplasms, 559–560
        Kaposi's sarcoma, 559
        non-Hodgkin's lymphoma, 560
    other, 560
        salivary gland disease, 560
        xerostomia, 560
    viral infections, 555–557
        cytomegalovirus, 557
        herpes simplex virus, 557
        human papillomavirus, 556–557
        oral hairy leukoplakia, 555–556
        varicella zoster, 557
lesions of, in Wegener's granulomatosis, 643–644
Orbital metastases, of distant carcinomas, 613

P

Papillomavirus, human, oral, in adolescents and adults with HIV and AIDS, 556–557
Paranasal sinuses, metastases of distant carcinomas to, 614
Paraneoplastic pemphigus, **577–584**
    clinical presentation, 579–580
    diagnostic work-up, 580
    epidemiology, 579
    histopathology, 580
    pathophysiology, 579
    treatment, 580
Parotid gland, metastases of distant carcinomas to, 615
Pemphigus vulgaris, **577–584**
    clinical presentation, 576–577
    diagnostic work-up, 577–578
    epidemiology, 575
    histopathology, 578
    pathophysiology, 575–576
    treatment, 578–579
Pemphigus, paraneoplastic, **577–584**
    clinical presentation, 579–580
    diagnostic work-up, 580
    epidemiology, 579

histopathology, 580
pathophysiology, 579
treatment, 580
Peutz-Jeghers syndrome, effects on oral cavity, 626–627
Psoriasiform cutaneous lupus erythematosus, 650
Psychiatric disorders, in adolescents and adults with HIV and AIDS, 550–551
Pulmonary disease, in adolescents and adults with HIV and AIDS, 546–547
Pulmonary manifestations, of Sjögren syndrome, 569

R

Reflux disorders, 623–624
    diagnosis, 624
    management, 624
    oral cavity features of, 623–624
Renal disease, in adolescents and adults with HIV and AIDS, 544–545
    in Wegener's granulomatosis, 642

S

Salivary gland disease, in adolescents and adults with HIV and AIDS, 560
Salivary glands, metastases of distant carcinomas to, 615
Schirmer test, in Sjögren syndrome diagnosis, 570
Scintigraphy, in Sjögren syndrome diagnosis, 570
Sialography, in Sjögren syndrome diagnosis, 570
Sialometry, in Sjögren syndrome diagnosis, 570
Sjögren syndrome, **567–575**
    clinical features, 566–569
        ophthalmologic findings, 567–568
        oral findings, 566–567
        other head and neck manifestations, 568–569
            ear, nose, and throat, 568
            larynx, 568
            thyroid, 568
        systemic manifestations, 568–569
            connective tissue disorders, 569
            gastrointestinal, 568–569
            hematology, 569
            neurologic, 569
            pulmonary, 569
    diagnosis, 569–571
        biopsy, 570–571
        Schirmer test, 570
        scintigraphy, 570
        sialography, 570
        sialometry, 570
    epidemiology and pathophysiology, 565–566
    treatment, 571–572
Skeletal disease, in adolescents and adults with HIV and AIDS, 548
Skin lesions, in adolescents and adults with HIV and AIDS, 540–542
    infectious, 540–541
    inflammatory, 542
    neoplastic, 541–542
    in Wegener's granulomatosis, 643
    metastases of distant carcinomas to head and neck skin, 617
Soft tissues, of oral cavity, metastases of distant carcinomas to, 612
Subacute cutaneous lupus erythematosus, 650
Submandibular gland, metastases of distant carcinomas to, 615–616
Surgery, oral and maxillofacial, in patients with leukemia, 604
Syphilis, oral, in adolescents and adults with HIV and AIDS, 559
Systemic lupus erythematosus, **651–662**
    description and prevalence, 649–650
    diagnosis, 653
    differential diagnosis, 653
    laboratory and imaging studies, 656
    management, 656–659
    morbidity and mortality, 653, 656
    physical findings, 651–653, 654, 655
    potential complications for oral and maxillofacial surgeons, 659
    variants, 650–651
        cutaneous, 650–651
            acute, 650
            chronic, including discoid, 650–651
            subacute, 650
        drug-induced, 651
        neonatal, 651
        systemic, 650

T

Temporal bone, metastases of distant carcinomas to, 614–615
Thrush. *See* Candidiasis, oral.
Thyroid, in Sjögren syndrome, 568
Tuberculosis, head and neck manifestations of, **635–642**
    bacteriology, 634–635
    diagnosis, 637–638
    epidemiology, 634
    history of, 633–634
    pathophysiology, 635–637
    treatment, 638–639
Tuberous sclerosis, effects on oral cavity, 626

U

Ulcerative colitis, effects on oral cavity, 628
Ulcerative gingivitis, necrotizing, in adolescents and adults with HIV and AIDS, 558

Index

Ulcers, oral, in adolescents and adults with HIV and AIDS, 560
    aphthous, 560
    neutropenic ulceration, 560
    See also Oral lesions.
Upper airway disease, in Wegener's granulomatosis, 643

V

Varicella zoster, oral, in adolescents and adults with HIV and AIDS, 557
Viral infections, oral, in adolescents and adults with HIV and AIDS, 555–557
    cytomegalovirus, 557
    herpes simplex virus, 557
    human papillomavirus, 556–557
    oral hairy leukoplakia, 555–556
    varicella zoster, 557

W

Wegener's granulomatosis, **643–649**
    diagnosis, 644–645
    differential diagnosis, 644
    etiology, 641
    eye disease in, 643
    general management, 645–646
    incidence/prevalence, 641
    initial clinical presentation, 641–642
    joint disease in, 643
    laboratory studies, 645
    lung disease in, 642
    nervous system disease in, 643
    oral histopathology, 644
    oral management, 646
    oral presentation, 643–644
    pathology, 644
    renal disease in, 642
    skin disease in, 643
    upper airway disease in, 643

X

Xerostomia, in adolescents and adults with HIV and AIDS, 560

Moving?

Make sure your subscription moves with you!

To notify us of your new address, find your **Clinics Account Number** (located on your mailing label above your name), and contact customer service at:

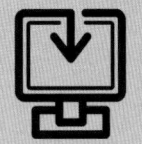

E-mail: elspcs@elsevier.com

800-654-2452 (subscribers in the U.S. & Canada)
1-407-563-6020 (subscribers outside of the U.S. & Canada)

Fax number: 407-363-9661

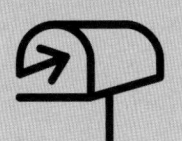

Elsevier Periodicals Customer Service
6277 Sea Harbor Drive
Orlando, FL 32887-4800

*To ensure uninterrupted delivery of your subscription, please notify us at least 4 weeks in advance of move.

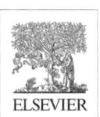

Statement of Ownership, Management, and Circulation
(All Periodicals Publications Except Requester Publications)

United States Postal Service

1. Publication Title	2. Publication Number	3. Filing Date
Oral and Maxillofacial Surgery Clinics of North America	0 0 6 - 3 6 2	9/15/08

4. Issue Frequency	5. Number of Issues Published Annually	6. Annual Subscription Price
Feb, May, Aug, Nov	4	$244.00

7. Complete Mailing Address of Known Office of Publication (Not printer) (Street, city, county, state, and ZIP+4)

Elsevier Inc.
360 Park Avenue South
New York, NY 10010-1710

Contact Person: Stephen Bushing
Telephone: 215-239-3688

8. Complete Mailing Address of Headquarters or General Business Office of Publisher (Not printer)

Elsevier Inc., 360 Park Avenue South, New York, NY 10010-1710

9. Full Names and Complete Mailing Addresses of Publisher, Editor, and Managing Editor (Do not leave blank)

Publisher: John Schrefer, Elsevier, Inc., 1600 John F. Kennedy Blvd. Suite 1800, Philadelphia, PA 19103-2899

Editor: John Vassallo, Elsevier, Inc., 1600 John F. Kennedy Blvd. Suite 1800, Philadelphia, PA 19103-2899

Managing Editor: Catherine Bewick, Elsevier, Inc., 1600 John F. Kennedy Blvd. Suite 1800, Philadelphia, PA 19103-2899

10. Owner

Full Name	Complete Mailing Address
Wholly owned subsidiary of Reed/Elsevier, US holdings	4520 East-West Highway, Bethesda, MD 20814

11. Known Bondholders, Mortgagees, and Other Security Holders Owning or Holding 1 Percent or More of Total Amount of Bonds, Mortgages, or Other Securities. If none, check box ☐ None

Full Name	Complete Mailing Address
N/A	

12. Tax Status (For completion by nonprofit organizations authorized to mail at nonprofit rates) (Check one)

☐ Has Not Changed During Preceding 12 Months
☐ Has Changed During Preceding 12 Months

13. Publication Title	14. Issue Date for Circulation Data Below
Oral and Maxillofacial Surgery Clinics of North America	August 2008

15. Extent and Nature of Circulation

		Average No. Copies Each Issue During Preceding 12 Months	No. Copies of Single Issue Published Nearest to Filing Date
a.	Total Number of Copies (Net press run)	3075	2900
b. Paid Circulation (By Mail and Outside the Mail)	(1) Mailed Outside-County Paid Subscriptions Stated on PS Form 3541	2020	1959
	(2) Mailed In-County Paid Subscriptions Stated on PS Form 3541		
	(3) Paid Distribution Outside the Mails Including Sales Through Dealers and Carriers, Street Vendors, Counter Sales, and Other Paid Distribution Outside USPS®	337	366
	(4) Paid Distribution by Other Classes Mailed Through the USPS (e.g. First-Class Mail®)		
c.	Total Paid Distribution (Sum of 15b (1), (2), (3), and (4))	2357	2325
d. Free or Nominal Rate Distribution (By Mail and Outside the Mail)	(1) Free or Nominal Rate Outside-County Copies Included on PS Form 3541	48	36
	(2) Free or Nominal Rate In-County Copies Included on PS Form 3541		
	(3) Free or Nominal Rate Copies Mailed at Other Classes Mailed Through the USPS (e.g. First-Class Mail)		
	(4) Free or Nominal Rate Distribution Outside the Mail (Carriers or other means)		
e.	Total Free or Nominal Rate Distribution (Sum of 15d (1), (2), (3) and (4))	48	36
f.	Total Distribution (Sum of 15c and 15e)	2405	2361
g.	Copies not Distributed (See instructions to publishers #4 (page #3))	670	539
h.	Total (Sum of 15f and g)	3075	2900
i.	Percent Paid (15c divided by 15f times 100)	98.00%	98.48%

16. Publication of Statement of Ownership

☐ If the publication is a general publication, publication of this statement is required. Will be printed in the **November 2008** issue of this publication. ☐ Publication not required

17. Signature and Title of Editor, Publisher, Business Manager, or Owner

John Tamucci - Executive Director of Subscription Services

Date: September 15, 2008

I certify that all information furnished on this form is true and complete. I understand that anyone who furnishes false or misleading information on this form or who omits material or information requested on the form may be subject to criminal sanctions (including fines and imprisonment) and/or civil sanctions (including civil penalties).

PS Form 3526, September 2006 (Page 2 of 3)